AF903040

ADVANCED TECHNIQUES IN LIPOSUCTION AND FAT TRANSFER

Edited by **Nikolay Serdev**

Advanced Techniques in Liposuction and Fat Transfer
Edited by Nikolay Serdev

Published by InTech
Janeza Trdine 9, 51000 Rijeka, Croatia

Copyright © 2011 InTech
All chapters are distributed under the Creative Commons Non Commercial Share Alike Attribution 3.0 license, which permits to copy, distribute, transmit, and adapt the work in any medium, so long as the original work is properly cited. After this work has been published by InTech, authors have the right to republish it, in whole or part, in any publication of which they are the author, and to make other personal use of the work. Any republication, referencing or personal use of the work must explicitly identify the original source.

Statements and opinions expressed in the chapters are these of the individual contributors and not necessarily those of the editors or publisher. No responsibility is accepted for the accuracy of information contained in the published articles. The publisher assumes no responsibility for any damage or injury to persons or property arising out of the use of any materials, instructions, methods or ideas contained in the book.

Publishing Process Manager Masa Vidovic

Technical Editor Teodora Smiljanic

Cover Designer InTech Design Team

Additional hard copies can be obtained from orders@intechopen.com

Advanced Techniques in Liposuction and Fat Transfer, Edited by Nikolay Serdev
p. cm.
ISBN 978-953-307-668-3

We are IntechOpen, the world's leading publisher of Open Access books

Built by scientists, for scientists

4,000+
Open access books available

116,000+
International authors and editors

120M+
Downloads

151
Countries delivered to

Our authors are among the
Top 1%
most cited scientists

12.2%
Contributors from top 500 universities

CLARIVATE ANALYTICS
BOOK CITATION INDEX
INDEXED

WEB OF SCIENCE™

Selection of our books indexed in the Book Citation Index in Web of Science™ Core Collection (BKCI)

Interested in publishing with us?
Contact book.department@intechopen.com

Numbers displayed above are based on latest data collected.
For more information visit www.intechopen.com

For EU product safety concerns:
IN TECH d.o.o., Prolaz Marije Krucifikse Kozulić 3, 51000 Rijeka, Croatia,
info@intechopen.com or visit our website at intechopen.com.

Meet the editor

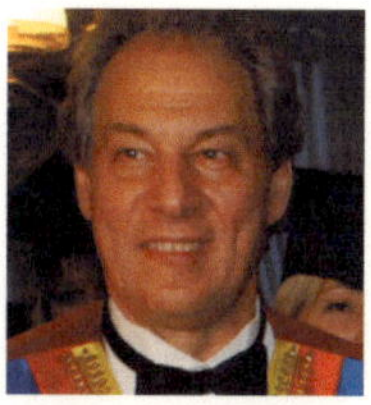

Nikolay P. Serdev, M.D., Ph.D., (b. April 26, 1948) is a Sofia, Bulgaria based board certified specialist in General Surgery and Cosmetic Surgery. He is both Professor and Director of the International University Program in Cosmetic Surgery at New Bulgarian University. Dr. Serdev is a graduate of the Sofia Medical University, and trained in General and then Cosmetic Aesthetic Surgery at the Military Medical Academy, and Aesthetic Surgery, Aesthetic Medicine Medical Center in Sofia, 1991-1996 he was a deputy head and acting head of the Burns Department in the Military Medical Academy and 2006-2008 National consultant in Cosmetic (Aesthetic) Surgery medical specialty at the Ministry of Health, Bulgaria.

Contents

Preface

Liposuction is the first cosmetic procedure to change beutification surgery from open extensive excision surgery into a more atraumatic closed one. It gave rise to the modern understanding of minimally scarring and minimally invasive surgery and changed the understanding and preferences of both patients and doctors. It also became the most common procedure in cosmetic surgery world-wide, practiced by an increased number of physicians from various specialties. The techniques of fat grafting, closely bound with liposuction, have found widespread application and fat stem cells seem to be changing the future of many areas in medicine.

Training became necessary in view of the constantly changing and developing character of medical science, and because of the progress in new devices emerging on the market.

Turning the pages, the reader will find a lot of information about advances, tips and tricks, and important milestones in the development of the different methods available, such as classic, power, ultrasound, laser and radio-frequency assisted liposuction etc. Most useful anesthesia techniques are described and discussed, and guidelines have been established for medical indications. Special attention is paid to good patient selection, complications and risks.

We have invited renowned specialists from all continents to share their valued expertise and experience. We will never be able to thank every single person or institution who helped in fulfilling our work. The difficult task of writing a comprehensive book about the status and science of the most desired and most practiced procedure in cosmetic surgery, in order to prevent dissatisfaction and misunderstandings, was marked with hard work and continuous improvements. It is a privilege to share our knowledge concerning contemporary advances in this area of medicine, and thus help people change and improve their lives. It is our greatest reward as well.

Prof. Dr. Nikolay Serdev
National Consultant of the Ministry of Health in the Specialty of
"Cosmetic (Aesthetic) Surgery" 2006-2008,
Medical Center "Aesthetic Surgery, Aesthetic Medicine" 11,
Bulgaria

Part 1

Liposuction: History and Techniques

1

Application of the Liposuction Techniques and Principles in Specific Body Areas and Pathologies

Diego Schavelzon et al.*
Argentina

1. Introduction

1.1 Three dimensional gluteoplasty

The buttocks have been a symbol of attraction, sexuality and eroticism since ancient times and therefore, they have an important role in defining the posterior body contour.

More and more people are talking about and understand the meaning and the role that buttocks play in modeling and physical beauty.

The three dimensional gluteoplasty (3-DGP) is an innovative technique that allows us to change volume, shape and firmness, not only in the buttocks but also in the adjacent regions such as the thighs and trochanters, becoming an ideal tool to answer the frequent reasons of consultation of our patients about this particular area of the body:

I want to reduce the volume of my buttocks

I want to lift my buttocks...

I want to improve the shape of my buttocks.

Numerous factors conspire against an ideal buttock.

First, the weight of the buttocks and the variations of fatty tissue component in addition to the presence of a strong lower groove skin adhesion called subgluteal fold or inferior gluteal groove, which is strongly influenced by the action of gravity, cause the appearance of ptosis with subsequent buttock deformity and that of the adjacent regions.

Other factors such as obesity, the lack of muscle activity (gluteal muscles), the aging process, a significant decrease in weight and extreme thinness play an important role in the development of gluteal ptosis.

The word ptosis comes from the Greek word meaning "falling" or "fall". From a medical perspective refers to prolapsus or caudal displacement, outside its natural site, of a tissue or organ.

The ophthalmologists were the first to use the term to define the upper eyelid drop, and by analogy, over time its use became widespread.

---

*Louis Habbema, Stefan Rapprich, Peter Lisborg, Guillermo Blugerman, Jorge A. D'Angelo, Andrea Markowsky, Javier Soto, Rodrigo Moreno and Maria Siguen
Centros B&S "Excelencia en Cirugía Plástica", Buenos Aires, Argentina
Medisch Centrum 't Gooi, The Netherlands
Department of Dermatology, Darmstadt Hospital,Germany
PrivatKlinik Lisborg & Parner,Österreich
Universidad Nacional del Nordeste, Corrientes, Argentina,

1.2 Gluteal Ptosis[(1)]

What does gluteal ptosis mean?

Gluteal ptosis refers to the excess skin and/ or adipose tissue of the gluteal region that exceeds the caudal inferior gluteal groove. The progression of gluteal ptosis is usually from medial to lateral.

What does pseudo-ptosis mean?

(Sad or long gluteus). When the buttock support system gradually loses its strength and its power to lift, the entire gluteus falls, and subgluteal groove descends moving distally. With the consequent loss of natural contour and shape the buttocks have.

It is critical to have a classification of gluteal ptosis, which serves to select the most appropriate technique in each case.

The extension in depth and length of the subgluteal groove is a key indicator of ptosis.

1.2.1 Gonzalez classification of gluteal ptosis

To determine the degree of ptosis the marking is done with the patient in standing position, with straight hips, and facing backwards. We identify the ischial tuberosity by palpation, and from there we draw a vertical line (Line T) and a second parallel to the first one (line M) corresponding to the midpoint of the posterior thigh [(1)] (Figure 1).

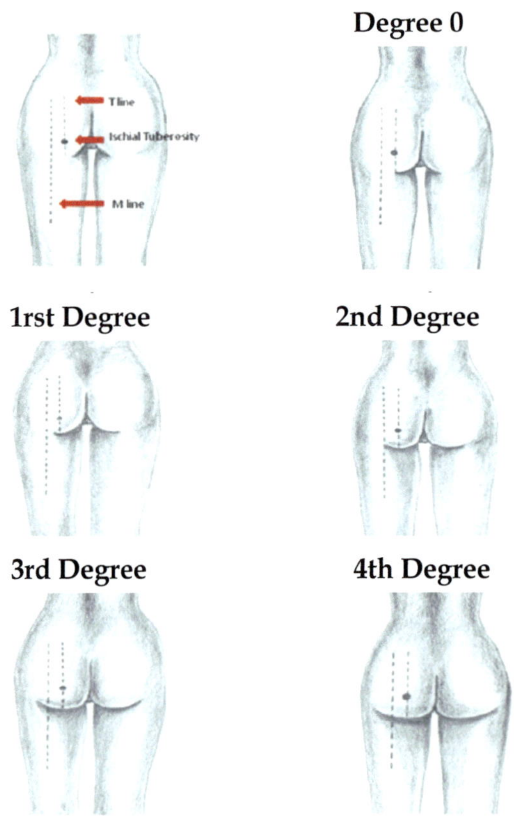

Fig. 1. Gonzalez classification of gluteal ptosis in degrees.

Degree 0 No ptosis.
1rst Degree Minimal pre-ptosis, subgluteal groove lies between the line T and M.
2nd Degree Moderate pre-ptosis, subgluteal groove reaches the M-line and there is ptotic tissue at line T.
3rd Degree Borderline Ptosis, subgluteal groove goes beyond the M-line, but without ptotic tissue.
4th Degree Real ptosis, adipose tissue is projected on the thigh. From here on the excess of ptotic tissue is measured in centimeters.
Since the creation of liposuction Dr. Illouz (2,3), Pierre Fournier (4) and others (Fig.2 y 3) pointed the buttocks as a taboo area for this technique, prohibiting the performance of liposuction due to the bad results they had obtained.

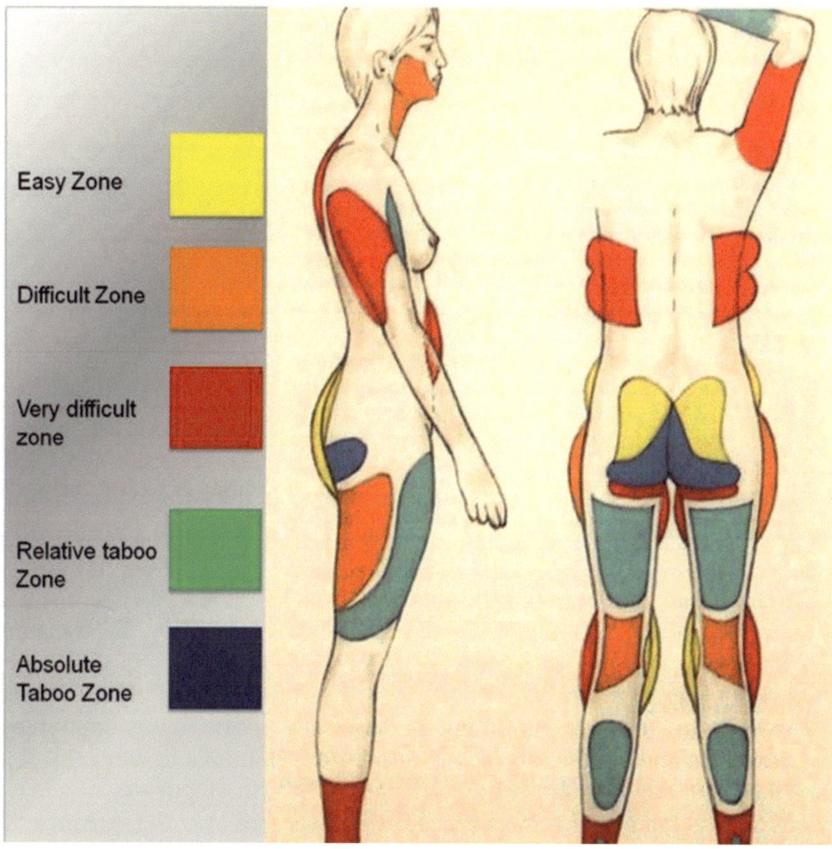

Fig. 2. Liposuction zones described by a Gottfried Lemperle in "Ästhetische Chirurgie". Note the zone shaded as "Absolute Taboo Zone". (10)

Despite technical advances and the arrival of tumescent local anesthesia (5) the rule continued to be applied until 2002, when evaluating photographic images, based on an anatomical study (6) (7) (8) (9) and a correct diagnosis of ptosis we started working the adipose tissue of buttocks with a concept of three-dimensional fat remodeling.
The results obtained were very promising, as for the first time we gave the buttocks a more harmonious shape with the rest of the body.

The three-dimensional technique has given indirect benefits to adjacent areas as well as to the trochanter and the "Banana fold", so called to the deposit of adipose tissue in the posterior thigh below and parallel to the inferior gluteal groove.
This fat deposit is a result of buttocks pressure on the subgluteal groove, transmitting that pressure on the posterior thigh fat layer thus creating this fold deformity [1].
There are multiple surgery techniques performed to correct this kind of defect, but all without much success because they are treating the defect and not its cause.

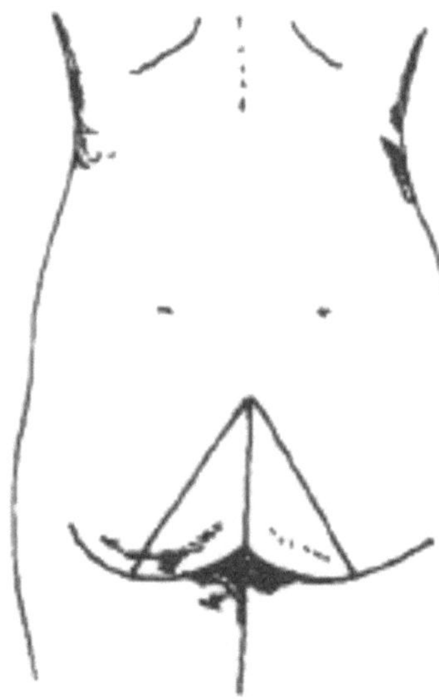

Fig. 3. The Bermuda short triangle. Its corners are the level of the ischial tuberosities and the upper edge of the intergluteal crease. [4]

1.3 Surgical technique

The preoperative marking is done with the patient in standing position. Then the marking is done comprising the surrounding tissue of inter-gluteal and sub-gluteal groove thus determining an L-shaped marking. This mark is divided into two zones, a vertical one which is parallel to the inter-gluteal groove in which the liposuction is done in both deep and superficial plane, and another horizontal to sub-gluteal groove in which the liposuction is only done deeply to avoid flaccidity and wrinkles in the skin. (Figure 4).
Two incisions are used to perform this procedure. One located over the sacrum and another on the trochanter area at the end of the sub-gluteal groove.
Later on the subcutaneous fat is infiltrated with tumescent solution at all levels with the B&S peristaltic pump [11] and a Klein needle [5], covering the areas previously marked until reaching tumescence and the area is stabilized.
Regularly it is needed only 500 to 1000 ml to achieve adequate tumescence point, due to the special characteristics of the gluteal fat (Fig. 5).
To obtain a more accurate and better skin contraction we then begin the treatment of fat through the use of an Nd: YAG 1064 laser assisted liposuction or bipolar radiofrequency assisted liposuction (RFAL) with the Body Tite® [12] . The action of laser or radiofrequency

energy on the adipocytes causes the rupture of cell membranes due to the abrupt rise of interstitial temperature, causing a characteristic noise known as "Popcorn Effect". Once the fat is processed, we proceed to evacuate the oil emulsion obtained, using a vibrating tube of 3 mm.

MAST (Manual Assisted Stabilization Tissue) is a very helpful maneuver in which an assistant presses on the buttock to prevent accompanying the movements of the tissues performed by the surgeon's cannula during the procedure, thus achieving a greater accuracy and reducing surgical time.

The lipo-aspirated volume usually does not exceed 100 ml per buttock, but the influence of those few milliliters into the final shape of the area is really important (Figure 6 y 7).

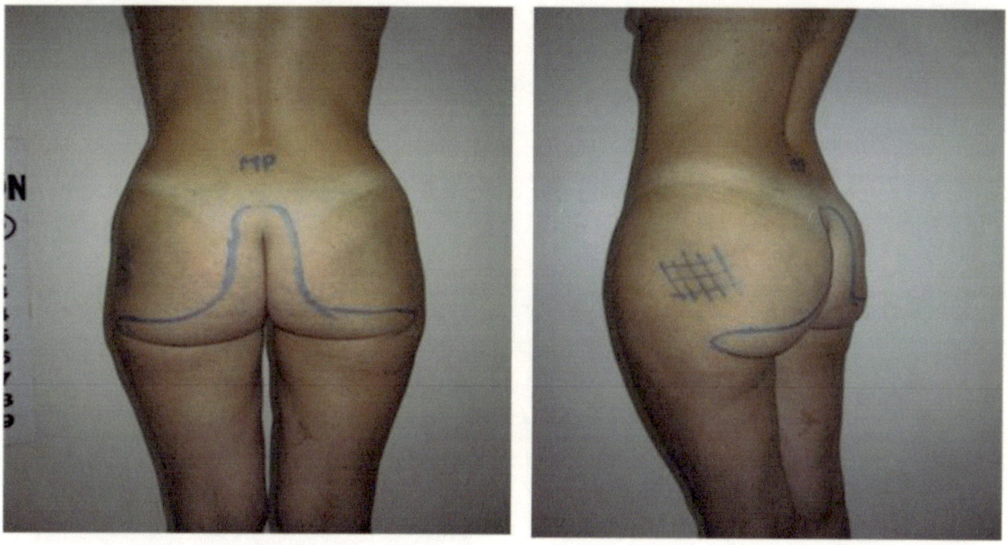

Fig. 4. Markings guiding the surgeon for areas and planes of fat removal. Front and lateral views.

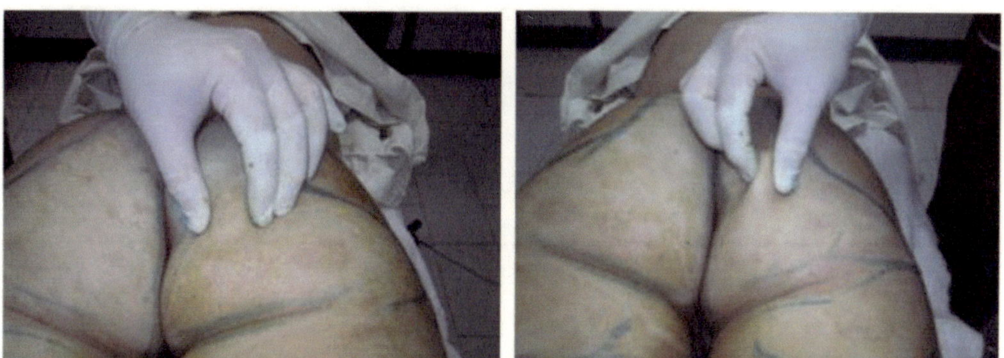

Fig. 5. Intra-operative views with tumescent anesthesia (left) and after liposuction (right).

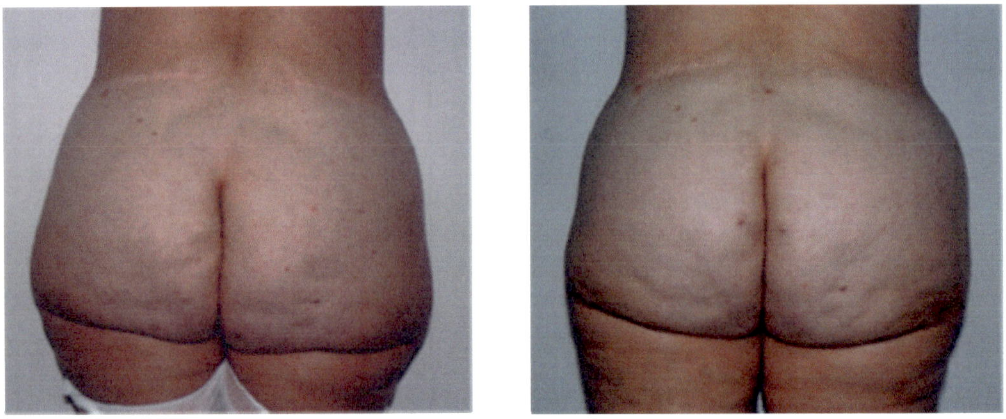

A) B)

Fig. 6. A Pre-operative view of a 42 year-old woman B. Post-operative view 1 month after a Three Dimensional Gluteoplasty (3-DGP).

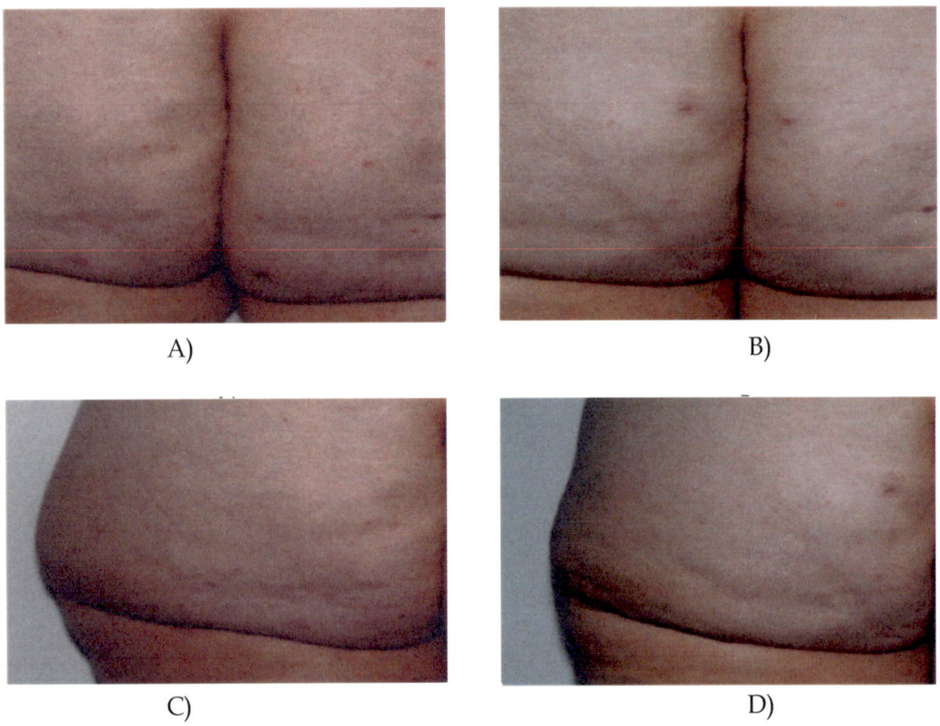

Fig. 7. A Preoperative view of ptosis and subgluteal crease B. Improvement in the inter-gluteal aspect and in the lower gluteal area. C. Preoperative view of the trochanteric area. D. Postoperative view of the trochanteric area without performing any type of procedure in this area, only the 3-DGP.

Our actual concept of three-dimensional remodeling buttocks includes the combination of several procedures as described below, in association with:

- Liposuction to the near buttocks areas.
- Enriched Adipose Micrografts with Autologous Plasma.
- Liposhifting superficial and deep subcision procedures.
- Sub-muscular gluteal implant.

1.3.1 Liposuction to the near buttocks areas

Liposuction of the adjacent buttock regions allows a much better result of the final shape. Liposuction in upper and lower back gives a good skin retraction due to its greater thickness and its fibrous tissue content, which produces a significant improvement in the posterior contour and therefore in the buttocks. Another region that responds to liposuction is the sacral region, thus enhancing and defining the buttocks.
In our practice the best results are obtained with RFAL (Body Tite®) (12) that allows us to achieve greater tissue retraction in less time.

1.3.2 Enriched Adipose Micrografts (EAM)

In some cases due to the marked ptosis we use adipose grafting, this theme is explained in "Enriched Adipose Micrografts with Autologous Plasma" (13,14) (Figure 8).

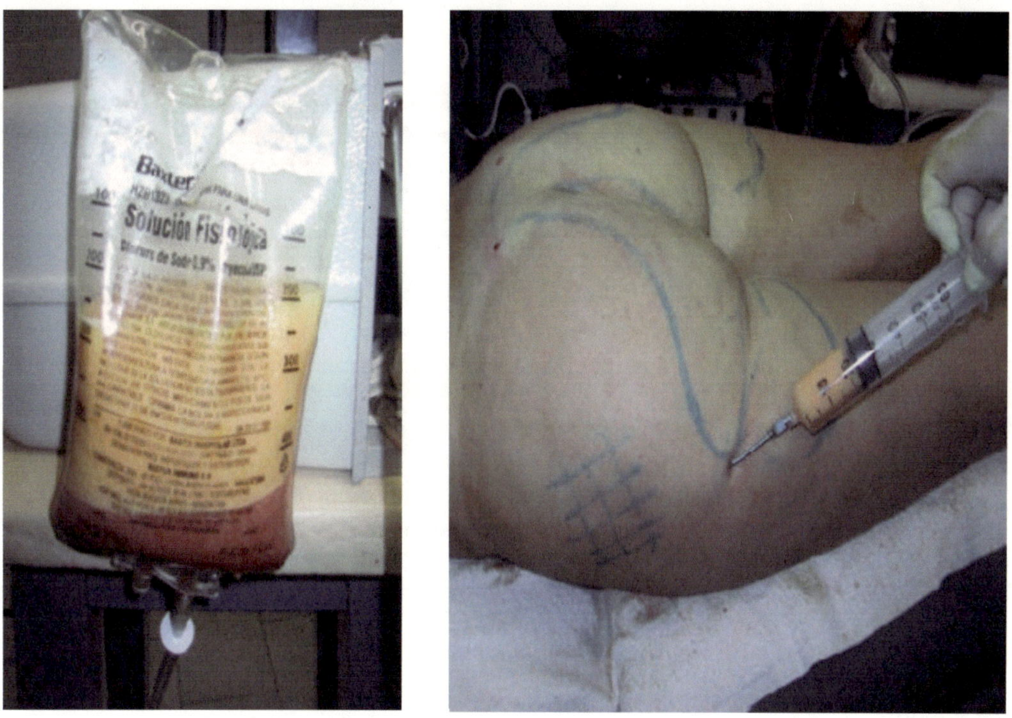

Fig. 8. View of the fat tissue post-liposuction. Lateral view of EAM technique in trochanteric depression.

1.3.3 Liposhifting and deep-superficial subsicion

Liposhifting technique allows us to repair irregularities and depressions found in the gluteal region.[14] For treatment of depressions or irregularities we cut the fibrous septa that cause adhesions of the skin to deeper layers. This allows for the formation of new tissue and replacement of fibrin by vascularized fibrous tissue.Superficially we use Nokor ® type needles; it has a tapered end similar to the scalpel blade. For the deeper plane we use a hook instrumental that only cuts when removed.

1.3.4 Buttocks implants

Where there is a lack of volume in the gluteal region that can not be resolved by the procedures previously described we opt for the placement of cohesive gel implants in a submuscular plane through an incision in the inter-gluteal groove [15].

1.4 Conclusion

There are different procedures to improve the gluteal area.

The Three Dimensional Gluteoplasty is a global useful technique not only to correct gluteal ptosis and to raise the subgluteal crease or correct skin asymmetry but also to reshape the buttock.

The result in this procedure depends on patient selection, and a correct technique development.

2. Liposuction treatment for lipedema

2.1 Introduction

Lipedema is a painful, hereditary disorder usually affecting women that involves accumulation of excess fatty tissue on the extremities. Characterstic symptoms include pain as well as sensitivity to touch and pressure. Patients also tend to bruise easily after minimal trauma. Over time, the disorder pregressively worsens [16, 17, 18].

2.2 Classification

The diagnosis is based on clinical appearance (Figure 12). Lipedema should be differentiated from lipohypertrophy and lymphedema [33]. Lipedema may be divided into three types : whole leg, thigh and lower leg lipedema. In about 30% of patients, there is also involvement of the arms [19, 20, 28].

2.3 Etiology and pathophysiology

The cause of lipedema is unknown. Hormones are certainly one factor, as lipedema occurs virtually exclusively in women. In addition, early signs of disease tend to appear with the onset of puberty or after pregnancy. During these stages, the disease may also be referred to as lipohypertrophy which may develop into lipedema. Full-blown symptomatic disease usually manifests in the third or fourth decade of life. In addition to hormonal factors, a genetic disposition may be presumed, as the disease often affects several women in the same family.

An important factor in the patho-physiology of lipedema is increased capillary leading to orthostatic edema. This, and not the amount of adipose tissue, is responsible for the increased sensitivity of the tissue to touch and pressure. The increased capillary fragility also explains the tendency to hematoma development.

Lymph drainage is undisrupted. Indeed, it is even increased in the early stages of lipedema. In later stages, the capacity of the lymphatic system is exhausted and can no longer ensure adequate drainage. This results in dynamic insufficiency. With decompensation of the lymphatic system, secondary lymphedema develops. In clinical terms this is known as lipolymphedema - with all related sequel including leg ulcers. There are no characteristic histological changes associated with the disease.

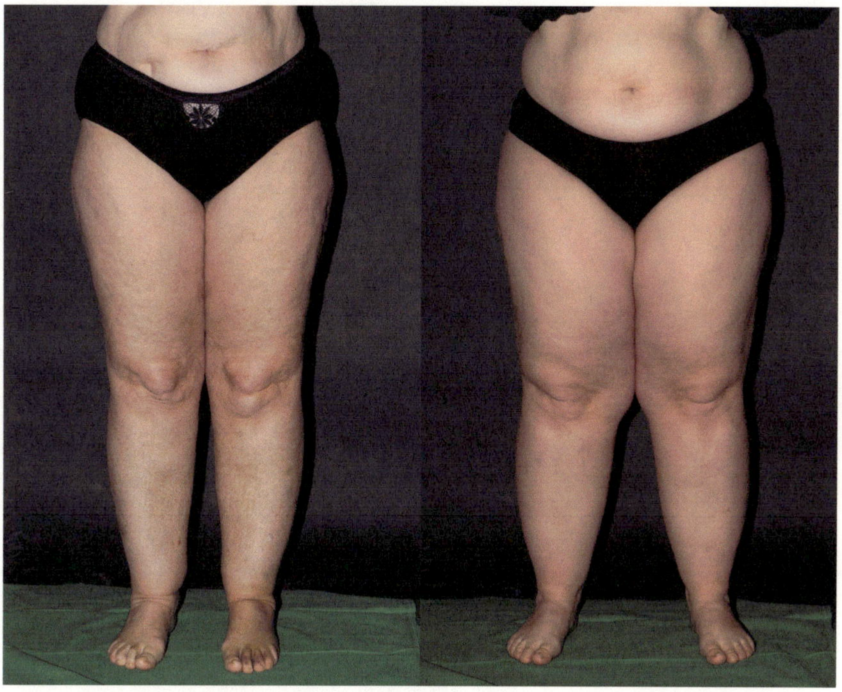

Fig. 12. Mother and her daughter with lipedema.

The disorder occurs in three stages :
Stage I: Thickening and softening of the subcutis with small nodules; skin is smooth
Stage II: Thickening and softening of the subcutis with larger nodules; skin texture is uneven.
Stage III: Thickening and hardening of the subcutis with large nodules, disfiguring lobules of fat on the inner thighs and inner aspects of the knees.

2.3 Therapeutic options

Complex physical therapy (CPT), which is widely recommended, is only effective against edema. Only some patients actually experience an improvement in symptoms, and then only for a short period of time following each treatment session.

The removal of excess fatty tissue using liposuction has been made possible by microcannulae and - in a more advanced form - with vibrating cannula under tumescent local anesthesia (Figure 13 and 14) [21, 22, 23, 24, 25, 29, 31, 32, 34].

The procedure of the liposuction in lipedema does not differ from aesthetic indications [26, 27, 28]. Stringent guidance of the cannula in longitudinal direction and aspects of safety have to be considered in the same way.

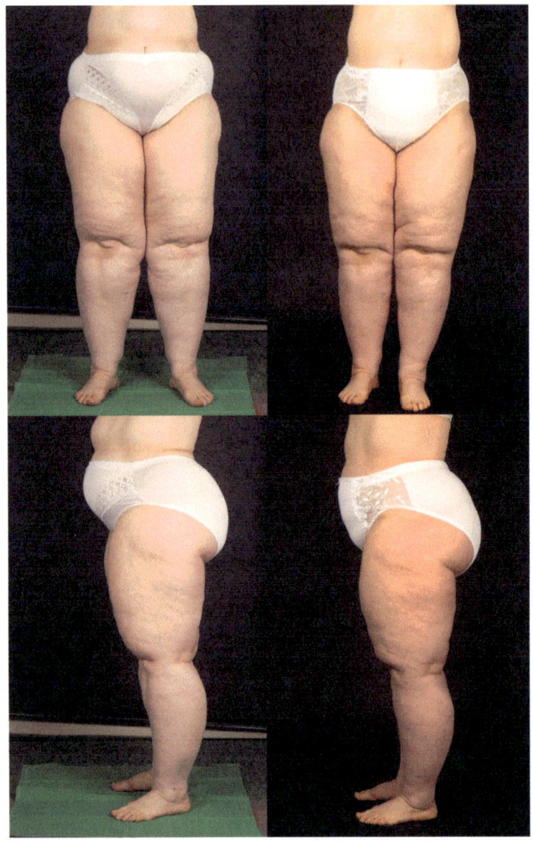

Fig. 13. Patient pre- and 6 months postoperative, 3 sessions

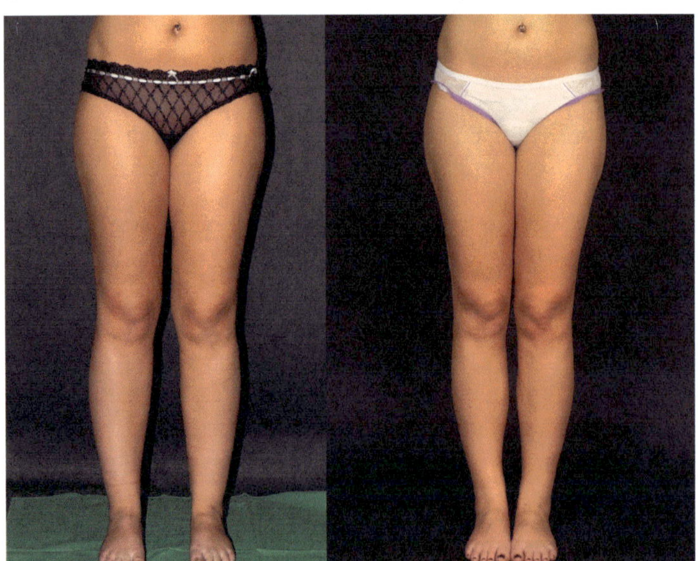

Fig. 14. Patient pre- and 6 months postoperative, 1 session lower legs

Just as much important is the postoperative complex physical therapy (CPT). CPT consists in manual lymph drainage (MLD) and compression therapy for 4-6 weeks or for the time of visible postoperative edema. The combination of liposuction and CPT is the optimal treatment to lipedema.

2.4 Results

A study with 25 patients demonstrated the effectiveness of liposuction against lipedema [35]. All patients were between 22 and 65 years old. Twenty patients had lipedema affecting the whole leg, 3 had lipedema of the thigh, and 2 had lower leg involvement only. Clinical examination pre- and postoperative included leg volume measurement using 3D imaging (Image3D, Bauerfeind) and self-assessment, based on a questionnaire with 15 criterias. They were assessed by the patient using a visual analogue scale (VAS) of 0 to 10. The survey was completed prior to beginning therapy and again at 6 months after the final liposuction treatment (Figure 15).

Questionnaire		Results		
Rate the level of pain on a scale of 1-10 (no pain to very severe pain)	keine – sehr starke; 0 1 2 3 4 5 6 7 8 9 10 (x at 5)	Mean VAS before liposuction	Mean VAS 6 months after liposuction	Significance
Are the affected areas painful?	keine – sehr starke; 0 1 2 3 4 5 6 7 8 9 10	7.2	2.1	p< 0.001
Are the affected areas sensitive to touch or pressure?	keiner – sehr stark; 0 1 2 3 4 5 6 7 8 9 10	6.4	1.9	p< 0.001
Do you bruise easily (hematoma)?	keine – sehr stark; 0 1 2 3 4 5 6 7 8 9 10	7.9	4.2	p< 0.001
Do you feel tension in your legs?	keines – sehr stark; 0 1 2 3 4 5 6 7 8 9 10	7.7	2.3	p< 0.001
Do you feel excessive warmth in the legs?	keines – sehr stark; 0 1 2 3 4 5 6 7 8 9 10	3.0	1.4	p< 0.008
Do you legs feel cold?	keines – sehr stark; 0 1 2 3 4 5 6 7 8 9 10	3.8	2.1	p< 0.120
Do you have muscle cramps?	keine – sehr häufig; 0 1 2 3 4 5 6 7 8 9 10	2.7	1.3	p< 0.043
Do your legs feel heavy?	keines – sehr stark; 0 1 2 3 4 5 6 7 8 9 10	8.4	3.6	p< 0.001
Do your legs feel tired?	keines – sehr stark; 0 1 2 3 4 5 6 7 8 9 10	8.4	3.5	p< 0.001
Do you something have swelling?	keine – sehr starke; 0 1 2 3 4 5 6 7 8 9 10	6.9	3.3	p< 0.001
Is there skin involvement?	keine – sehr starke; 0 1 2 3 4 5 6 7 8 9 10	3.5	1.3	p< 0.001
Is there itching?	keiner – sehr stark; 0 1 2 3 4 5 6 7 8 9 10	4.2	1.9	p< 0.001
Do you have difficulty walking?	gar nicht – sehr stark; 0 1 2 3 4 5 6 7 8 9 10	4.6	1.6	p< 0.001
How much does the condition affect your quality of life?	keine – sehr stark; 0 1 2 3 4 5 6 7 8 9 10	8.7	3.6	p< 0.001
How satisfied are you with the appearance of your legs?	sehr zufrieden – sehr unzufrieden; 0 1 2 3 4 5 6 7 8 9 10	9.5	5.0	p< 0.001
Total score	(maximum 150)	92.0	39.0	p< 0.001

Fig. 15. Questionnaire and results.

In most patients about 6000 ml tumescent solution (0,05% prilocaine) was infiltrated per session, with a maximum of 7000 ml and a minimum of 2000 ml. Liposuction was performed with vibrating cannula of 4 mm diameter. Patients were treated in 1 to 5 sessions (mean 2,5). The following regions on the body were combined and treated symmetrically:

- Medial aspects of the thighs and inner aspects of the knee
- Lateral aspects of the thighs and hip in the same or an additional session
- For larger-volume thighs the anterior aspects were also treated
- Lower legs

Three sessions at 4-week intervals were generally needed. The therapy usually began with the medial aspects of the thighs and knees or with the area that was causing the greatest discomfort. For each session the aspirated volume was an average of 2482 ± 968 ml and the pure fat component was on average 1909 ± 874 ml respectively 77%.

3D imaging showed a reduction in leg volume of 18.0 ± 3.8 to 16.8 ± 3.5 l. This corresponds to an average reduction of leg volume of 1.2 ± 1.0 l or 6.9 %.

The results of self-assessment of symptoms indicate a significant or highly significant improvement in all areas. With regard to pain, the chief symptom of lipedema, there was an improvement of 7.2 ± 2.2 to 2.1 ± 2.1 (Figure 16). There was also significant improvement in sensitivity to pressure, which is typical of lipedema, and bruising. The results showed also a highly improvement of quality of life (Figure 17).

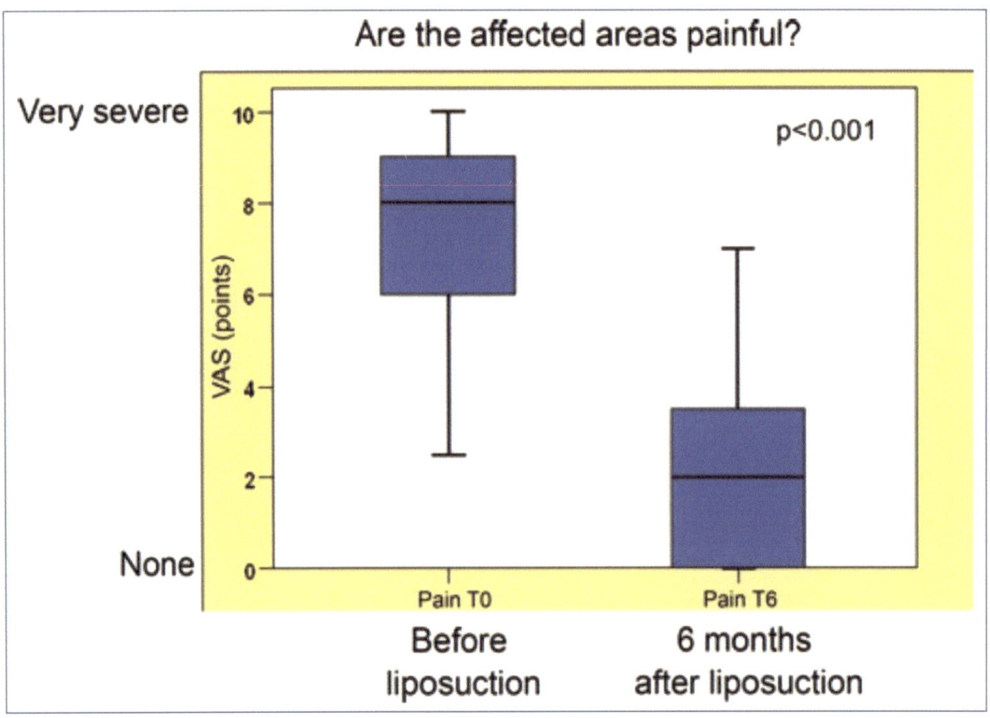

Fig. 16. Significant reduction of pain before and 6 month post liposuction

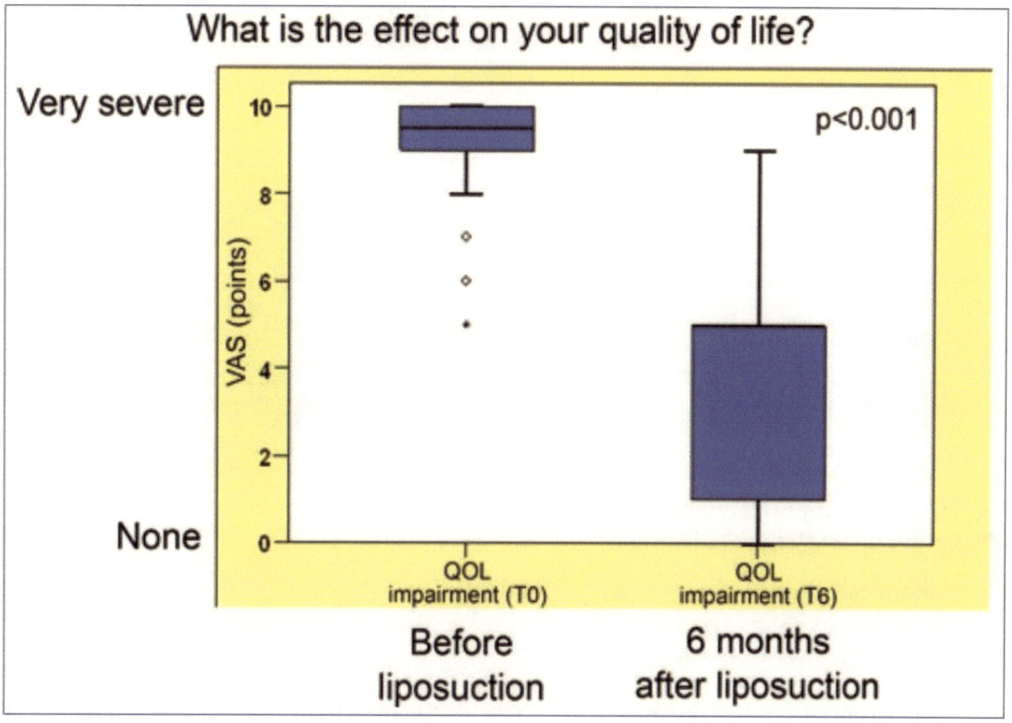

Fig. 17. Significant improvement of quality of life before and 6 month post liposuction.

2.5 Conclusion

When performed by an experienced practitioner, tumescent liposuction is a safe and effective method of treatment for lipedema. The results of therapy are better in younger patients with early-stage disease compared with more severe disease in older patients. CPT, before and after liposuction, is an important part of therapy.

3. Medial thigh lift combining energy assisted liposuction and dermal flaps suspension to the adductor tendon

3.1 Introduction

The medial thigh area remains a troublesome region for body contouring in patients with lipo-dystrophy and/or skin flaccidity. Liposuction has proven to be effective in patients with excess of fat deposits without a significant degree of skin laxity. The skin in this particular body area is often thin and inelastic and in most circumstances where skin laxity is present liposuction alone fails. To contour and tighten the inner thigh, it is necessary to combine liposuction with skin excision to achieve acceptable cosmetic results (36).

Adverse results associated with current inner thigh lifting (37) surgery include pigmented or hypertrophic scars, flattening of the vulva as result of excess of traction created by the lower flap on the vulvae tissues, caudal wound migration that cannot be hidden when using swimming suits (Figure 18), and recurrence of the inner thigh ptosis that may require additional corrective surgery (38).

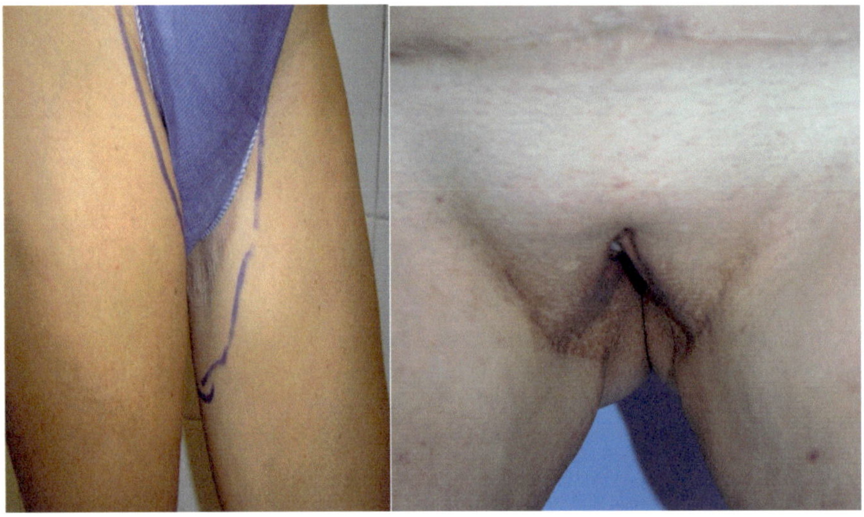

Fig. 18. Caudal wound migration that cannot be hidden when using swimming suits. Scar traction producing vaginal distortion

The anatomical absence of a well-defined and strong superficial fascial structure to anchor the inferior flap in a stable position and the histological skin characteristics of the inner thigh are two of the main reasons for poor results.
The purpose of this paper is to present the authors' technique of inner thigh lift using a new resection design of the dermoadipose flap. This technique allows an effective anchoring of the inferior flap of the inner thigh into the adductor major tendon at the pubic bone insertion . This new approach creates a strong and stable anchoring place for the inferior inner thigh flap. In the authors' experience this technique has proved safe and effective with a decreased morbidity and satisfactory cosmetic results.

3.2 Anatomy

The skin in the medial thigh has a minimal dermal component and has an average thickness of 0.03 mm.
The subcutaneous tissue of this area is separated in two layers by a poorly defined superficial fascia [39]. The thickness and quality of the fascia varies considerably from patient to patient and identification of this structure can be difficult at the time of surgery when tumescent local anesthesia is used.
The adductor muscle tendon added to the gracillis tendon is a fibrous structure, a finger thick in diameter that inserts on the ischiopubic portion of the pelvic bone (Figura.19).
It is easily identifiable and there are no significant anatomical structures located behind the tendon. The superficial fascia covers the tendon.

3.3 Patient selection

Correct patient selection and evaluation of their expectations are paramount. The strategy to treat these patients who frequently require various body lifting and liposuction procedures is planned at the initial visit. Evaluation of the degree of skin laxity and its quality, the overall extent of deformity of the inner thigh and the extent of lipodystrophy is relevant [40].
An important aspect of the initial physical examination is the evaluation of the lower

abdomen and pubis. In the presence of significant lower abdomen fat deposits and skin excess along with a ptotic and enlarged fat pubic area, these parts should be treated before the performance of the inner thigh lift procedure (41).

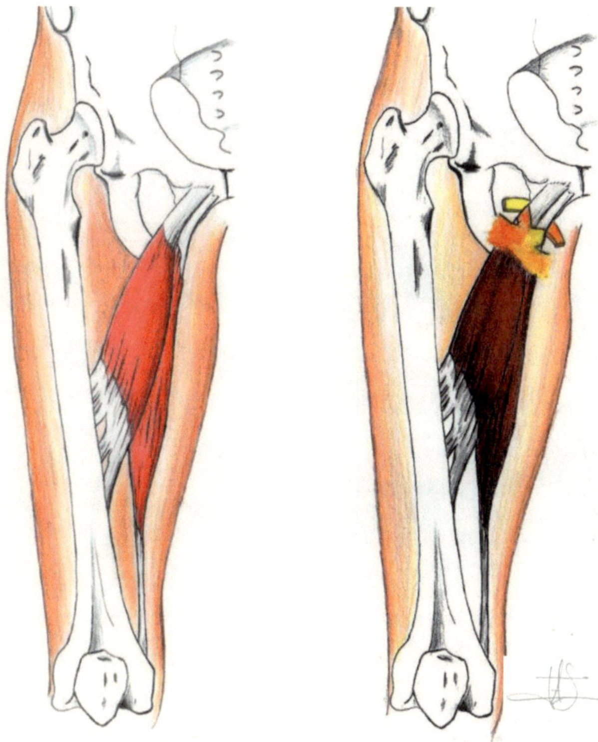

Fig. 19. Anatomy of the adductor muscles. Notice the situation in which the dermal flap is fixed to the tendon.

In our experience a conservative approach to the inner thigh area using energy-assisted liposuction (Ultrasound, Laser or Radiofrequency) without skin resection has resulted in satisfactory improvement in 50 % of our patients.
When the liposuction fails to achieve adequate cosmetic results the inner thigh lift surgery is performed 3 to 6 month after the initial liposuction. Most of our patients undergoing inner thigh lift are females between the ages of 35 and 75. We have found that in men the presence of hair in the inner thigh skin makes difficult to create a dermal flap free of hair follicles.
The Mathes (42) and Kenkel classification has been very useful in deciding what patients are good candidates for the authors' inner thigh lift procedure.
A standard comprehensive preoperative work up is performed in all patients. In patients at high risk for DVT active preventive maneuvers at surgery such as sequential compression and the use of compression socks are used. Contraceptive pills are discontinued.

3.4 Surgical technique

A Clorexidine soap shower is routinely performed just before the patient is moved to the operating room. Standard preoperative photographs are taken. Using a good quality pen, the patient is marked in the standing position with the knees apart. Using the "pinch test" we determine the degree of redundant skin that needs to be removed and the amount of fat that will be suctioned by liposuction (43). Marking the patient in a resting position may result in over-resection of the inner thigh lower flap. The marking of the outer border of the ellipsoid-shaped skin incision is then completed (Figure 20).

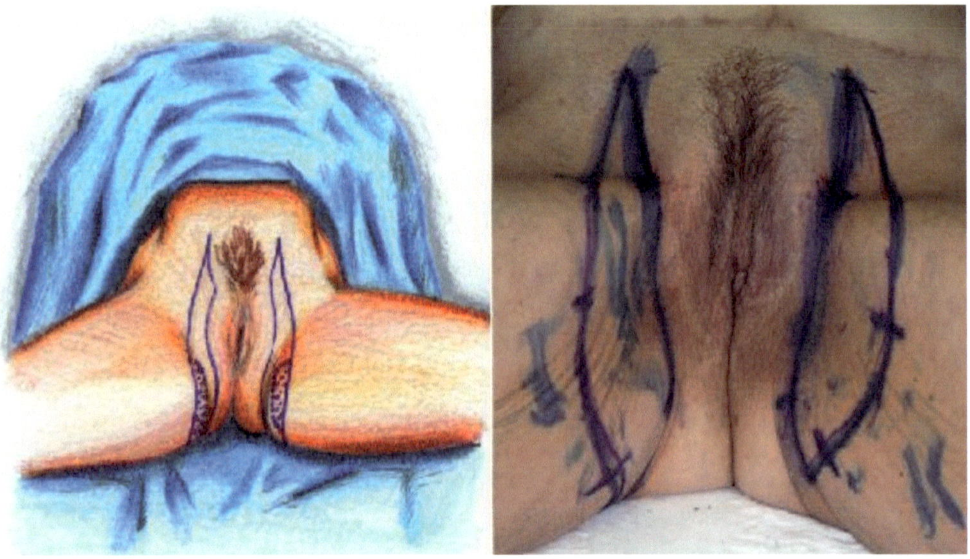

Fig. 20. Marking of the skin to be resected, the dotted area corresponds to the dermal-adipose flap.

Our patients prefer the scars placement on the sides of their pubis instead of the inguinal sulcus because it is easier to cover it with their underwear or beach garments. The medial incision of each side is marked in a vertical way in one of the lateral borders of the mons pubis and advanced vertically to the adductor tendon projection on the skin (Figure 21).

From the adductor tendon projection to the ischion projection the skin incision is placed in the sulcus that exists between the labia major lateral aspect and the inner thigh. We avoid the extension of the skin incision beyond the point of projection of the ischion at the buttock's fold. Care is taken to keep enough skin on the labia side in order to avoid distortions and preserve the normal anatomy of this area. (Fig. 18)

The extent of the ellipsoid skin excision ranges from to 2 cm to 5 cm at the central area of the ellipse to be excised.

With the patient in the prone position we mark the dermal-adipose fixation flap.

The dermal-adipose fixation flap is 1 cm. wide and 8 to 10 cm. long, with a central area 2 cm wide just in the projection of the vector that we want to create during the flap elevation.

The patient is then placed in a frog-leg position with both feet in contact. Standard sterilization preparation is completed and local tumescent anesthesia is infiltrated (44). A 0.06% solution of Lidocaine is infiltrated in the area to undergo liposuction and 0.12 % Lidocaine is infiltrated on the area of skin resection. Following the completion of the liposuction using the Avelar approach (65), the epidermis is removed from the skin of the dermal-fat flap preserving as much dermis as possible. This step is carefully performed because this small flap is the anchor of the lower inner thigh flap and holds the lower flap in place under tension following the completion of the surgery.

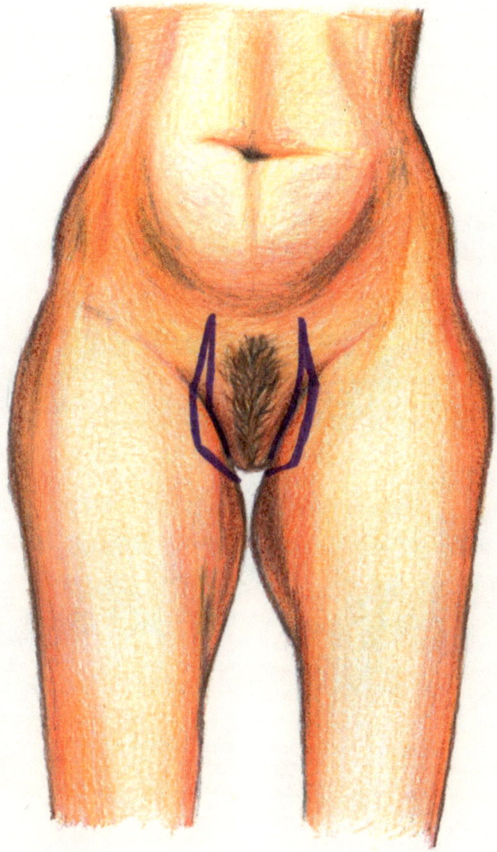

Fig. 21. Front view of the marking with the patient standing.

The rest of the skin ellipsoid area is then removed.
During surgery deep dissection of the femoral triangle area is avoided to prevent potential serious bleeding and lymphatic trauma.
At the dermal-fat flap two strips 1 cm wide and 4 cm long are performed.
Using blunt dissection with a Halsted forceps a tunnel is created under the adductor major tendon. With the same forceps the end of each dermo-adipose strip flap is grasped and both ends are then passed under the tendon. The two flaps are then wrapped around the tendon. The flaps are fixed to the tendon suturing them to each other and to the tendon with 2/0 permanent multifilament sutures. The excess of the flaps is resected.
The superficial fascia of Colles is identified. Anchoring sutures using 2/0 Vicryl , are placed to approximate the Colles' fascia with the subdermal layer of both superior and inferior skin flaps (Figure 22).
Superficial subcutaneous sutures are placed with 3-0 Monocryl sutures and sterile Micropore tape is placed on the skin to reduce the tension on the inner thigh suture line.
All patients receive single IV doses of antibiotics (Cefazoline) during the procedure.
Drains are not routinely placed. Compression garments are used for 3 weeks. Early ambulation starts the night of the surgery and is encouraged to reduce the risk of DVT. The majority of patients are discharged the day of the surgery.

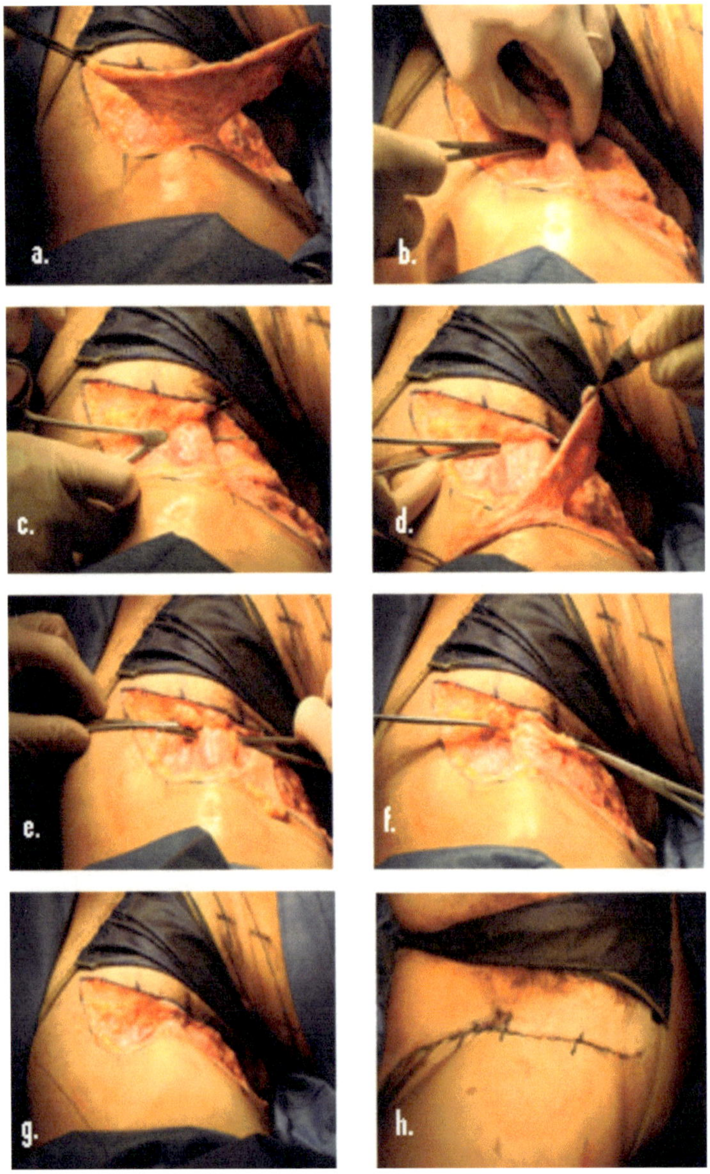

Fig. 22. Consecutive steps from the carving of dermal-adipose flap, tendinous tunnel creation and subsequent fixation

3.5 Discussion

Most of the current medial thigh lift techniques are based on Lockwood's (45, 46) concept of supporting the thigh tissues with sutures (44, 47). The authors' technique introduces a more substantial approach to support the flap while reducing distortions of the vulva and mons pubis (Figure 18). This technique also avoids the T incision. The success in this procedure depends on patient selection, surgical planning and patients' realistic expectations (Figure 23).

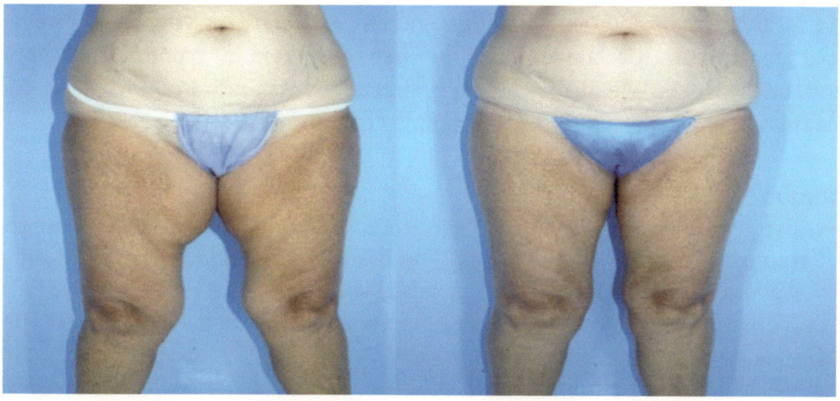

Fig. 23. Pre-and postoperative photographs of Medial Thigh Lift combining liposuction and Dermal Flaps Suspension to the Adductor Tendon

4. Breast reduction by liposuction

4.1 Introduction

Several techniques for breast reduction by excision under general anesthesia are available. Extensive scarring, necrosis of the nipple-areolar complex and postoperative pain are common sequellae, contributing to a long recovery time. The potential for breast-feeding following surgical reduction may be impaired.

Breast reduction by liposuction using tumescent local anesthesia (TLA) and powered cannulas eliminates most of the complications of the excisional technique. There is no need for hospitalization, the downtime is minimal and there are no disfiguring scars. Therefore, this technique could be the preferred treatment modality in a selected group of patients.

Patient satisfaction is high, which can be explained by the significant volume reduction (average 50%) in combination with a ptosis reduction, short downtime and minimal scarring. However, secure and careful patient selection is critical.

4.2 Patient selection

The content of fat in the breast increases with age. This is independent from the BMI. For that reason, older women are good candidates for breast reduction by liposuction as this technique reduces the fat amount only. The breasts of younger women as an average contain less fat and more glandular tissue, which diminishes the amount of fat that can be aspirated. The Body Mass Index (BMI) could be used to indicate the amount of fat in the breasts in younger women. However, the BMI cannot be used as an absolute selection criterion, because patients with fatty legs and a high BMI as a consequence, as we see in patients with lipedema, do not necessarily have a high percentage of fat in the breasts.

With the exception of post-menopausal women, patients who desire more that 50% reduction in breast size are not good candidates for breast reduction by liposuction using TLA. Moderate lifting and conservation of the original shape of the breasts are realistic goals; however, patients who are more concerned about breast lifting than volume reduction should not have breast reduction using TLA. The ideal candidate is one who refuses excision and will accept any degree of breast reduction that is possible with liposuction using TLA. All patients should understand and accept the relative unpredictability of the

amount of fat that can be removed with liposuction, especially in younger women. There is no reliable benchmark for the amount of size reduction a patient may expect with liposuction. Bra size is unreliable because it is affected by the individual wearing it.
A personal history of breast cancer is an absolute contraindication.

4.3 Technique

A preoperative mammogram should be performed to identify malignant or benign tumors, and the mammogram serves as a baseline. The mammogram should be repeated yearly to detect post-operative calcification, although this is very unlikely.
Photo-documentation and precise measurements for volume and ptosis are performed (Figure 24).
Preoperative antibiotics are administered.
Preoperative markings are made with the patient in the upright position (Figure 25). They may extend under the armpit in case the lateral extension of the breast should be treated as well.
Local anesthesia is given to 8 skin sites on each breast.
Sharp needles are introduced to start the infiltration of the tumescent solution in the breast using a peristaltic infiltration pump (Table 1). The needles are regularly re-positioned in the breast tissue as tumescence is obtained in each area (Figure 26). The infiltration is initiated in the deepest plane, just above the muscle layer. Also the more superficial layers, including the most superficial subdermal plane, are meticulously infiltrated.
After completion of the infiltration, at least 30 minutes is dedicated to the even diffusion of the solution through the breast tissue and to develop adequate anesthesia and vasoconstriction. A second infiltration can then be performed to achieve profound tumescence. The total volume of tumescent solution infiltrated will be 150-200 percent of the measured breast volume (eg. 1500-2000 ml) will be infiltrated when the breast volume was measured as 1000 ml by water displacement.
Incisions are made in the lateral and medial infra-mammary crease. Liposuction is then started using a powered blunt cannula with a 3 mm diameter. A criss-cross pattern is performed through the various layers of the breast. The entire procedure is performed from the infra-mammary incisions only. Most of the fat lies deeply, but the layers close to the surface must also be suctioned in case the maximum amount of fat has to be removed. The surgeon must avoid aggressive suction from the upper pole of the breast. Otherwise, irregularities may be created and/or the breast may take on an unnatural shape which may become visible when wearing garments with low necklines.
After suction of the second breast, one hour should be allowed for separation of infranatant and supranatant in the canister before calculating the final volume of tissue removed.
Excessive suction under the nipple should not be performed in order to avoid necrosis and loss of sensation.
One breast is suctioned completely before the other is begun. When breasts are of equal size, care must be taken to remove the same amount of fat from each breast. The breasts are wrapped in a special absorbent material and an elastic garment which allows tight but adjustable compression. A second more tight compression band can be applied for 1 day to prevent extensive hematoma.

4.4 Postoperative period

The patient may shower on the morning after surgery. Compression is continued for 2-4 weeks. The incisions may still have some drainage. During the first days, relatively firm

compression is maintained in order to prevent seroma and edema. After the first or second week a sport-bra is used. Mild activity can be resumed after two days. Solid masses will be noticed in the weeks following treatment. It takes about four months for complete resolution of the masses. The surgical procedure itself is generally easier on the patient than they expect. Normal office work can be resumed within a few days of surgery, but intense physical activity must be delayed because of sensitivity of the breasts during motion.
Postoperative visits are scheduled after 6 and 16 weeks. At these times, photodocumentation and measurements of volume and ptosis are repeated.

4.5 Expected benefits of the procedure

The goal of breast reduction by liposuction is a reduction in volume with negligible scars, minimal risk of complications and conservation of the original shape of the breasts.
Patients are concerned that breasts will look like "empty bags". Surgeons who practice liposuction using TLA with powered microcannulas are aware of the considerable retraction of subcutaneous tissues on other body areas, especially on the abdomen and neck. A similar phenomenon is seen after liposuction of the breast. This can be explained by reduction in breast weight, the irritation of the connective tissue in the subcutaneous layer and subsequent contraction during healing and contraction of Cooper's ligaments. Induction of scar tissue results in further contraction. The "empty bag" phenomenon does not occur even when 50 percent or more of the breast volume has been removed. The average lifting effect is 3 cm and rises with age (Table 2).
Experience demonstrates that in properly selected cases, a 20-70 percent reduction can be achieved. Patients who have had 30 percent or more of the breast volume removed are usually very satisfied also because they feel that their breasts are the same shape as before surgery but without the feeling of being heavy.
Preoperative back and shoulder pain usually disappears or diminishes substantially when 30 percent or more of the breast volume has been removed.

4.6 Considerations

If the patient wishes a reduction in ptosis and/or a change in breast shape, liposuction is not the correct procedure. If volume reduction is the goal, then liposuction should be considered (Table 3).
If long scars and general anesthesia are rejected, a second opinion focusing on breast reduction by excision may be unnecessary. The short recovery period and minimal risk of complications may be major deciding factors for patients who chose breast reduction by liposuction (Figure 27,28).
If the breast size has increased over the years, discounting the effect of pregnancy and hormonal treatment, the amount of fat in the breasts has probably increased. This may suggest that a considerable reduction is possible with liposuction. When excessive weight is gained during puberty, the breast probably contain a great deal of fat. A considerable reduction by liposuction is possible in these patients. When large breasts are caused by glandular hypertrophy, liposuction will probably be less successful. When the development of larger breast are associated with a gain in body weight, a successful reduction by liposuction is likely.
There is no reason to pretend that glandular tissue might be damaged. The evaluation of specimens taken from the supranatant fat showed only minor fragments of ductuli in a small minority of younger patients. It is extremely unlikely that lactation will be impaired by this minimal damage.

4.7 Side effects and complications

Most patients develop a temporary loss of sensation around the nipple. The breasts are usually sensitive for at least several weeks following surgery. Hematoma may develop in the hours or days following surgery. Drainage must be followed by firm compression. Other side-effects and complications are similar as those in liposuction using TLA in other body areas.
Postoperative mammograms rarely reveal any new calcifications.

4.8 Conclusion

Breast reduction by liposuction using TLA and powered cannulas is a safe and effective treatment modality in properly selected patients. Complications are minor and infrequent, and patients are able to return to normal daily activities within 3-4 days after the procedure. Sports and heavy physical activities can be gradually resumed, and patient satisfaction is excellent.

NaCl 0.9%	1000 mL
Lidocaine	500 mg
Epinephrine	1 mg
Sodium bicarbonate 8.4%	10 mL

Table 1. Solution as used in breast reduction under tumescent local anesthesia.

	Average	Spread
Age (years)	46	16-77
Ptosis reduction (cm)	3	0-7,0
Supranatant Fat Removed per breast (mL)	550	80-2275
Breast Volume Removed (%)	54	24-87
TLA infiltrated per breast (mL)	1925	650-4900

Table 2. Data on 200 women after breast reduction by liposuction using Tumescent Local Anesthesia.

Women who refuse breast reduction by excision
Women who will accept a reduction of 50% or less
Women > 40 years of age
Unoperated large breasts
Large breasts after surgical reduction
Asymmetry in volume of the breasts
Patients who prefer local anesthesia over general anesthesia
Patients with (relative) contra-indications for general anesthesia

Table 3. Good candidates for breast reduction by liposuction using Tumescent Local Anesthesia.

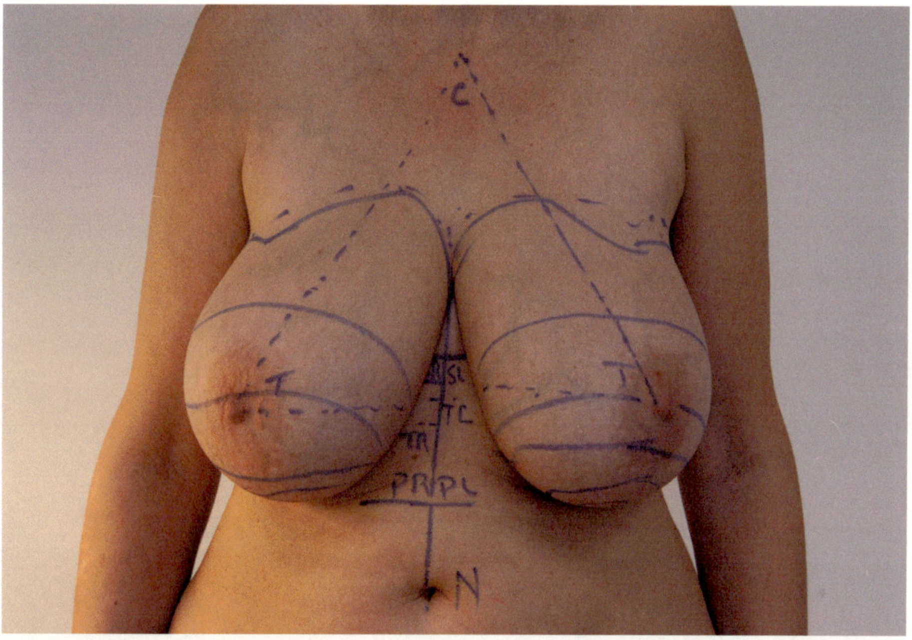

Fig. 24. Preoperative measurements, S representing position of inframammary fold, P representing lowest projection of breast and T representing projection of the nipple. L represents Left, R represents Right.

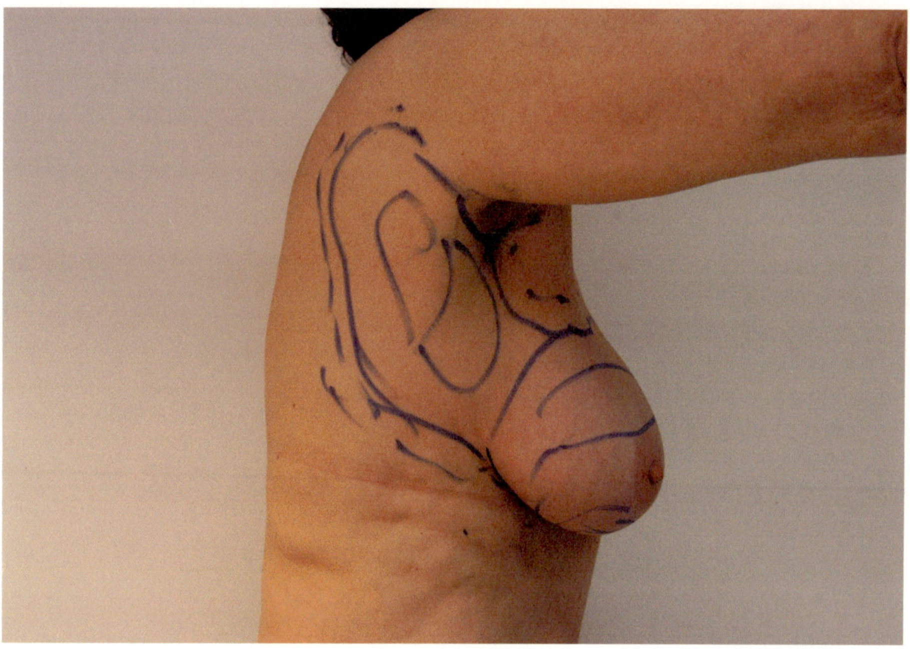

Fig. 25. Markings guiding the surgeon for areas and planes of fat removal side view with axillary tail.

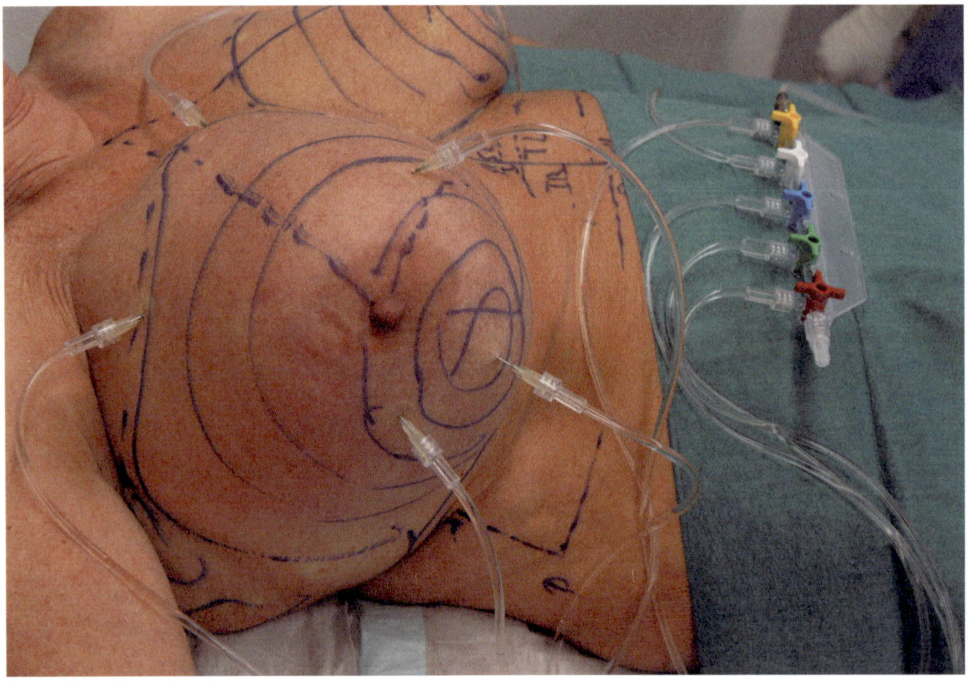

Fig. 26. Five infiltration needles are used during infiltration.

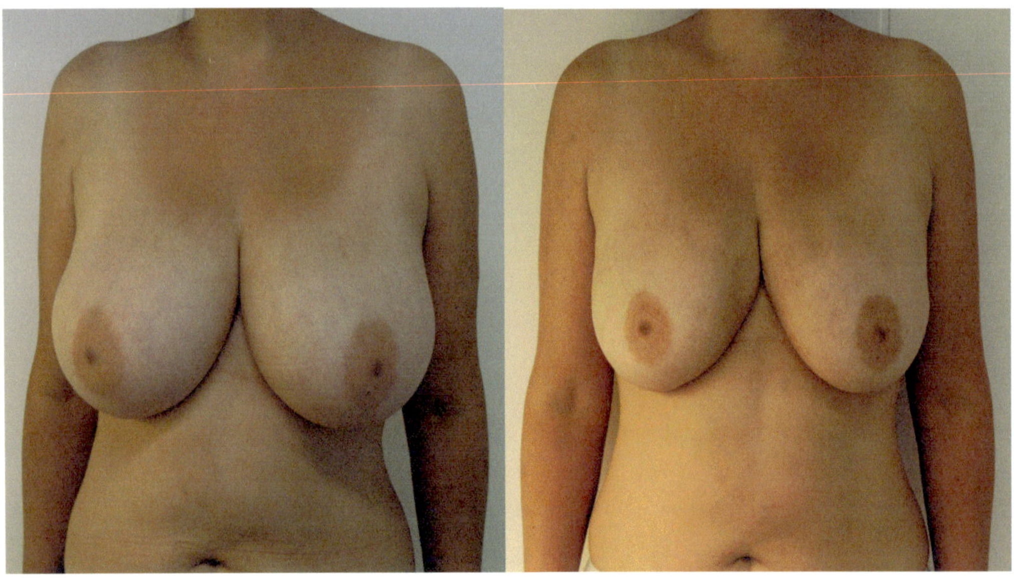

Fig. 27. A: Before liposuction of the breast in a 42 year-old woman. B: 4 months after liposuction: volume reduction 675 ml supranatant fat per breast (56%) and ptosis reduction 3,7 cm (50%).

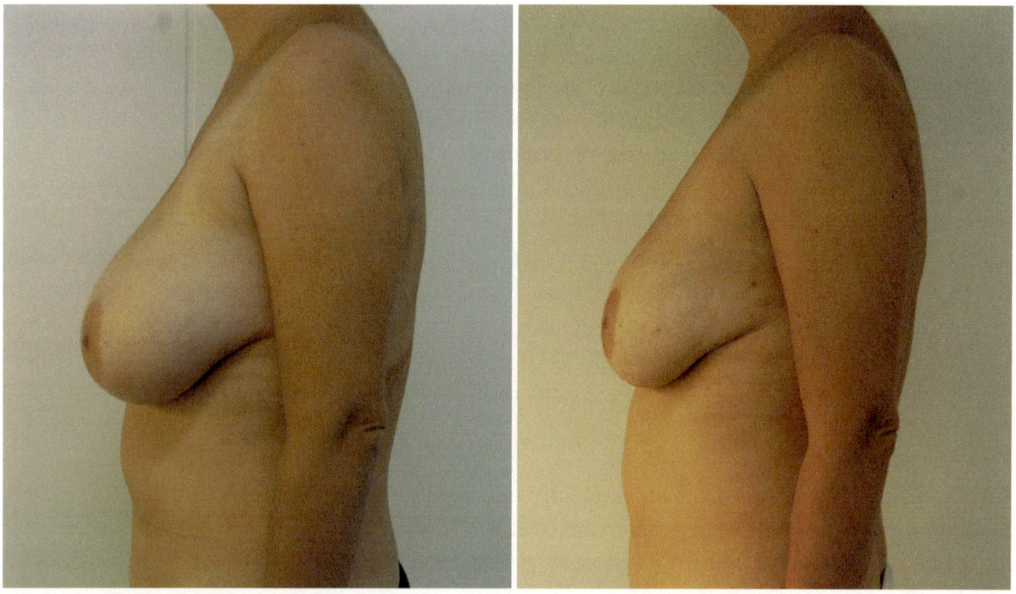

Fig. 28. From axillary tails additional 200 ml supranatant fat aspirated. A Posoperative view.

5. Safety combination of liposuction and abdominoplasty with B&S technique

5.1 Introduction

Tummy tuck, or abdominoplasty, is the fifth most frequently requested cosmetic procedure. More than 116,000 abdominoplasty surgeries were performed in the United States alone during the year 2010 (48).

The abdominoplasty with simultaneous liposuction is a procedure that has become a save and effective solution for the abdominal contouring and flaccidity. The history of abdominoplasty goes back to the late eighteen hundreds in the Johns Hopkins Hospital where it was described as a conjunct procedure for large abdominal wall hernias, and through out the twentieth century it had evolved into a procedure with acceptable aesthetic results.

Although this procedure is becoming more popular, classical abdominoplasty is related to a relatively high complication rate. General and local complications include pulmonary thrombo-embolism, seroma, hematoma and necrosis of the dermal-fat flap.

According to a national survey, postoperative mortality in a national survey was 0.2% in 1972 (49) and decreased to 0.04% by 1989 (50). The last national survey had no mortalities in over 11,000 procedures (51). Factors leading to the decrease in the incidence of wound healing problems were: undermining the flap in an inverted "V" fashion, avoiding operating on active smokers, avoiding excess tension on the flap closure, limited flap thinning and avoiding excessive flap liposuction.

Although major complications have diminished in recent decades, wound complication rates remain high—up to 30 % (50, 51, 52, 53, 54).

After the creation and publishing of the blunt-tipped liposuction by Yves-Gerard Illouz (56), the history of the abdominoplasty was changed completely and new combinations of surgeries emerged. Through out the past three decades there has been a series of publications and creations of new surgical techniques related to the association of liposuction and abdominal surgery, including proposals for reduction of abdominal flap dissection to decrease the complications statistics.

During the 1990s, the combination of liposuction and abdominoplasty gained much popularity (55, 57, 58, 59). The increased use of tumescent anaesthesia in particular, enabled the procedure to be performed ambulatory—often in a physician's office setting (60, 61, 62, 63, 64). Despite these developments, wound complications such as seromas, dehiscence and necrosis still remained high (58, 59, 60).

Juarez Avelar, MD, postulated that large-scale undermining of the abdominal flap involving the rupture of the lymphatic and perforator blood supply caused wound complications. To reduce these complications, he developed a new surgical technique that avoids wide undermining, which he presented at the 36th Brazilian Congress of Plastic Surgery in 1999(65, 66). Blugerman then modified this specific technique by including the use of tumescent anaesthesia (67).

This technique with the combined use of liposuction in abdominoplasty under the tumescent local anesthesia has been proved to be an effective technique to reduce complications. The tumescent infiltration used for liposuction of the abdominal wall creates an internal ex-sanguination and vasoconstriction which eliminates all stagnant blood that can be injurious for the flap, reduces in an important manner the vascular injury and the blood loss. Also the liposuction of the superior portion of the abdomen and flanks makes it possible to do a selective undermining of the flap thus preserving the vascularity and sensitivity of the flap. Adding to this, liposuction of the flap and contiguous areas greatly improve the cosmetic outcome.

Nowadays we have combined the use of laserlipolisys and radiofrequency assisted liposuction (60) with the abdominoplasty in patients with different indications, such as vascular fragility or cutaneous flaccidity correspondingly, bringing better results with lower risks.

The purpose of this article is to demonstrate the safety and effectiveness of this relatively new abdominoplasty technique.

6. Patients and methods

Between April 2002 and December 2010, 852 patients underwent surgery to remove excess abdominal skin and fat. All of these patients had surgery in well-equipped office facilities on an outpatient basis. Of those patients, 97% were female and ranged in age between 20 and 82; the average age was 47.

Indications for abdominoplasty were localized adiposities with flaccid, poor-quality skin.

Patients were premedicated with 3–5 mg of midazolam, sedated with propofol and locally infiltrated with 0.05–0.1% of tumescent solution (lidocaine, epinephrine, and sodium bicarbonate). The concentration and volume of tumescent solution was adapted to allow maximal volume infiltration of the treated areas and did not exceed 50 mg lidocaine/kg.

Liposuction with powered cannula (PAL) was then performed on the entire abdominal region, starting at the deep and ending at the superficial levels. Under the skin to be resected, a radical liposuction was performed to remove as much fatty tissue as possible. On the upper abdomen a moderate liposuction was performed. The skin of the lower abdomen was then resected very superficially (Fig.29).

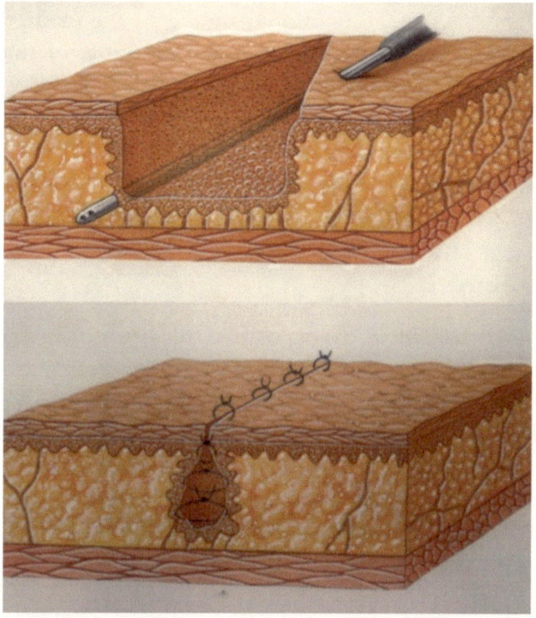

Fig. 29. The original concept of this procedure, consisting in radical liposuction of the area where the desepithelization will be done with subsequent plication.

Caution was given to specifically resect only the dermis and preserve the subcutaneous structures. For umbilicus transformation, undermining was performed restrictively and only in the medial plane to preserve the para-median perforating neurovascular bundles (Fig. 30) and to enable umbilicus re-implantation.

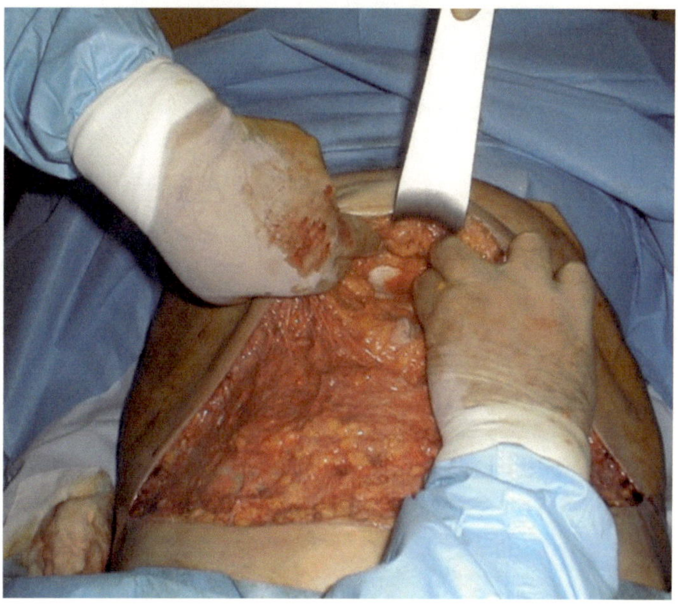

Fig. 30. Medial plane undermining, thus preserving the abdominal wall perforators.

In cases with rectus diastasis (n=27), the undermining of the median plane was continued superiorly until the xiphoid. When necessary, small amounts of tumescent solution were infiltrated under the rectus fascia, enabling the diastasis to be closed with strong nylon sutures under direct vision.
Wound closure was performed directly, without further undermining, by folding over the subcutaneous structures. No drains were used. Patients were mobilized immediately after the operation and then given non-steroid antiphlogistic to control their postoperative pain.

7. Results and follow-up

Full abdominoplasty with umbilicus transposition was performed in 556 patients. Mini-abdominoplasty with liposuction was performed in 296 patients. There were no intra-operative complications. There were no cases of skin necrosis. Wound infections were observed in 13 patients (5,2%). One patient was admitted to hospital for minor wound care. There were no cases of skin necrosis and no seromas were aspirated. One patient developed a suture fistula with a resulting wound dehiscence (4 cm diameter), and achieved secondary healing under ambulatory care. Two patients reported prolonged pain (more than one week), and only one patient required more than one week to resume normal activity (Fig. 31).

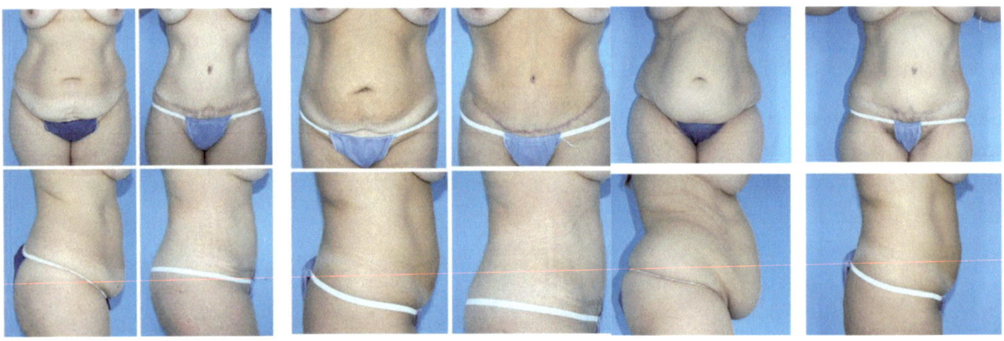

Fig. 31. Pre-operative results of 3 different patients.

8. Conclusion

Classical abdominoplasty with wide-flap undermining certainly achieves the best aesthetic result with low scarring. The aesthetic result may be improved by combining it with liposuction, although not always considered to be safe (68). The elimination of general anaesthesia may reduce systemic complications, as was demonstrated by Rosenberg (69). The rate of local complications however remained high, so Avelar temporarily refrained from performing the procedure (65).
Conventional abdominoplasty with wide undermining results in profound devascularisation of the abdominal flap, (70, 71) explaining complications such as skin and/or fat necrosis. Furthermore, wide undermining creates a large wound surface that is prone to seroma. Lymph drainage is also impaired by separating the perforating vessels that are exasperating the problem. The trend towards inverted "V" type undermining certainly acknowledges the need to preserve better flap perfusion. Decreased sensibility in the hypo-gastric region is also a problem not to be underestimated after wide undermining (71).

The principle of minimal undermining combined with extended liposuction, as originally proposed by Avelar (65), appears to solve most of these problems (Fig 32).

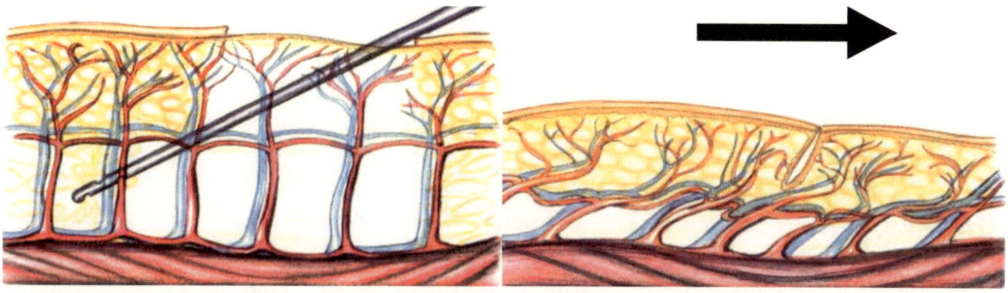

Fig. 32. Extended liposuction with minimal undermining described by Avelar (65).

Performing abdominoplasty in sedonalgesia using the tumescent solution on an outpatient basis appears to be a safe procedure. Further studies are required to confirm the low complication rates.
Liposuction of the upper abdomen is, of course, not comparable to wide undermining; but the aesthetic compromise of a slightly higher scar seems acceptable in view of the low complication rate.

9. References

[1] Gonzalez R. Buttocks Reshaping, Indexa, 219:291

[2] Illouz Y, et al. Lipoaspiration Hipocrates, 201:208

[3] Illouz Y. Une nouvelle technique pour les lipodystrophies localisées. Rev Chir Esthet.

[4] Fournier P. Liposculpturing: The Syringe Technique. "The Bermuda Triangle" 185:190. Arnette Blackwell.

[5] Klein J. Tumescent Technique. Tumescent Anesthesia and Microcanular Liposuction. Mosby , Chap 1 :23.

[6] Rouviere H, et al. Human Anatomy. 11 Ed. Elsevier, 412:413

[7] Jacob . S Atlas of Human Anatomy Elsevier ,160:162

[8] Latarjet et al. Human Anatomy Panamericana, 715:731

[9] Moore K. Clinical Orientation of Anatomy. Panamericana; 731:732

[10] Liposuction zones described by a Gottfried Lemperle in "Ästhetische Chirurgie" ecomed medizine

[11] D. Bergfeld, et al. Technik der Infiltration. Tumeszenz-Localanästhesie: praktische Awendung. Springer,. 50.

[12] Blugerman G, Schavelzon D, Paul MD. A safety and feasibility study of a novel radiofrequency assisted liposuction technology. Plast Reconstr Surg. 2010;125(3):998-1006

[13] Blugerman G. et al. Actual methodology for autologous fat graft. Actas del XXIII Brasilian Congress of Plastic Surgery

[14] Yamaguchi Ch. Proc. Minimal Invasive Aesthetic Procedures 381:425 Santos

[15] Gonzalez R. Buttocks Reshaping. Indexa : 95:160

[16] Allen EV, Hines EA. Lipedema of the legs. Proc Mayo Clin 1940; 15: 184-7.

[17] AWMF. Leitlinien der Deutschen Gesellschaft für Phlebologie (DGP): Lipödem. AWMF-Leitlinien-Register Nr. 037/012. 2009.
[18] Schmeller W, Meier-Vollrath I. Lipödem - Aktuelles zu einem weitgehend unbekannten Krankheitsbild. Akt Dermatol 2007; 33: 1–10.
[19] Herpertz U. Ödeme und Lymphdrainage. Diagnose und Therapie von Ödemkrankheiten. Schattauer, Stuttgart, New York, 2003.
[20] Herpertz U. Krankheitsspektrum des Lipödems an einer Lymphologischen Fachklinik - Erscheinungsformen, Mischbilder und Behandlungsmöglichkeiten. Vasomed 1997; 5: 301-7.
[21] Meier-Vollrath I, Schneider W, Schmeller W. Lipödem: Verbesserte Lebensqualität durch Therapiekombination. Deutsches Ärzteblatt 2005; 102: A-1061-67.
[22] .Schmeller W, Meier-Vollrath I. Erfolgreiche operative Therapie des Lipödems mittels Liposuktion. Phlebologie 2004; 33: 23–9.
[23] Schmeller W, Meier-Vollrath I. Moderne Therapie des Lipödems: Kombination von konservativen und operativen Maßnahmen. Lymph-Forsch 2004; 8: 22–6.
[24] Schmeller W, Meier-Vollrath I. Tumescent liposuction: a new and successful therapy for lipedema. J Cutan Med Surg 2006; 10: 7–10.
[25] Schmeller W, Meier-Vollrath I. Das Lipödem: neue Möglichkeiten der Therapie. Schweiz Med Forum 2007; 7: 150–5.
[26] Kaufmann R, Landes E, Podda M. Dermatologische Operationen. 3. Auf- lage, Thieme Verlag, Stuttgart, New York, 2005.
[27] Rompel R, Petres J. Operative Dermatologie. 2. Auflage, Springer Verlag, Heidelberg, 2007.
[28] Cornely ME. Lipödem und die Differentialdiagnosen. Journal für Lymphologie 2001; 1: 32–3.
[29] Rapprich S, Loehnert M, Hagedorn M. Therapy of lipoedema syndrome by liposuction under tumescent local anaesthesia. Ann Dermatol Venereol 2002; 129: 1S711.
[30] Sattler G, Bergfeld D, Sommer B. [Liposuction]. Hautarzt 2004; 55: 599–604.
[31] Sattler G, Hasche E, Rapprich S et al. Neue operative Behandlungsmöglichkeiten bei benignen Fettgewebserkrankungen. Z Hautkr 1997; 72: 579–82.
[32] Sattler G, Rapprich S, Hagedorn M. Tumeszenz-Lokalanästhesie - Untersuchung zur Pharmakokinetik von Prilocain. Z Hautkr 1997; 7: 522–5.
[33] Herpertz U. Die häufigsten Beinödeme. Differenzierung zwischen Phlebödem, Lymphödem und Lipödem. Phlebologie 2001; 30: 48–52.
[34] Langendoen SI, Habbema L, Nijsten TE, Neumann HA. Lipoedema: from clinical presentation to therapy. A review of the literature. Br J Dermatol 2009; 161(5): 980–6.
[35] Rapprich S, Dingler A, Podda M. Liposuction is an effective treatment for lipedema - results of a study with 25 patients. Journal of the GermanSociety of Dermatology. JDDG;2010• 8 - 1-8
[36] Lewis JR Jr. Correction of ptosis of the thighs: the thigh lift. Plast Reconstr Surg 1966; 37(6):494–8.
[37] Candiani P, Campiglio GL, Signorini M. Fascio-fascial suspension technique in medial thigh lifts. Aesthetic Plast Surg 1995; 19(2): 137–40.
[38] Ersek RA, Salisbury AV. The saddle lift for tight . Aesthetic Plast Surg 1995; 19(4):341–3.
[39] Spirito D. Medial thigh lift and DE.C.LI.VE. Aesthetic Plast Surg 1998; 22(4):298–300.

[40] Hurwitz DJ. Single-staged total body lift after massive weight loss. Ann Plast Surg 2004;52(5): 435–41.
[41] Pitanguy I. Surgical reduction of the abdomen, thighs and buttocks. Surg Clin North Am 1971; 51(2):479–89.
[42] Mathes DW. Current Concepts in Medial Thighplasty. Clin. Plastic. Surg '35 (2008) 151-163
[43] Vilain R, Dardour JC. Aesthetic surgery of the medial thigh. Ann Plast Surg 1986; 17(3):176–83.
[44] Le Louarn C, Pascal JF. The concentric medial thigh lift. Aesthetic Plast Surg 2004; 28(1):20–3 [Epub 2004 Mar 25].
[45] Lockwood TE. Fascial anchoring technique in medial thigh lifts. Plast Reconstr Surg 1988; 82(2):299–304.
[46] Lockwood T. Lower body lift with superficial fascial system suspension. Plast Reconstr Surg 1993; 92(6):1112–22 [discussion: 1123–5]
[47] Planas J. The "Crural Meloplasty" for lifting of the thighs. Clin Plast Surg 1975; 2:495–503.
[48] American Society of Plastic Surgeons, National Plastic Surgery Statistics 2010, ASPS 2011.
[49] Grazer FM, Goldwyn RM. Abdominoplasty assessed by survey, with emphasis on complications. Plast Reconstr Surg. 1977;59(4): 513-517.
[50] Teimourian B, Rogers WB III. A national survey of complications associated with suction lipectomy: a comparative study. Plast Reconstr Surg. 1989;84(4):628-631.
[51] Matarasso A, Swift RW, Rankin M. Abdominoplasty and Abdominal Contour Surgery: A National Plastic Surgery Survey.Plast Reconstr Surg. 2006;117(6):1797-1808.
[52] Manassa EH, Hertl CH, Olbrisch RR. Wound healing problems in smokers and nonsmokers after 132 abdominoplasties. Plast Reconstr Surg. 2003;111(6): 2082-2089.
[53] Hensel JM, Lehman JA Jr, Tantri MP, Parker MG, Wagner DS, Topham NS. An outcomes analysis and satisfaction survey of 199 consecutive abdominoplasties. Ann Plast Surg. 2001;46(4):357-363.
[54] Chaouat M, Levan P, Lalanne B, Buisson T, Nicolau P, Mimoun M. Abdominal dermolipectomies: early postoperative complications and long-term unfavorable results. Plast Reconstr Surg. 2000;106(7): 1614-1618.
[55] Matarasso A. Abdominoplasty: a system of classification and treatment for combined abdominoplasty and suction-assisted lipectomy. Aesthetic Plast Surg. 1991;15(2):111-121.
[56] Avelar J., Illouz Y., Lipoaspiração, Hipócrates 1986
[57] Shestak KC. Marriage abdominoplasty expands the mini-abdominoplasty concept. Plast Reconstr Surg. 1999;103(3):1020-1035.
[58] Cardenas-Camarena L, Gonzalez LE. Large-volume liposuction and extensive abdominoplasty: a feasible alternative for improving body shape. Plast Reconstr Surg. 1998;102(5):1698-1707.
[59] Dillerud E. Abdominoplasty combined with suction lipoplasty: a study of complications, revisions, and risk factors in 487 cases. Ann Plast Surg. 1990;25(5):333-343.

[60] Kryger ZB, Fine NA, Mustoe TA. The outcome of abdominoplasty performed under conscious sedation: six-year experience in 153 consecutive cases. Plast Reconstr Surg. 2004;113(6):1807-1817.
[61] Namias A, Kaplan B. Dermatol Surg. Tumescent anesthesia for dermatologic surgery. Cosmetic and Noncosmetic Procedures. 1998;24(7):755-758.
[62] Byrd HS, Barton FE, Orenstein HH, Rohrich RJ, Burns AJ, Hobar PC, Haydon MS. Safety and efficacy in an accredited outpatient plastic surgery facility: a review of 5316 consecutive cases. Plast Reconstr Surg. 2003;112(2): 636-646.
[63] Cochran TA. Abdominal lipectomy as an office procedure. J Med Assoc Ga. 1991;80(11):631-633.
[64] Abramson DL. Tumescent abdominoplasty: an ambulatory office procedure. Aesthetic Plast Surg. 1998;22(6):404-407.
[65] Avelar JM. A new technique for abdominoplasty-closed vascular system of subdermal flap folded over itself combined with liposuction. Revista Brasilera de Cirurgia 1999;88/89:3-20.
[66] Avelar JM. Abdominoplasty without panniculus undermining and resection: analysis and 3-year follow-up of 97 consecutive cases. Aesthet Surg J. 2002 Jan;22(1):16-25.
[67] Blugerman G. Modified abdominoplasty, a new South American technique. Vortrag auf dem Kongress der Deutschen Gesellschaft für Ästhetische Chirurgie, Heidelberg 2002. 19a.
[68] Matarasso A. Abdominal dermolipectomies: early postoperative complications and long-term unfavourable results (Discussion). Plast Reconstr Surg. 2000;106(7):1619-1623.
[69] Rosenberg MH, Palaia DA, Bonanno PC. Abdominoplasty with procedural sedation and analgesia. Ann Plast Surg. 2001;46(5):485-487.
[70] Mayr M, Holm C, Hofter E, Becker A, Pfeiffer U, Muhlbauer W. Effects of aesthetic abdominoplasty on abdominal wall perfusion: a quantitative evaluation. Plast Reconstr Surg. 2004;114(6):1586-1594.
[71] Graf R, de Araujo LR, Rippel R, Neto LG, Pace DT, Cruz GA. Lipoabdominoplasty: liposuction with reduced undermining and traditional abdominal skin flap resection. Aesthetic Plast Surg. 2006 Jan-Feb;30(1):1-8.
[72] Kolker AR. Improving esthetics and safety in abdominoplasty with broad lateral subcostal perforator preservation and contouring with liposuction. Ann Plast Surg. 2008 May;60(5):491-7.
[73] Heller JB, Teng E, Knoll BI, Persing J. Outcome analysis of combined lipoabdominoplasty versus conventional abdominoplasty. Plast Reconstr Surg. 2008 May;121(5):1821-9.
[74] Farah AB, Nahas FX, Ferreira LM, Mendes Jde A, Juliano Y. Sensibility of the abdomen after abdominoplasty. Plast Reconstr Surg. 2004;114(2): 577-583.

2

Liposuction and Fat Graft to Enhance Facial Contour in Reconstructive Surgery - Nine Years Experience with the Use of Peridural Cannula

Claudia Gutiérrez Gómez,
Marcia Pérez Dosal and Alexander Cardenas Mejia
Postgraduate Course in Plastic and Reconstructive Surgery Universidad Nacional Autonoma de México/General Hospital "Dr. Manuel Gea González ", México City Mexico

1. Introduction

Correction of severe facial contour abnormalities still is a challenge to plastic surgeons. The aim of plastic surgical treatments is to restore a harmonious and symmetrical appearance. Some of the entities that cause this abnormalities include: Parry Romberg syndrome, lupus, Melkerson Rosenthal syndrome, Morphea, trauma's sequel, embolization sequel, trauma, hemifacial microsomy, etc. (Gutiérrez " et al". 2007,2009).

The free fat graft has been used since 1889, with the open ceiling technique, in 1893 Neuber recommended the use of fat grafts size lesser than an almond (Neuber 1893).In 1910 Lexer start the use of fat graft in aesthetic surgery and in 1925 reports the first case of facial contour reconstruction in a patient with Parry Romberg syndrome.(Lexer 1910) Peer reports lost of fat tissue as much as 50% (Peer 1950,1956) later it was used the fat obtained by liposuction ; absorption of the graft was the main problem and several different procedures have been described to minimize this phenomenon .Illouz in 1990 demonstrated that 80% of the injected fat graft was resorbed (Illouz 1990) .In 1994 it started the " atraumatic purified" technique preconized by Coleman. Being the last one the one with better results in preserving volume because of a more viability of the adipose tissue and long lasting results. He recommends to avoid chopping, washing, manipulation, freezing, high negative pressure during extraction with a vacuum or high positive pressure during placement. Exposure to dry air will cause fat to desiccate rapidly.(Coleman 1995,1997,2002).

Fat grafts collected by liposuction can be subcutaneously reinjected for correction of depressed or irregular areas. The live fat tissue is revascularized at the transplantation site within 48 hours,during which time it is fed by diffused materials from plasma. Explantation of adipose tissue as performed during the procedure of autologous fat transfer confers stress to preadipocytes and adipocytes. Disruption of blood supply during fat harvesting may result in hipoxia and apoptosis of the heterogeneous population of cells present in adipose tissue. Preadipocytes play an important role in soft tissue augmentation, because these adipocyte precursor cells have a higher survival rate under ischemic conditions than mature adipocytes and even have the ability to proliferate and differentiate into mature adipocytes. (Asken 1990;Guerrerosantos "et al". 1996; Latoni "et al".2000;Rieck & Schlaak 2003; Sadick &

Hudgins 2001.) Easy of technique, unlikelihood of scar formation, low morbidity, and low cost have increased the popularity of this operation. Fat grafts collected by liposuction can be subcutaneously reinjected for correction of depressed or irregular areas.
Fat should be harvested as an intact tissue small enough to pass through a small- lumen cannula, eliminating the need to later reduce the size of the parcel of fat by washing, chopping or straining. To obtain predictable results harvested subcutaneous tissue should be refined so the material infiltrated is mainly viable fatty tissue; via centrifugation, oil, blood, water and extracellular components should be removed without causing significant damage to the fat to be transplanted (Coleman 2001).

2. Patients and methods; Patient data

During the last nine years we have been injecting the fat graft with a peridural cannula in 73 patients for fat graft in the face.With ages from 5 to 61 years old, with a media of 28.3 years. They were females in 75.4% (55 cases) and male in 24.6% (18 cases). The ethiology of the deformities were Parry Romberg Syndrome 71.2% (52 cases), Morphea in 6 cases (8.2%), trauma sequel 4 cases (5.4%), hemifacial microsomia, lupus and post tumor resection sequel in 9 cases (3 each group; 4.1% each). Depression after embolization of vascular anomaly 1 case (1.3%), Number 7 facial cleft 1 case (1.3%).With a total of 132 procedures realized (about 1.8 per patient). Table 1.

ETHIOOGYL	# CASES	%
PARRY ROMBERG	52	71.2
MORPHEA	6	8.2
TRAUMA SEQUEL	4	5.4
HEMIFACIAL MICROSOMIA	3	4.1
TUMOR RESECTION SEQUEL	3	4.1
LUPUS	3	4.1
EMBOLIZATION SEQUEL	1	1.3
7 FACIAL CLEFT	1	1.3

Table 1. Etiology of facial contour deformity in 73 cases.

3. Surgical technique

All the procedures were done under general anesthesia and meticulous sterile technique. The donor sites were abdomen and flanks in all patients.The donor sites were infiltrated with lidocaine 0.5% with 1:100,000 epinephrine in a Ringer's lactate solution; in a ratio of 1 ml of solution for each cubic centimeter of fat harvested using a blunt cannula for infiltration. After 10 minutes we use a two holed cannula with blunt tip (shaped like a bucket handle), the other end of the cannula is attached to a 10cc syringe. The distal openings of the harvesting cannula are the same size as the entrance lumen of the syringe to avoid damage of the fatty tissue. The plunger of the syringe is gently manipulated to provide about 1 or 2 cc of negative pressure space in the barrel of the syringe while the cannula is pushed through the harvest site. After the fat has been harvested, the cannula is removed from the syringe and replaced with a plug which is twisted on to create a seal to prevent spillage during the centrifuging process. The plunger is removed from the proximal end of the syringe. Then the syringes are centrifuged at 3000 rpm for 3 minutes. The upper oil is discharged, and also the lower portion (composed by blood, water and lidocaine). Then the middle portion of the syringe which is composed primarily of potentially viable parcels of fat tissue is transfered to 1cc syringes with a disposable three lines key , with a gentle aspiration from the 1 cc syringes. The recipient areas are not infiltrated to avoid deformity of the recipient areas. Only the sites were the peridural cannula will be placed are infiltrated with 0.5% lidocaine with 1:200,000 epinephrine with a 27 gauge needle, incisions 1 or 2 mm long are made with a No. 15 Bard Parker blade. The incisions will be placed depending of the areas to be injected 1 cm inside the scalp (for forehead), in the external canthus, below the lobule, lip commissure, alar base (for cheek, lip and chin), in nasion for the nose.The fat transfer is done with a peridural cannula (18G BD Tuohy 17g x 89mm). Although it has a blunt point (Huber-Tuohy-Hustead point). The bevel's sharp point of the peridural cannula is unsharpened as shown in figure 1.

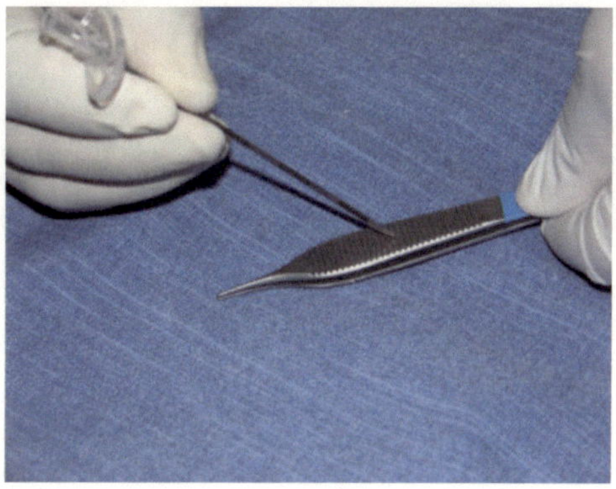

Fig. 1. Peridural cannula (18G BD Tuohy 17g x 89mm).Although it has a blunt point (Huber-Tuohy-Hustead point) The bevel's sharp point of the peridural cannula is unsharpened on the lateral side of Adson forceps' handle.

The adipocytes are deposited in crossing lines in the desired areas being left during the take out of the cannula. The patient is discharged from the hospital 24 hours later with ketorolac in case of pain, amoxicillin clavulanic acid for seven days and cold for 2-3 days. The patients come to control every three months the first year and new lipoinjection if needed is realized 12 months after de last procedure, if they do not need more volume they are seen every 6 months for 5 years.

4. Results

Most of the patients had not had previous treatments 65 cases (89%), except 8 (10.9%).A total of 132 procedures realized in the first group about 1.8 per patient; in the second group (previous treated patients) 8 patients, had previous microsurgical corrections with 41 previous surgical procedures in this group about 5 procedures per patients . We injected 4755 cc fat tissue which represent about 65.4 cc per patient. The follow up was between 1 and 8 years. Complications the most common was under correction in 14 cases (19.1%), visible irregularities 5 (6.8%): oral mucosa perforation 2 (2.7%), granuloma 1 (1.3%) fat migration 2 (2.7%). We present some representative cases with long follow up.

5. Case reports

5.1 Case 1

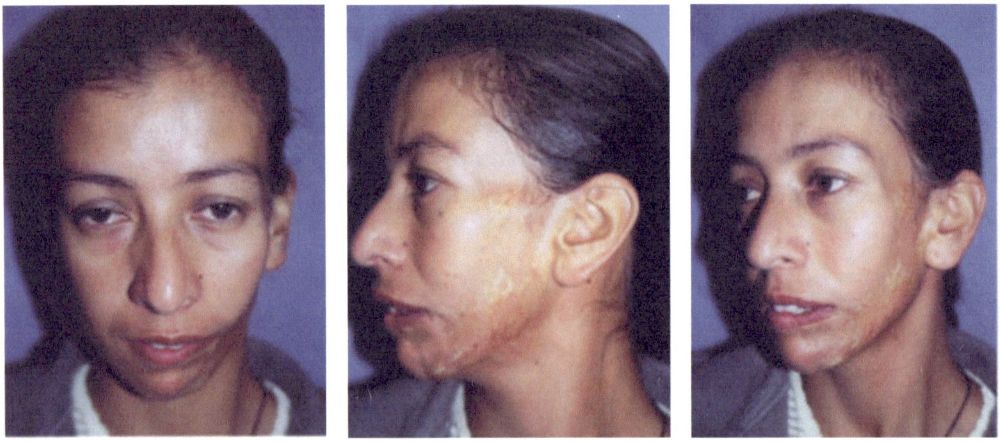

Fig. 2. 23 year-old girl had Morphea left side of the face, preoperative front, ¾ and lateral left views.

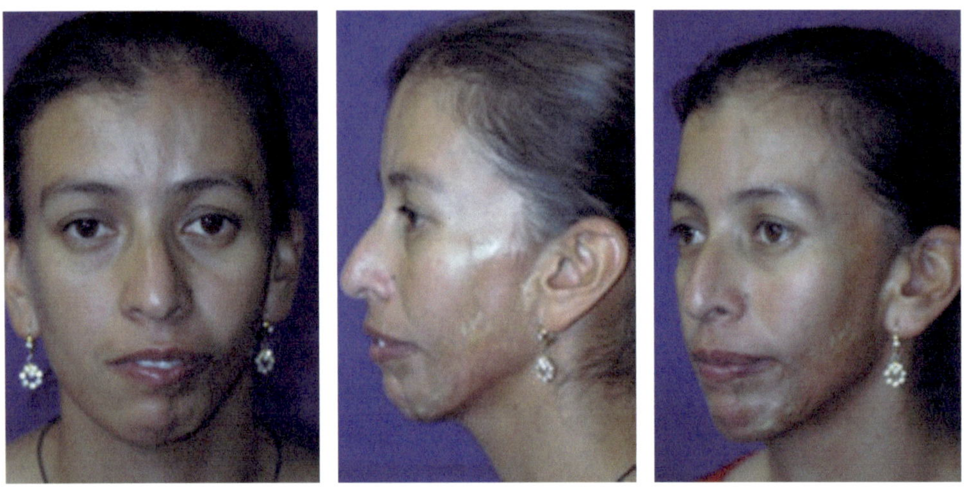

Fig. 3. Postoperative frontal ¾ and lateral left views after two lipoinjection procedures. Twelve months after the last one.

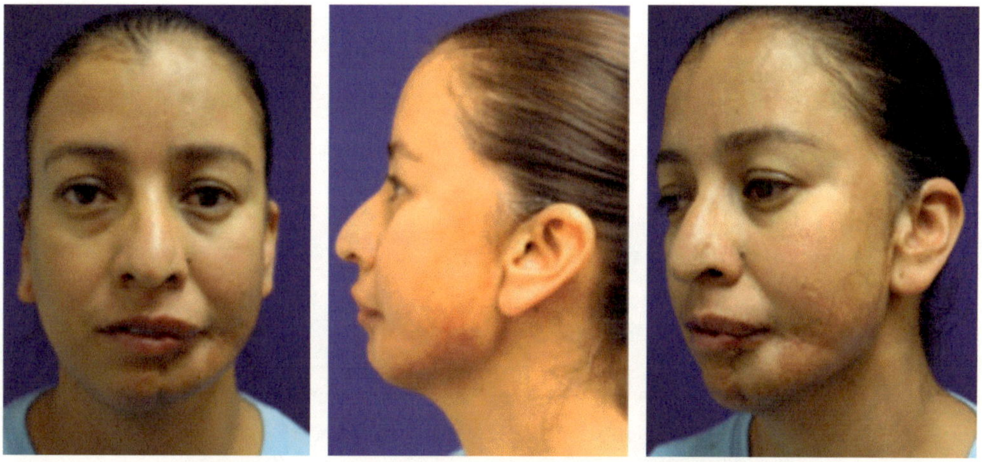

Fig. 4. Postoperative frontal, left ¾ and lateral views after 6 lipoinjection with a total volume of 163 cc 3 years after the last one. We can see that she increased her body weight in last years with proportional increase of the transplanted fat tissue.

5.2 Case 2

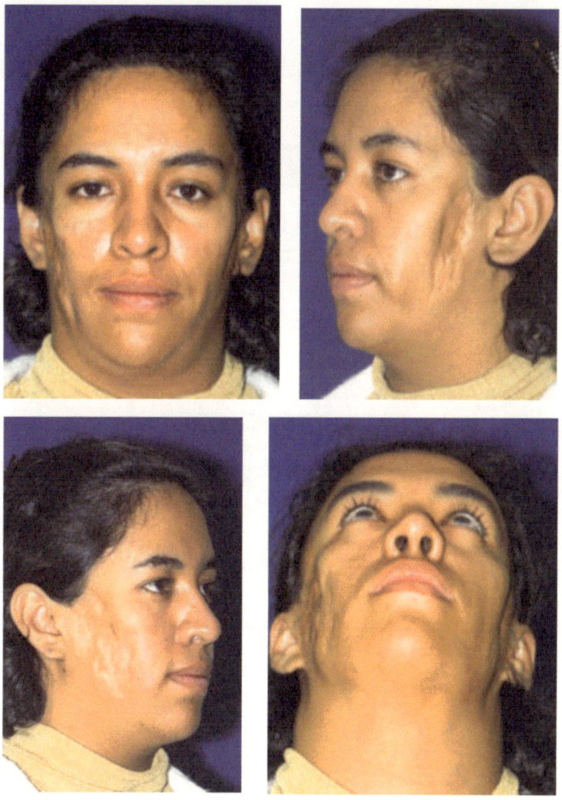

Fig. 5. 30 year old woman severe bilateral cheek atrophy secondary to discoid Lupus. Preoperative front ¾ right ,3/4 left and basal views.

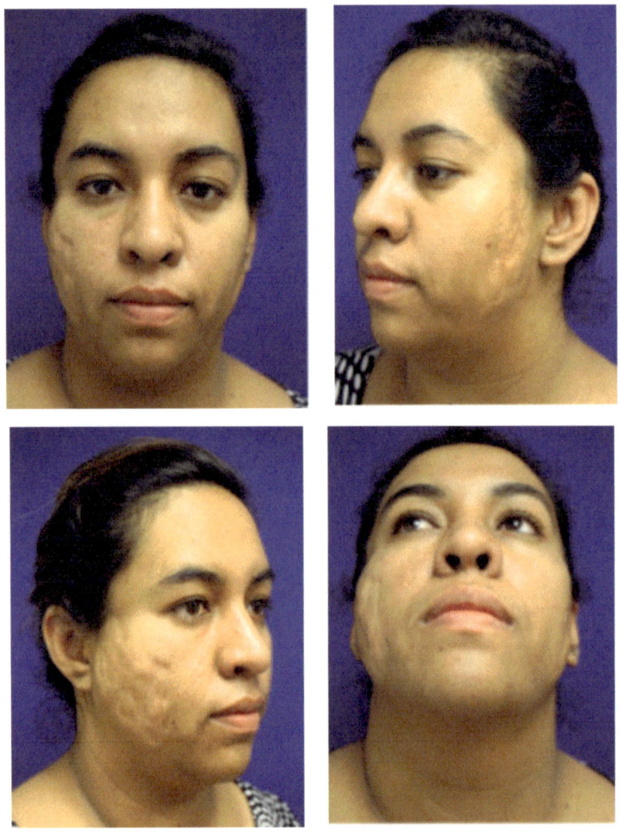

Fig. 6. Postoperative front, ¾ right, ¾ left and basal views post three lipoinjection procedures with a total volume of 147 cc fat graft two years follow up since the last procedure.

5.3 Case 3

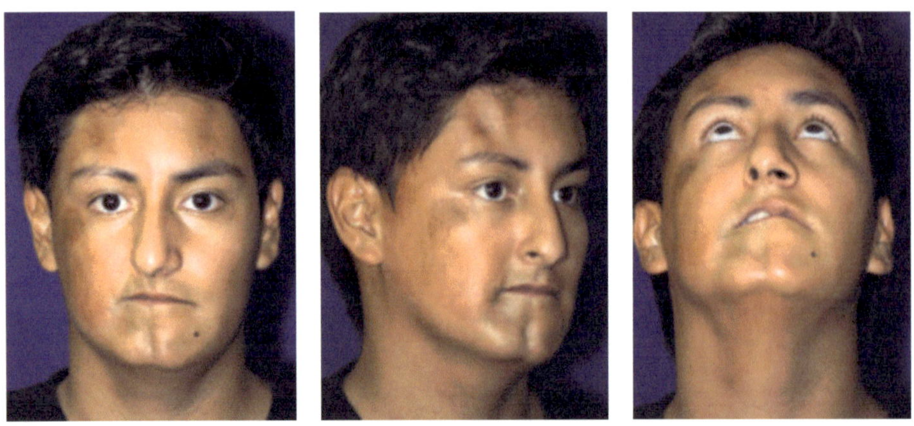

Fig. 7. 19 year old man with right face atrophy secondary to Parry Romberg syndrome. Front, ¾ right and basal preoperative views.

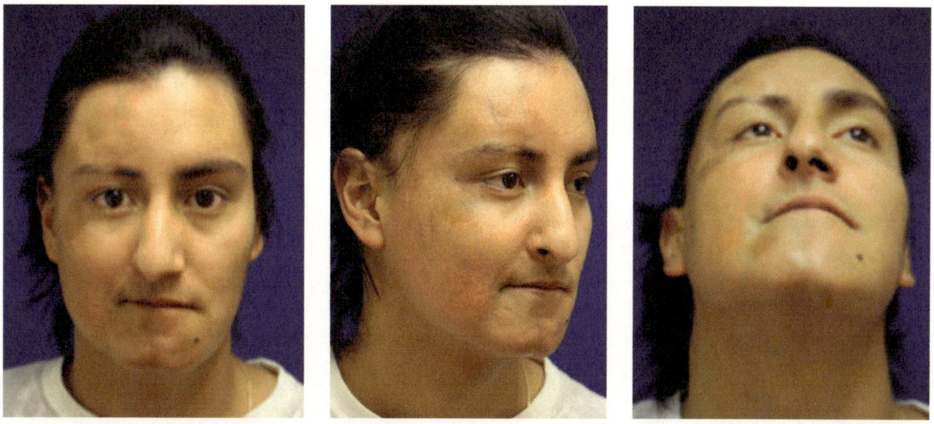

Fig. 8. Front, ¾ right and basal postoperative views after 4 procedures and a total volume of fat graft 132.5 cc, one year after the last procedure.

5.4 Case 4

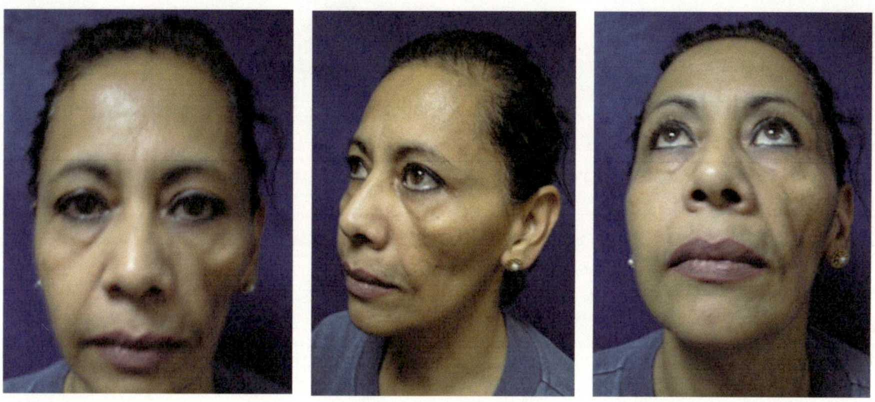

Fig. 9. 51 year old woman with Parry Romberg syndrome.Front ¾ left and basal preoperative views.

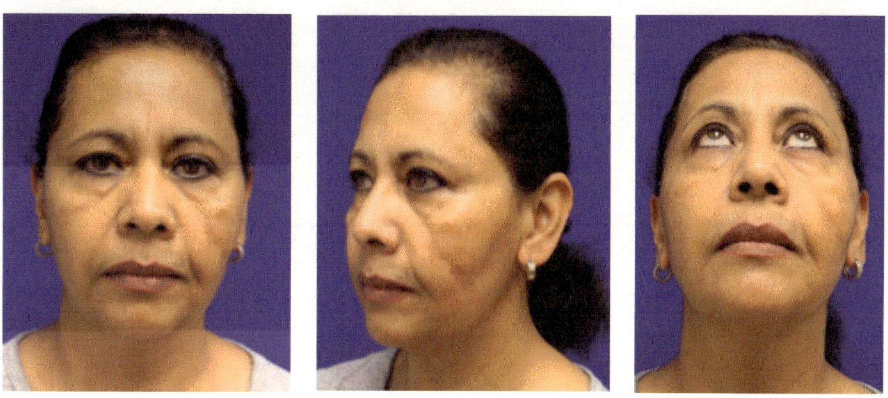

Fig. 10. Front ¾ left and basal postoperative views after two procedures and a 56 cc fat grafted, two years after the last procedure..

5.5 Case 5

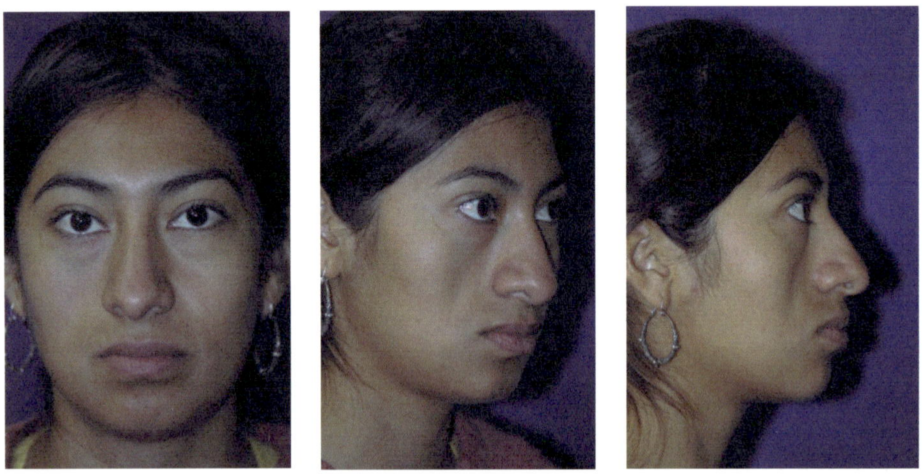

Fig. 11. 23 year old woman with right Parry Romberg syndrome front ,¾ and lateral preoperative views.

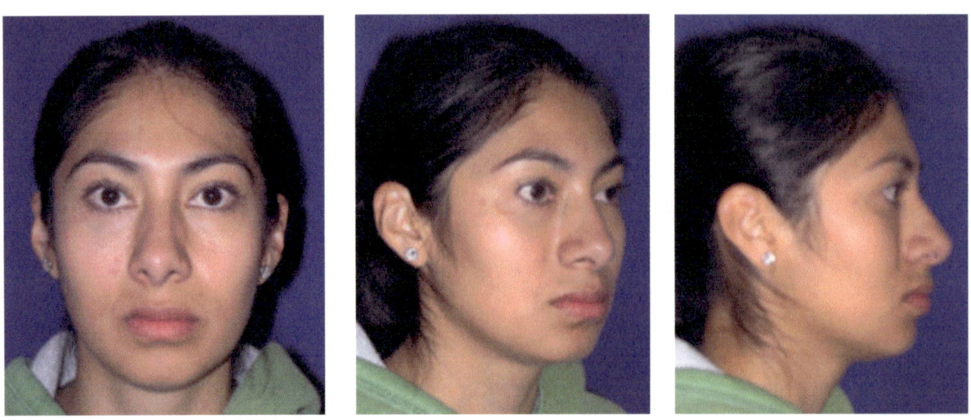

Fig. 12. Front, ¾ and lateral postoperative views after two procedures with a total of 18cc fat graft, two years after the last procedure.

5.6 Case 6

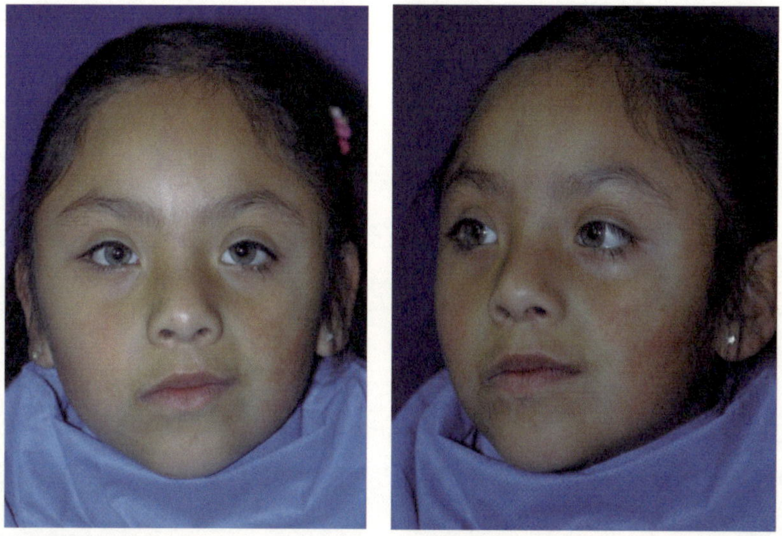

Fig. 13. 6 year old girl with left Hemifacial microsomia , front , and ¾ preoperative views.

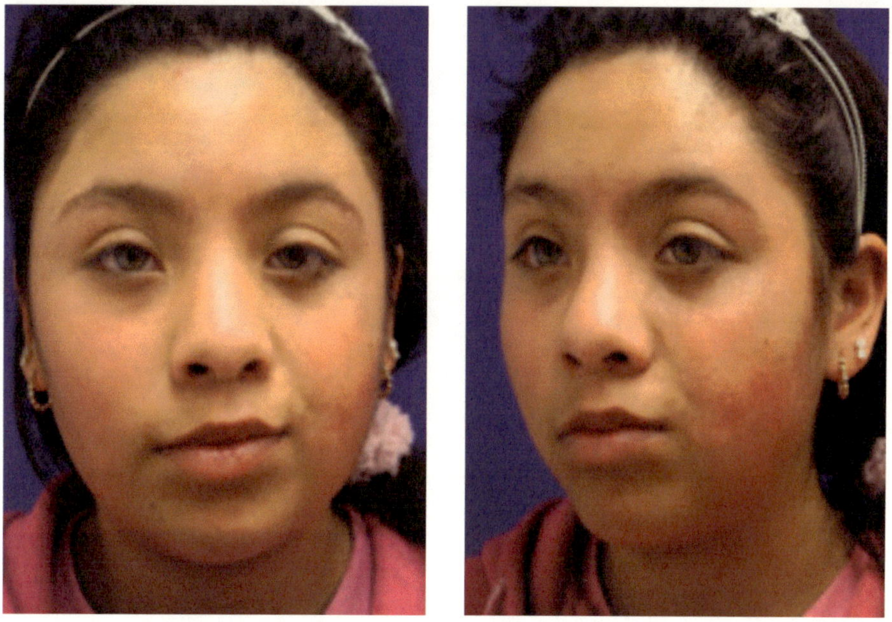

Fig. 14. Front and ¾ postoperative views after 3 lipoinjection procedures with a total 46 cc fat graft 3 years after the last lipoinjection.

5.7 Case 7

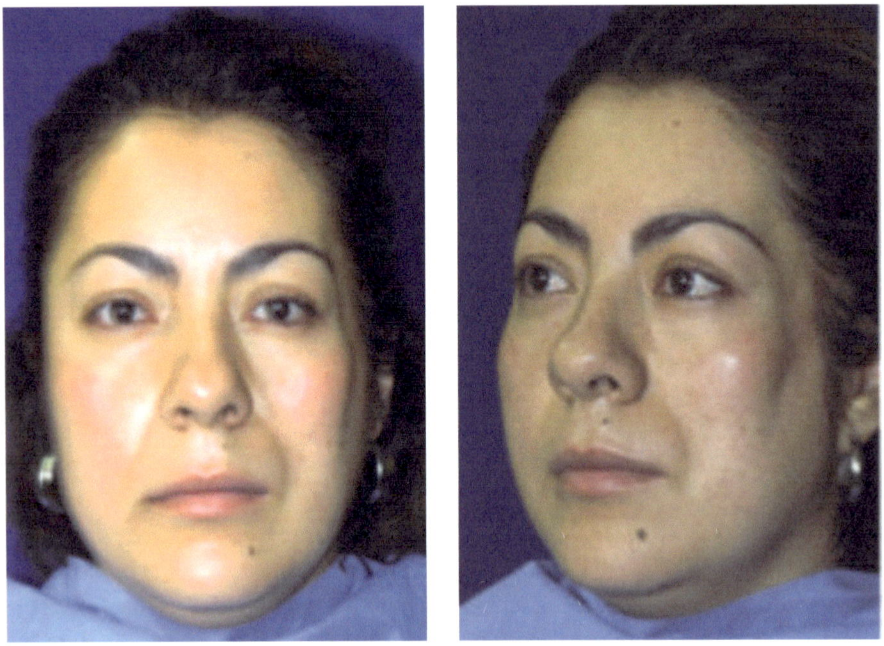

Fig. 15. 37 year old woman with left face Parry Romberg syndrome preoperative front and ¾ views.

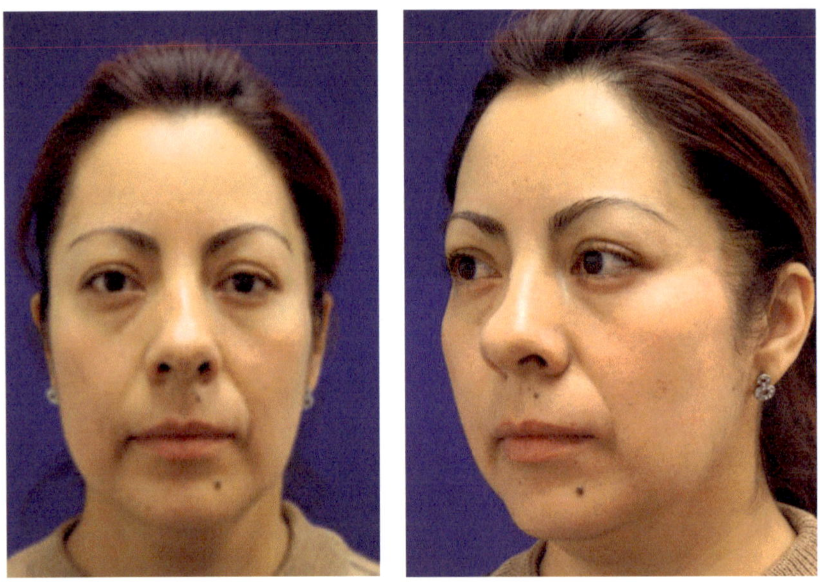

Fig. 16. Front and ¾ left postoperative views after 2 procedures a volume of 42 cc of fat graft injected. Four years after the last procedure.

5.8 Case 8

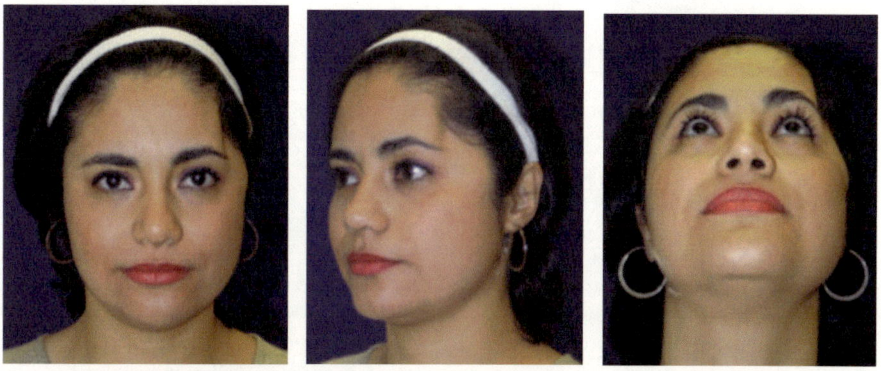

Fig. 17. 33 year old woman with sequel of temporal lobectomy with a left fronto temporal depression, front, ¾ and basal views.

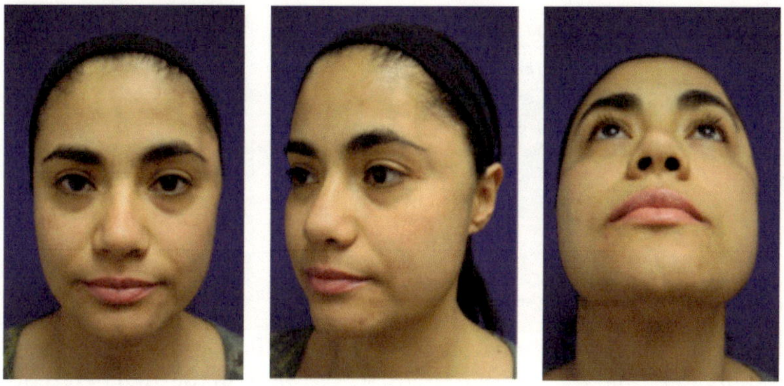

Fig. 18. Postoperative front, ¾ left and basal views after 61 cc fat grafted in two procedures, two years after the last one.

5.9 Case 9

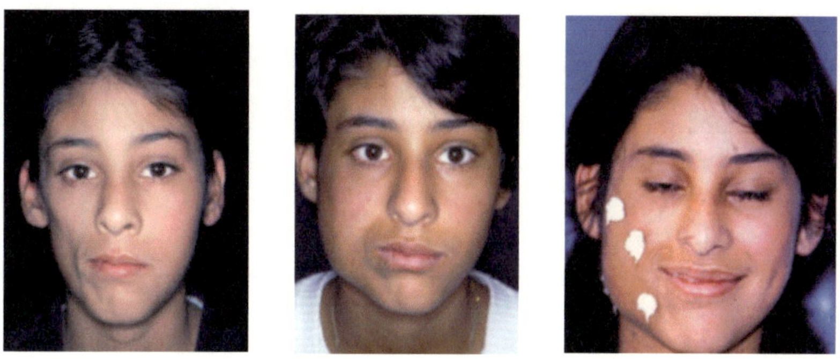

Fig. 19. 14 year old girl with right Parry Romberg syndrome. She had early reconstruction with scapular free flap at the age of fourteen. She had a transient braquial plexus injury after 12 hours of surgery. She had some other procedures in the later two years; rhinoplasty , piriform fossa cartilage graft, flap resuspension, flap defatting and chin implant. A total of five previous procedures.

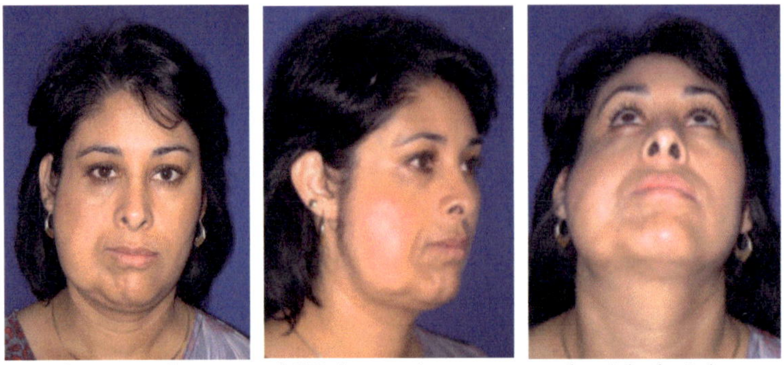

Fig. 20. 23 years later at the age of 37 the patient returned with facial asymmetry more pronounced than the one she presented in the preoperative. We can see that she increased her body weight in last years with disproportional increase of the transplanted flap's fat tissue. Front, ¾ right and basal views.

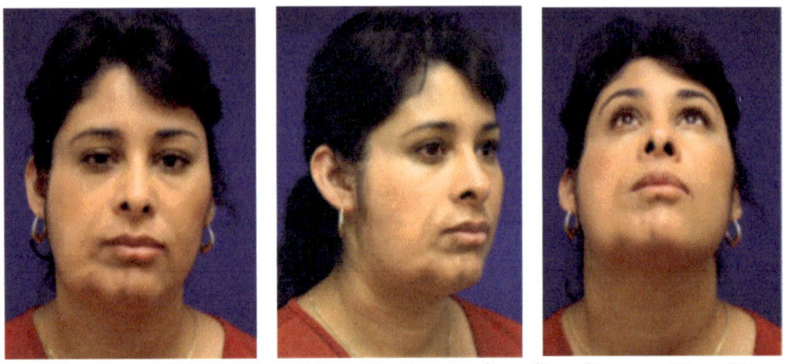

Fig. 21. Postoperative front, ¾ right and basal views after flap liposuction 33cc, resuspension of the flap and lipoinjection 52 cc, with a residual deformity in the jowl to be corrected.

6. Conclusion

The long lasting results presented permit us to evaluate inevitable known absorption of fat tissue injected. The time between each procedure (one year) let us know the final result of the fat grafted. As we can see in our patients the fat grafted behaves as the body fat when the patient increases the body weight with years. The use of peridural cannula is a safe and convenient instrument for fat grafting. In small deformities one procedure could be enough to solve it, specially if there is health tissue nearby as in trauma. The modification presented using the peridural cannula which is available in any Medical Centers also provides the advantage of being disposable. The number of procedures required depends of the size of the deformity and the tissue left one year after the fat grafted which will depend on the receptor tissue conditions (thin skin or scarring tissue) and this method will not permit transplant great volumes if there is not good skin conditions. As much as we know that small volume will survive better than great volume. The use of peridural cannula for lipoinjection is a reliable, safe and reproducible method. The period between each procedure was 12 months, this is time enough to evaluate absorption of the grafted fat, and there is no need of overcorrection. The complications reported with this method are similar to the ones reported with other methods.

7. Discussion

Free flaps has been considered as the gold standard for reconstruction in great defects (Inigo "et al". 1993;Wojcicki & Zachara 2011;Yu-Feng "et al". 2008). Unfortunately the long follow up as case 9 demonstrate that the behavior of the free flaps is more unpredictable than fat graft due to the gravitational force and the disproportional volume increase in relation to body weight changes. And the different match color when skin is required. Case one illustrates a great defect which was solved satisfactory with fat graft and when the patient increases her body weight the volumes is proportional to the normal side.

8. Acknowledgment

Residents Xitlali Baron, Jordi Espel, Fernando Francis, Roberto López and Guillermo Sánchez for their help in taking care of the patients.

9. References

Asken, S. (1990). Microliposuction and autologous fat transplantation for aesthetic enhacement of the aging face. *J. Dermatol Surg Oncol*, Vol.16, pp. 965-972, ISBN 0148-0812

Coleman, SR. (1995). Long-term survival of fat transplants: controlled demonstrations. *Aesthetic Plast Surg 1995*, Vol.19, pp.421-425, ISSN 1432-5241

Coleman, SR. (1997). Facial recontourig with lipostructure. *Clin Plast Surg*, Vol. 24, pp. 347-367, ISSN 1558-0504

Coleman, SR. (2001). Structural fat grafts: the ideal filler. *Clin Plast Surg*, Vol.28, (January 2001), pp. 111-119, ISSN 1558-0504

Coleman, SR. (2002). Hand rejuvenation with structural fat grafting. *Plast Reconstr Surg* Vol.110, (December 2002), pp.1731-1745, ISSN 0032-1052

Guerrerosantos, J., González-Mendoza, A., & Masmela, Y. (1996). Long-term survival of free fat graft in muscle: an experimental study in rats. *Aesthetic Plast Surg*. Vol.20, (September 1996), pp. 403-408, ISSN 1432-5241

Gutiérrez C, Hayakawa V, Franco A, Reyes L.(2007)Lipoinyección para reconstrucción del contorno facial en S. de Parry Romberg, esclerodermia y secuelas de trauma. Una alternativa práctica utilizando cánulas para bloqueo peridural.Rev Cir Plást ; 17 (3): 168-175 ,ISSN 1405-0625

Gutierrez C y Cols. (2009)Corrección de deformidad en olán en S. Melkerson Rosenthal. Cirplástiberolatinoam Vol 35 No. 1 enero-marzo pp79-84,ISSN 1405-0625

Illouz, Y.G. (1990). Fat Injection: A four year clinical trial in lipoplasty, In: *The theory and practice of blunt suction lipectomy*, Brown, pp. 148-152, Little,Boston

Inigo, F., Rojo, P., & Ysunza, A. (1993). Aesthetic treatment of Romberg's disease: experience with 35 cases. *Br JPlastSurg*, Vol.46, No.3, (April 1993), pp.194-200, ISSN 0007-1226

Latoni, J.D., Marshall, D.M., & Wolfe, S.A. (2000). Overgrowth of fat autotransplanted for correction of localized steroid-induced atrophy. *Plast Reconstr Surg*, Vol.106, (December 2000), pp. 1566-1569, ISSN 1529-4242

Peer, L.A.(1946) Plast Reconstr Surg 1955 Sep;16(3):161-8. Cell survival theory versus replacement theory. ISSN 1075-1270

Peer, L.A. (1956). The neglected free fat graft its behavior and clinical use. *Am J Surg* Vol.92, No.1, (July 1956), pp.40-47, ISSN 1879-1883

Rieck, B., & Schlaak, S. (2003). Measurement in vivo of the survival rate in autologous adipocyte transplantation. *Plast Reconstr Surg,* Vol.11, (June 2003), pp.2315-2323, ISSN 1529-4242

Sadick, N.S., & Hudgins, L.C. (2001). Fatty acid analysis of transplanted adipose tissue. *Arch Dermatol*, Vol.137, (June 2001), pp. 723-727, ISSN1538-3652

Wojcicki, P., & Zachara, M. Treatment of Patients with Parry-Romberg Syndrome. *Ann of Plast Surg*, Vol.66, No.3, (March 2011), pp. 267-72, ISSN1536-3708

Yu-Feng, L., Lai, G., & Zhi-Yong, Z. (2008). Combined Treatments of Facial Contour Deformities Resulting from Parry –Romberg Syndrome, *J Reconstr Microsurg*, Vol.24, No.5, (July 2008), pp. 333-342, ISSSN 1098-8947

3

Novel Liposuction Techniques for the Treatment of HIV-Associated Dorsocervical Fat Pad and Parotid Hypertrophy

Harvey Abrams[1] and Karen L. Herbst[2]
[1]Wilshire Aesthetics, Los Angeles, California
[2]University of California, San Diego
and the Veterans Affairs San Diego Healthcare System, San Diego, California
USA

1. Introduction

Liposuction since its beginning has been used primarily for contouring localized deposits of fat to give its recipients an improved cosmetic appearance. The most common areas to which liposuction techniques have been applied are the abdomen, flank region, thighs, and submental neck. Since the advent of the tumescent technique in the late 1980s, including the use of local anesthesia and small diameter cannulas, the safety of liposuction has been established. Along with safety has come the application of the liposuction technique to medical conditions including non-fatty tissues, such as the removal of salivary gland tissue in the treatment of axillary hyperhidrosis and the combined glandular and fatty tissue of gynecomastia.

This chapter will examine the application and efficacy of the liposuction technique in treating two common and related conditions found in human immunodeficiency virus (HIV) positive patients: the dorsocervical fat pad and bilateral parotid hypertrophy in the broader context of HIV lipodystrophy. The procedures described herein avoid general anesthesia and utilize the awake patient as a participant in the procedure to optimize reduction of the hypertrophic tissue. In the case of the dorsocervical fat pad, the positioning of the patient in the seated upright position results in a more effective and complete suctioning than in the traditional prone position. A bonus is that this position is more comfortable for the surgeon, in reducing operating room fatigue. In the case of parotid hypertrophy, using an established technique such as liposuction, can be shown to provide an excellent reconstructive and cosmetic result while providing a better safety profile than other treatment options. Our experience in the use of these procedures indicates that patients rate their experience and satisfaction with the procedures as very high.

Current procedural terminology (CPT) and international classification of disease (ICD) codes are provided to improve insurance provider reimbursement for patients.

2. Lipodystrophy

Since the advent of highly active antiretroviral therapy (HAART), people with HIV infections and acquired immunodeficiency syndrome (AIDS) are living longer and better lives(Taiwo et al. 2010). A side effect attributable to HAART is the development, in some patients, of a complex of signs and symptoms collectively referred to as lipodystrophy. HIV lipodystrophy is manifested by a constellation of anthropometric changes, including lipoatrophy of the face, extremities, and buttocks(Tien and Grunfeld 2004) as well as lipohypertrophy in the upper back, commonly called "buffalo hump" or dorsocervical fat pad. Fat loss in the face and extremities conveys a falsely cachectic appearance to patients who are otherwise healthy. Patients with lipodystrophy also commonly have increased abdominal adiposity, chest adiposity, and increased glandular breast tissue, the latter known as gynecomastia. While some patients have only lipoatrophy(Grunfeld et al. 2010), others over time develop signs and symptoms of lipohypertrophy as well. Many patients have associated internal and metabolic abnormalities such as diabetes, advanced coronary disease, and cardiomyopathy.(Carr et al. 1998; Domingo et al. 1999; Safrin and Grunfeld 1999; Murata et al. 2000; Petit et al. 2000)

Another less recognized feature of lipodystrophy is bilateral parotid hypertrophy. (Sooy, 1987) Enlargement of the parotid glands, the largest of the salivary glands, is commonly seen in HIV positive patients(Tall et al. 1985) and is often referred to in the HIV community as "chipmunk cheeks" as it imparts a fullness to the lateral check area. While HAART is often cited as its causation, as with lipodystrophy, its etiology is unknown.

The first part of this chapter will focus on the lipohypertrophy of the dorsocervical fat pad and a novel method of removing it with liposuction under local tumescent anesthesia. The second part of this chapter will focus on the removal of the lateral portion of the hypertrophied parotid gland in an equally novel but different approach using a technique borrowed from liposuction.

3. Dorsocervical fat pad

3.1 Background

The dorsocervical fat pad represents a subcutaneous, non-encapsulated accumulation of adipose tissue with a striking fibro-connective tissue component. The authors prefer the term "dorsocervical fat pad" to "buffalo hump" as it is more descriptive and accurate medical terminology, while the latter potentially denigrates already the situation for the cosmetically-embarrassed or depressed patient.(Steel et al. 2006; Crane et al. 2008) Aside from dramatic changes in appearance leading to depression and social withdrawal, patients with dorsocervical fat pads may complain of headaches, difficulty with sleep, decreased range of motion, and an inability to fully extend the neck due to the physical size of the mass.

There is general agreement in the medical community that liposuction is a safe and effective method of reducing the size of the dorsocervical fat pad.(Ponce-de-Leon et al. 1999; Piliero et al. 2003) The authors of this article have seen poor outcomes for many patients after attempted removal of the fat by direct surgical excision. The poor outcomes include only minimal reduction of the size of the fat pad while leaving long and unsightly scars. We have also seen suboptimal results in patients in which liposuction was performed in an effort to reduce the fat pads. One of the main reasons for the poor outcomes associated with liposuction of the dorsocervical fat pad is that these patients have all been placed in the prone position during the liposuction procedure. In the prone position, the dorsocervical fat pad recedes between the scapula and is harder to access. Neck extension in the prone position further anatomically distorts the cervical fat pads. This can be observed simply by placement of the patient in the prone position and visibly noting the dorsal surface region. The dorsocervical fat is flattened and less demonstrable in the prone position as compared to the upright, anatomic position. Access is further impeded by the placement of the occiput in the prone position. The cephalad portions of the lesion are inaccessible to cannula insertion, rendering significant sections of the fat pad inoperable in the prone position. This is especially true for patients with lipodystrophic fat accumulation in the posterior neck and occipital scalp region, in which neck flexion is essential to cannula insertion. In this article, we propose an alternate positioning of the patient, which we feel gives far superior results. The patient is awake and seated in an upright position with the legs dangling off the edge of the operating table. With this technique, the surgeon stands behind the patient, allowing the surgeon greater access to all of the tissue. Having a patient awake allows his/her assistance in the positioning, providing a more complete removal of tissue and, therefore, a more successful outcome.

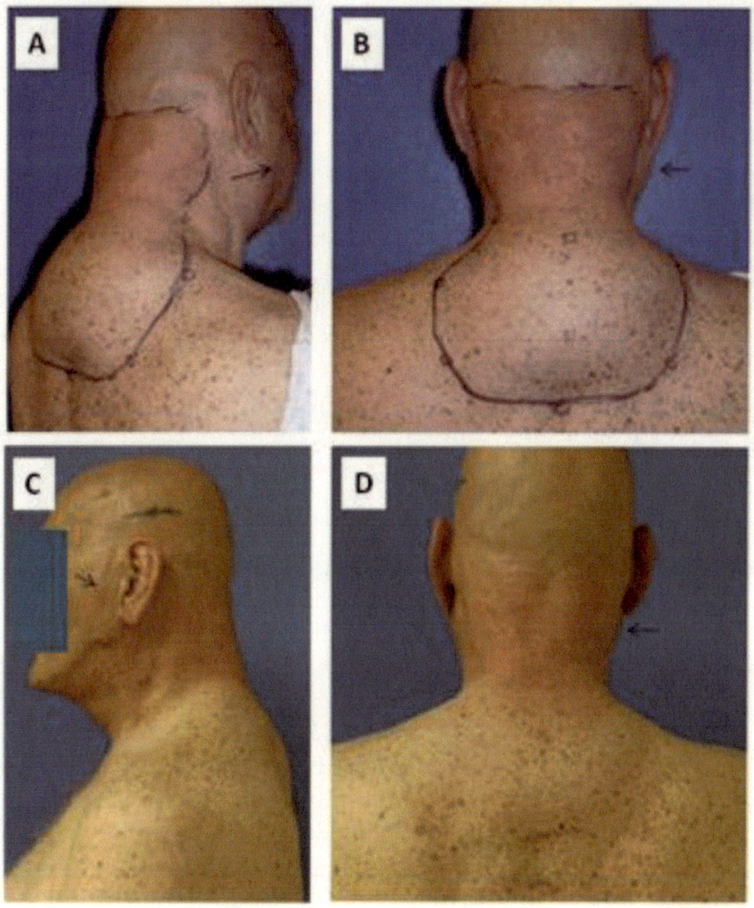

Fig. 1. HIV infected man on HAART with a dorsocervical fat pad before and after lipoaspiration. A. Outlined dorsocervical fat pad prior to aspiration with black arrow pointing to parotid hypertrophy, B. Outlined dorsocervical fat pad with incision circles prior to aspiration with black arrow pointing to parotid hypertrophy, C. Postsurgical resolution of parotid hypertrophy and improved dorsocervical fat pad, D. Much improved dorsocervical fat pad and parotid hypertrophy (arrow).

Physical examination of the dorsocervical fat pad

Physical examination of the patient with a dorsocervical fat pad reveals a fatty tissue buildup on the upper back which can be generally categorized as small, medium, large and extreme. There is no measurement guide to enable classification into these size categories. The fat accumulation in the dorsocervical area is subcutaneous and causes no changes to the skin itself, therefore, the overlying skin appears normal. Palpation reveals fat pads that are rather discrete, firm and immobile (unlike lipomas). Palpation often reveals that these masses extend into the posterior neck and nuchal regions of the occipital scalp. (Figure 1) Extension into the posterior neck and scalp deforms the normal dorsocervical angle and imparts a somewhat equine appearance to the neck. Rarely is there any pain associated with palpation, although patients report symptoms caused by these fat pads such as difficulty lying down, interference with sleep, and pain radiating to the shoulders and arms. Social withdrawal symptoms may be present, especially for patients with large, noticeable fat pads. These lesions are usually so characteristic, that it is not necessary to get any kind of diagnostic or radiographic confirmation with computed tomography (CT) or magnetic resonance imaging (MRI).

3.2 Novel method for liposuction of the dorso-cervical fat pad

The patient is prepared for local, tumescent liposuction in the pre-operative area. While in the pre-operative room the patient disrobes and puts on a hospital gown. Photographs are taken with the patient's back to the camera in silhouette to document the pre-operative size and location. With the patient in a seated position, and legs dangling off the edge of the exam table, the entire back and posterior neck are cleaned with alcohol. The peripheral border of the dorsocervical fat pad is outlined with a pen in a continuous line (Figure 1). Five small circles are made approximately 2 cm from the outer boundary of the fat pad in a clockwise manner at 1, 4, 6, 8 and 11 o'clock although this may vary slightly per patient (Figure 1B; Figure 2B). These are the entrance points for both the infusion and suction cannulae. Ordinarily five incision sites (ports) are used but for smaller fat pads, three may be sufficient. Each of the circled sites is injected with 1 cc of lidocaine 1% and epinephrine 1:100,000. The patient is pre-medicated with hydrocodone 5 mg and alprazolam 0.5 mg by mouth for pain and anxiety relief, and with lincomycin 600 mg I.M. for antibiotic prophylaxis.

The patient is then escorted into the operating room and instructed to sit on the edge of the operating table allowing the surgeon to position him/herself behind the patient (Figure 2A, 2C). During the surgery, the patient's vital signs are continuously monitored using pulse oximetry, sphygmomanometry and electrocardiography. A medical stand with pillow is placed in front of the patient to lean on for support. The patient is prepped and gowned in a standard sterile fashion. The surgeon makes 3 mm incisions into the previously anesthetized peripheral circular sites using a #11-blade surgical scalpel. Tumescent fluid consisting of lidocaine and epinephrine buffered with sodium chloride (see below) is infiltrated liberally throughout the entire fat pad and allowed to sit for 15 to 30 minutes in order to achieve maximal vasoconstrictive effect.

The tumescent fluid is prepared in the operative suite as follows: 1-2 vials of 50 mL lidocaine 1% and epinephrine 1:100,000 and 10 cc of sodium bicarbonate 8.4% are added to 1,000 mL of 0.9% saline solution. Using two 50 mL vials of Lidocaine 1% and epinephrine 1:100,000 results in a lidocaine concentration of 0.1%. Infusing 1,000 to 1,500 cc allows for adequate tumescence without undue risk of lidocaine toxicity.

Using a 3 mm Becker, or similar cannula, thorough and meticulous liposuction is carried out using all 5 of the peripheral incisions points (ports) employing a crisscross pattern over the entire expanse of the fat pad. The cannula is shifted every 16th of an inch angling up and over the entire breadth of the fat pad. For example, lipoaspiration will begin horizontal at the 6 o'clock port each time angling a 16th of an inch in a more vertical position going up and down, to and fro until the 12 o'clock position then working down on the opposite side again shifting every 16th of an inch. This same method is used at all incision sites. The neck and the occipital scalp can be accessed using these same incision sites provided a cannula of sufficient length is used (Figure 2E).

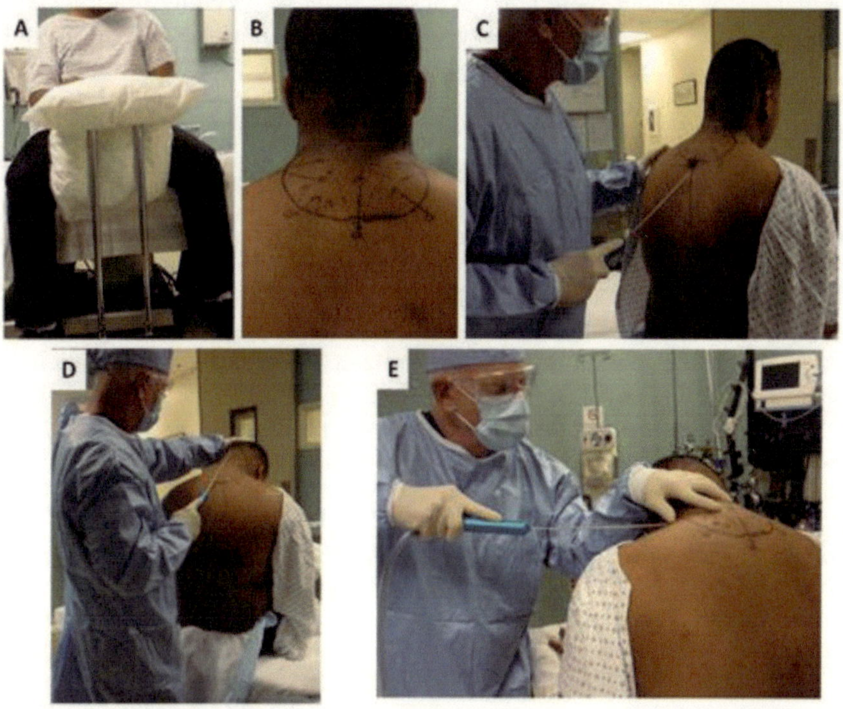

Fig. 2. HIV infected man undergoing apiration for dorsocervical fat pad. A. The patient was placed in the sitting position with his feet dangling over the edge of the bed with a pillow rest, B. The dorsocervical fat pad is outlined as are the incision ports, C. The surgeon is able to stand straight up during the aspiration procedure, D. The patient participates in the procedure by flexing the neck, E. The surgeon is able to access all of the dorsocervical fat pad with the assistance of the patient.

During the procedure the patient is asked to bend at the waist when the more cephalad parts of the dorsocervical fat pad are being aspirated and when the surgeon is using the superior ports. The patient position on the table can be angled at any time using the help of an assistant to make the suction more effective and comfortable to the surgeon and to remove as much tissue as possible to avoid recurrence. The patient's head may also be bent

in a flexed position when suctioning the lesions that extend more superiorly into the posterior neck, occipital and post auricular scalp regions (Figure 2D, 2E).
The fat entering the suction tubing from the dorsocervical fat pad appears yellow in color, although some admixture of blood is common. When the fat pad becomes flattened, the aspiration phase is over. The incision sites are closed using #5-0 nylon sutures, approximately two sutures per site. Antibiotic ointment and sterile dressings are applied to the incision sites. The patient is transferred to the post-anesthesia care unit (PACU) where vital sign monitoring is continued. Compression garments are not usually necessary, but the surgeon may recommend them for larger fat pads (25 cm in size and/or situated high onto the posterior head). The patient is discharged after 30 minutes of observation to the care of a family member or friend, at the discretion of the surgeon. Because patients have been pre-medicated with sedatives, they are not allowed to drive themselves home.
After discharge, the patient returns home and is asked to generally rest for 1-2 days. The patient may shower after 2 days and engage in their activities of daily living at this time except for those activities requiring rigorous physical effort such as running or weight-lifting. The sutures are removed after five days and no dressings are generally needed after this time. Exercise can generally be resumed in one week. Patients follow-up in one month and are usually discharged from the office at that time.

3.3 Outcomes after dorsocervical fat pad lipoaspiration of the awake patient

In a recent detailed survey by the authors of one woman and eighteen men with an average age of 52±1.8 (mean±sem) years seeking lipoaspiration treatment for HIV-related dorsocervical fat pad, prior to surgery, on a scale of 0-5, five being very affected, 3 being somewhat affected, 1 being a little affected, and zero being not affected, patients felt their appearance was very affected (4.8±0.1), they experienced discomfort (3.5±0.4), their lives were changed somewhat due to the dorsocervical fat pad (3.7±0.4), they had some depression (3.4±0.4) and social withdrawal (3.6±0.4), the fat pad interfered a little, to somewhat during sleep (2.7±0.5), and their posture was somewhat to very affected (3.8±0.4). Within a year after lipoaspiration, by paired student's t-test, there was a 82.1±6.2% improvement in appearance (average rating 0.9±0.3; $P<0.0001$), a 76.3±7.9% improvement in discomfort (0.4±0.1; $P<0.0001$), a 54.4±12.6% improvement in how their lives were changed by the dorsocervical fat pad (1.4±0.25 $P=0.0006$), a 72.9±7.5% improvement in feelings of depression (0.7±0.3; $P<0.001$), a significant 81.9±6.3% improvement in social withdrawal (0.5±0.2; $P<0.0001$), a significant decrease of 59.7±10.2% in sleep disturbance (0.3±0.1; $P=0.0001$) and a 61.1±10% improvement in posture (1.3±0.4; $P=0.006$). Eighteen of the patients graded the procedure as completely successful (5/5) and one graded the procedure as 4/5. One person had an infection after the procedure, one had slight pigmentation at the site of the scar and one felt the area was lumpy (2.5/5). On a scale of none (0), to moderate (2-3) to significant (5), patients rated swelling after the procedure at 2.7±0.3, bruising at 2.0±0.3, and discomfort at 2.6±0.4. These data suggest excellent effectiveness of this novel procedure and impressive patient satisfaction and improvement in their quality of life.

4. HIV-related parotid hypertrophy

4.1 Background

The most common HIV-associated salivary gland condition relates to the parotid glands. Originally described in 1985,(Ryan et al. 1985) HIV-associated salivary gland disease affects

1-5% of the infected population(Shanti and Aziz 2009; Schiodt et al. 1989) and usually involves diffuse enlargement of both parotid glands, known as bilateral parotid hypertrophy, although unilateral involvement has been seen. Also known as HIV-associated lymphoepithelial cysts of the parotid gland, they can occur as the initial manifestation of HIV infection or at any stage of the disease. (Shanti and Aziz 2009) While bilateral enlargement is most common, patients with unilateral hypertrophy are also seen.(Tao and Gullane 1991; Ortega et al. 2008) Patients present with a bulging or widening of the lateral cheek area, sometimes giving a chipmunk cheek-like appearance. (Figure 3A) The degree of enlargement varies widely from patient to patient, from a barely discernable widening of the cheek, to an extremely large and disfiguring effect. Facial wasting is common in patients with parotid hypertrophy and generally accentuates the enlarged appearance of the glands.

Histologically, the enlarged parotid is characterized by a marked squamous epithelium-lined cystic dilation of the salivary glands surrounded by a lymphoid hyperplasia containing enlarged germinal centers.(Tao and Gullane 1991) Other salivary glands can also be enlarged by uniform follicular hyperplasia or reactive lymphadenopathy with follicular hyperplasia.(Shugar et al. 1988; Rosenberg et al. 1992) A diffuse form of salivary gland enlargement can also occur that is characterized histologically by atrophy of the gland parenchyma, lymphocytic infiltration, and replacement of ducts by solid islands of epithelial and myoepithelial cells.(Heymsfield et al. 1990) While patients rarely have overt symptoms due to gland enlargement, gland hypoplasia can occasionally lead to obstruction of the salivary duct and dryness of the mouth that mimics Sjögren's syndrome.(Schiodt et al. 1992) Rarely, patients report tenderness to touch. (Mandel and Surattanont 2002) Once the parotid gland is enlarged, it tends to persist in size, rarely decreasing.(Schiodt et al. 1992)

Many patients with parotid hypertrophy seek care because of a desire for cosmetic improvement especially when the glands are disfiguring. These patients may become reclusive and exhibit other social withdrawal types of behavior; depression is not uncommon. (Beitler et al. 1999)

Prior to the procedure to lipoaspirate the hypertrophied parotid gland as described in this chapter, it is important that the surgeon consult with the patient's primary care physician often in consultation with an ear, nose and throat (ENT) surgeon to rule out parotid hypertrophy due to HIV from other etiologies including bacterial infection with *mycobacterium* or *pneumococcus*,(Hanekom et al. 1995) viral infections with *paramyxovirus* (mumps)(McQuone 1999), autoimmune disease such as with Sjögren's syndrome and rare manifestations including cancers such as carcinoma, Kaposi's sarcoma(Burket et al. 2008), bilateral Warthin's tumors, bilateral cystic pleomorphic adenomas,(Som et al. 1995) or lymphoma,(Wotherspoon and Isaacson 1996)sarcoidosis, necrotic intraparotid lymph nodes and bilateral first branchial cleft cysts (intraparotid).(Michelow et al., 2011) Evaluation of the parotid gland may include imaging such as CT or MRI.(Chapnik et al. 1990)

4.2 Treatment options for parotid hypertrophy

The options to reduce the size of the parotids in HIV-positive patients are: 1) direct surgical excision with a high rate of recurrence; 2) radiation therapy; and 3) a modification of a liposuction technique as described in this chapter. It is the experience of the authors that direct surgical excision and radiation therapy are fraught with complications and often have a high rate of recurrence. Complications of direct surgical excision include those associated with general anesthesia, infection and fistula formation. Radiation therapy complications include the loss of taste, dryness of the mouth, thrush and radiation dermatitis. Although rare, formation of malignant tumors can occur, usually ten years out from radiation treatment using higher dose treatment modalities.(Beitler et al. 1999) It is the experience of the authors that the most favorable outcome results from using a tumescent liposuction technique that successfully reduces the size of the parotids to a normal appearance without resultant complications. (see Methodology)

4.3 Physical examination of the parotid glands

Physical examination reveals a patient with discernable enlargement of the lateral cheeks. Palpation allows the parotid gland to be easily appreciated. The size of the parotid hypertrophy varies from patient to patient but is generally felt just anterior to the tragus of the ear extending inferiorly and wrapping around the earlobe crease near the sternocleidomastoid muscle. Sometimes the parotid may feel like a hypertrophied masseter muscle but it is the wrapping of the parotid around the earlobe crease that differentiates the enlarged parotid from muscle. It is also important to note that palpation is of the superficial aspect of the gland. The deeper portions of the gland that envelop the facial nerve cannot be palpated. While the enlarged glands are usually not tender, care should be taken on initial palpation as occasionally, some of the glands are tender to touch.

4.4 Methodology for suction-assisted partial parotidectomy

The patient is prepared for local, tumescent liposuction in the pre-operative area. While in the pre-operative room the patient disrobes and puts on a hospital gown. Photographs are taken with the patient facing the camera and in silhouette to document the pre-operative size and location. After photography, the patient is placed in a supine position and the entire face and neck are cleaned with alcohol. The peripheral border of the hypertrophied parotid gland is outlined with a pen in a continuous line and the incision sites are marked on the sideburn and on the earlobe crease. Depending on how far down the gland extends, a third incision site may be placed anterior to the sternocleidomastoid muscle. Each of the circled sites is injected with 1 cc of lidocaine 1% and epinephrine 1:100,000. The same procedure is repeated on the other side immediately after. The patient is then pre-medicated with hydrocodone 5 mg and alprazolam 0.5 mg by mouth for pain and anxiety relief, and lincomycin 600 mg I.M. for antibiotic prophylaxis.

The pre-treated patient is brought to the operating room and placed in a supine position and prepped and draped in a sterile manner. Tumescent solution is very slowly infiltrated with a small diameter 1-2mm infiltration cannula throughout the entire parotid gland. Approximately 100cc of tumescent fluid is used on each side. Both glands are treated during the same surgical session. After the tumescent fluid is infused, a suction-aspiration technique using 2-3 mm cannulas with an aggressive tip is used to suction the lateral aspect of the parotid (Figure 3B). Generally shorter length cannulas are used with the parotids to gain better suction control. Parotid tissue can be seen entering the suction tubing as white fleshy tissue with a wet tissue appearance. Occasionally this tissue is often intermixed with yellow fat, tumescent fluid and blood if patients with lipodystrophy have infiltration of fat into the parotid gland. The patient is asked to turn his/her head when needed to facilitate access to the glands to be aspirated (Figure 3C). The surgeon's to-and-fro motions are to be continued until it is felt that enough superficial glandular tissue has been removed to restore a normal appearance to the lateral face. During this procedure, we again note that only the superficial part of the parotid is removed. When suctioning over the anterior portion of the check, it is important to maintain a superficial position in order not to compromise the integrity of the facial nerve. Many patients in conjunction with parotid hypertrophy have submental fat accumulation. Removal of the parotid gland is often combined with a submental fat aspiration during the same procedure.

Generally, no sutures are needed and the incision sites are left open to heal spontaneously. This allows for drainage of the tumescent fluid and generally prevents hematoma and seroma formation. All patients receive a universal chin compression garment in the operating room and afterwards, the patient is transferred to the PACU. In place of a compression garment, an ace bandage may also be used. All compression should include the submental aspect of the neck. After approximately one hour of observation, patients are discharged to the care of a responsible family member or friend; the patient is never allowed to drive home.

During the recovery period, the patient and usually rests for 4-5 days at home while continuously wearing the compression garment. The patient returns to the office for a follow-up visit at which time the patient is examined for possible infection, hematomas, seromas, etc. The patient may resume activities of daily living at this time except for those that require rigorous physical effort. Exercise can generally be resumed in 2-3 weeks depending on the patient's signs and symptoms such as tenderness, swelling and bruising which are common following surgery of the head and neck is common. It is recommended that symptoms completely resolve before resuming any strenuous activity especially heavy lifting and running.

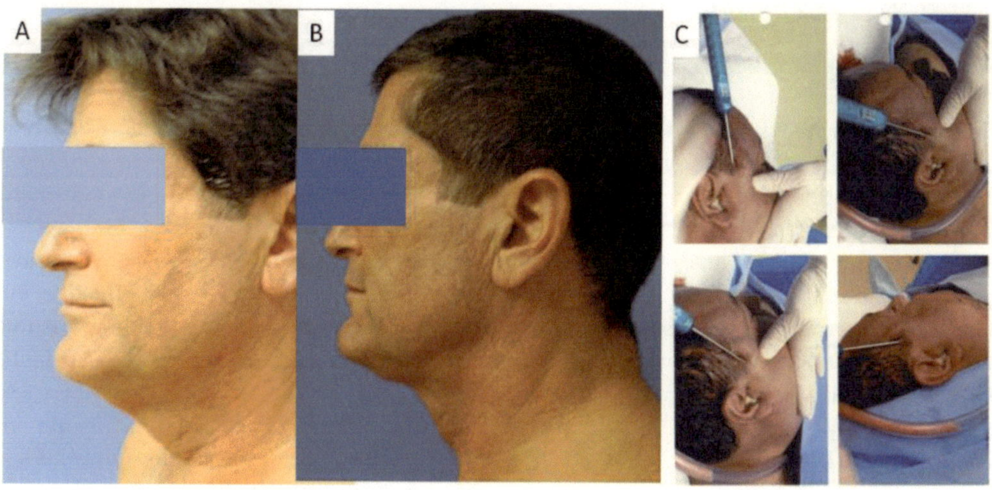

Fig. 3. Surgical lipospiration technique for parotid hypertrophy in HIV-infected men on HAART. A. Pre-surgical parotid hypertrophy, B. Post-surgical resolution of parotid hypertrophy, C. Angling techniques enabled by awake positioning of the patient.

4.5 Outcomes after parotid lipoaspiration

In a recent detailed survey by the authors of one woman and eleven men with an average age of 53.5±2 years seeking lipoaspiration treatment for parotid hypertrophy, three had prior radiation treatment, two had previous surgery and two had both previous radiation and surgery. Prior to surgery, on a scale of 0-5, five being very affected, 3 being somewhat affected, 1 being a little affected, and zero being not affected, patients felt their appearance was very affected (4.65±0.2), they experienced discomfort (4.0±0.5), a significant change in their lives due to the parotid hypertrophy (4.3±0.4), some depression (3.9±0.4) and social withdrawal (3.9±0.4) and a little problem with chewing (1.4±0.4). Within a year after lipoaspiration, by paired student's t-test, there was a 76.8±4.7% improvement in appearance (average rating 1.08±0.2; P<0.0001), a 69±8.6% improvement in discomfort (1.09±0.3; P<0.0001), a 72.5±7.9% improvement in how their lives were changed by parotid hypertrophy (1.08±0.2; P<0.0001), a 60±10% improvement in feelings of depression (1.5±0.3; P<0.001), a 73.9±5.4% improvement in social withdrawal (1.09±0.3; P<0.00001) and a 45±12.5% improvement in chewing (0.9±0.1; P=0.006). After the surgery, two patients had minor infections at the surgical site, two patients continued to complain of xerostomia due to prior radiation with no new cases of xerostomia, one patient developed thrush, and four patients had some discoloration of the skin at the surgical incision sites. When asked about regrowth of the parotid tissue, ten had none and two had some regrowth. Nine of the patients graded the procedure as completely successful, two said it was somewhat successful and one graded the surgery in-between somewhat and completely successful. In a larger number of patients (n=72) treated with the tumescent suction technique under local anesthesia, follow-up questionnaires were obtained in 43 patients. In these 43 patients using a scale of 0 to 5, with 0 being 'no success' and 5 being 'highly successful', the rate of success was on average (±sem) 4.8±0.1. In this larger sampling of patients, there were no incidents of infection, no disturbance in chewing, no complaints of dry mouth and no incidents of recurrence at 3 year follow-up.

5. Discussion

HIV dorsocervical fat pad and HIV-related parotid hypertrophy are frequently seen in clinical practice. The use of novel liposuction techniques in the treatment of these conditions as described in this chapter are advances that result in better outcomes, i.e., better cosmetic results, lower recurrence rates and fewer complications than previously used techniques.

With respect to HIV-related dorsocervical lipodystrophy, tumescent liposuction under general anesthesia, with the patient in the prone position has been shown to be effective, but recurrence is commonly seen, with only partial removal of tissue. It is reasonable to assume that optimal tumor clearance is essential, not only in creating an acceptable cosmetic outcome but also for maintaining long-term results. Due to the fibrous nature of these lesions, aspiration is typically difficult and more laborious as compared to aspiration of non-dystrophic fat.(Davison et al. 2007)It is imperative for the surgeon to position him/herself with respect to the patient in a strategic manner that will facilitate optimal lesion visualization and rigorous cannula dissection while preserving comfort for both the surgeon and the patient. Working with an intubated patient under general anesthesia limits access to the superior portions of the fat pad and those portions in the posterior neck and scalp. For example, when the patient is lying prone under anesthesia, the mass of the dorsocervical fat pad tends to disappear between the scapulae making it difficult access the entire depth of the tissue. We can speculate that the high rate of recurrence may be due to incomplete tissue removal when the patient is in the prone position. We use standard liposuction procedures for suction of the fat pad but position the patient awake and upright with the surgeon behind the patient. The patient participates by bending and twisting to allow for suction-assisted removal of the maximum amount of tissue. With our method of positioning, the patient can round the shoulders exposing the mass of the tissue. This provides a better cosmetic result, improves patient satisfaction, and decreases the rate of recurrence. Having a cooperative awake patient also eliminates the complications of general anesthesia, which are well known. Since 1997, the authors have treated over 1400 patients with dorsocervical fat pads with the patients seated upright and awake. During this period of time, it appears that less than 10% of these patients have had a recurrence. Difficulty with patient follow-up, however, makes it impossible to be completely accurate with our statistics.

With respect to lipoaspiration of the hypertrophied parotid gland, the goal of the parotid reconstructive procedure is to restore the patient to a more normal appearance; not to remove the entire gland. The procedure is limited to the removal of only that portion of the parotid lying superficial to the facial nerve. Local tumescent anesthesia achieves adequate anesthesia in all patients undergoing suction aspiration for parotid reduction. Using this procedure, our data suggest that patient satisfaction is high and quality of life is improved with minimal complications. Since the tissue being removed during the suction-assisted partial parotidectomy is not primarily fat, the procedure cannot technically be called liposuction. The authors suggest the term "glandular aspiration" or "adeno-suction" to more accurately characterize the operative procedure to reduce parotid size.

We feel the novel positioning during our procedures with patients that are awake and participate in the procedure, should be the standard of care for HIV-related dorsocervical fat pad and parotid hypertrophy. We welcome other surgeons to replicate these procedures in a similar fashion and report their results so as to add to the general experience with these procedures. Our hope is that improvements can be made based on the work we have accomplished to date.

5.1 ICD-9 and CPT Coding

An important issue for patients relates to insurance reimbursement for the correction of HIV-lipodystrophy and parotid hypertrophy. Using standard liposuction codes (15887 liposuction, truncal and 15886 liposuction, facial) are met with consistent denials from insurance companies as these codes imply procedures performed for cosmetic purposes. Insurance carriers understandably do not reimburse for cosmetic procedures such as liposuction performed to eliminate "love handles" or abdominal fat to provide a trimmer waistline. However, the conditions as described in this chapter are clearly reconstructive as they are intended to correct a deformity caused by a disease. State health and safety codes clearly define the difference between cosmetic and reconstructive procedures (e.g., California Health and Safety Code Section 1367.22). Although during the procedures, the equipment and techniques are the same as in cosmetic liposuction, we feel it is justified to code these procedures for reimbursement of HIV lipodystrophy and HIV partial parotidectomy as partial excisions, excisions and radical excisions as appropriate to the individual patient (refer to Table 1 for guidance in diagnostic and procedure coding decisions). We hope the health insurance industry can broaden their understanding of the damaging effects of people living with HIV lipodystrophy and parotid hypertrophy and reimburse as they would for other reconstructive procedures such as breast reconstruction following mastectomy or cleft palate surgery

CPT Code	Description
21555	Excision, tumor, soft tissue of neck or anterior thorax, subcutaneous; ≤3 cm
21557	Radical resection of tumor (e.g., malignant neoplasm), soft tissue of neck or anterior thorax; <5 cm
21558	Radical resection of tumor (eg, malignant neoplasm), soft tissue of neck or anterior thorax; ≥5 cm or greater
21930	Excision, tumor, soft tissue of back or flank, subcutaneous; 3 cm or greater
21935	Radical resection of tumor (eg, malignant neoplasm), soft tissue of back or flank; ≤5 cm
21936	Radical resection of tumor (eg, malignant neoplasm), soft tissue of back or flank; ≥5 cm
42410	Excision of parotid tumor or parotid gland; lateral lobe, without nerve dissection (parotidectomy)
2011 ICD-9	**Description**
042	Human immunodeficiency virus (HIV) disease
272.6	Lipodystrophy; a collection of rare conditions resulting from defective fat metabolism and characterized by atrophy of the subcutaneous fat; includes total, congenital or acquired, partial, abdominal infantile, and localized lipodystrophy.
235	Parotid hypertrophy (neoplasm of uncertain behavior of major salivary glands)

Table 1. Reimbursement codes for the surgical management of the HIV positive patient.

6. Summary

The main goal of lipoaspiration of the dorsocervical fat pad and parotid hypertrophy as part of HIV infection and HAART treatment is to improve patient outcomes and safety. It is also important to preserve the comfort of the surgeon while providing a cost effective procedure that is affordable by the patient and covered by insurance. These lipoaspiration procedures described here avoid general anesthesia and include the patient as a direct participant in the procedure to ensure maximal removal of adipose tissue in the dorsocervical fat pad, and accurate removal of glandular tissue in the case of parotid hypertrophy. Our experience in the use of these procedures is that patients rate their experience and satisfaction with the procedures as very high.

7. References

Beitler JJ, Smith RV, Brook A, Edelman M, Sharma A et al. (1999) Benign parotid hypertrophy on +HIV patients: limited late failures after external radiation. Int J Radiat Oncol Biol Phys 45(2): 451-455.

Burket LW, Greenberg MS, Glick M, Ship JA (2008) Burket's oral medicine. Ontario: B.C. Decker, Inc. 586 p.

Carr A, Samaras K, Chisholm DJ, Cooper DA (1998) Pathogenesis of HIV-1-protease inhibitor-associated peripheral lipodystrophy, hyperlipidaemia, and insulin resistance. Lancet 351(9119): 1881-1883.

Chapnik JS, Noyek AM, Berris B, Wortzman G, Simor AE et al. (1990) Parotid gland enlargement in HIV infection: clinical/imaging findings. J Otolaryngol 19(3): 189-194.

Crane HM, Grunfeld C, Harrington RD, Uldall KK, Ciechanowski PS et al. (2008) Lipoatrophy among HIV-infected patients is associated with higher levels of depression than lipohypertrophy. HIV Med 9(9): 780-786.

Davison SP, Timpone J, Jr., Hannan CM (2007) Surgical algorithm for management of HIV lipodystrophy. Plast Reconstr Surg 120(7): 1843-1858.

Domingo P, Matias-Guiu X, Pujol RM, Francia E, Lagarda E et al. (1999) Subcutaneous adipocyte apoptosis in HIV-1 protease inhibitor-associated lipodystrophy. Aids 13(16): 2261-2267.

Grunfeld C, Saag M, Cofrancesco J, Jr., Lewis CE, Kronmal R et al. (2010) Regional adipose tissue measured by MRI over 5 years in HIV-infected and control participants indicates persistence of HIV-associated lipoatrophy. Aids 24(11): 1717-1726.

Hanekom WA, Chadwick EG, Yogev R (1995) Pneumococcal parotitis in a human immunodeficiency virus-infected child. Pediatr Infect Dis J 14(12): 1113-1114.

Heymsfield SB, Smith R, Aulet M, Bensen B, Lichtman S et al. (1990) Appendicular skeletal muscle mass: measurement by dual-photon absorptiometry. Am J Clin Nutr 52(2): 214-218.

Mandel L, Surattanont F (2002) Bilateral parotid swelling: a review. Oral Surg Oral Med Oral Pathol Oral Radiol Endod 93(3): 221-237.

McQuone SJ (1999) Acute viral and bacterial infections of the salivary glands. Otolaryngol Clin North Am 32(5): 793-811.

Michelow P, Dezube BJ, Pantanowitz L Fine needle aspiration of salivary gland masses in HIV-infected patients. Diagn Cytopathol 2011:Epub ahead of print.

Murata H, Hruz PW, Mueckler M (2000) The mechanism of insulin resistance caused by HIV protease inhibitor therapy. J Biol Chem 275(27): 20251-20254.

Ortega KL, Ceballos-Salobrena A, Gaitan-Cepeda LA, Magalhaes MG (2008) Oral manifestations after immune reconstitution in HIV patients on HAART. Int J STD AIDS 19(5): 305-308.

Petit JM, Duong M, Duvillard L, Piroth L, Grappin M et al. (2000) HIV-1 protease inhibitors induce an increase of triglyceride level in HIV-infected men without modification of insulin sensitivity: a longitudinal study. Horm Metab Res 32(9): 367-372.

Piliero PJ, Hubbard M, King J, Faragon JJ (2003) Use of ultrasonography-assisted liposuction for the treatment of human immunodeficiency virus-associated enlargement of the dorsocervical fat pad. Clin Infect Dis 37(10): 1374-1377. .

Ponce-de-Leon S, Iglesias M, Ceballos J, Ostrosky-Zeichner L (1999) Liposuction for protease-inhibitor-associated lipodystrophy. Lancet 353(9160): 1244.

Rosenberg ZS, Joffe SA, Itescu S (1992) Spectrum of salivary gland disease in HIV-infected patients: characterization with Ga-67 citrate imaging. Radiology 184(3): 761-764.

Ryan JR, Ioachim HL, Marmer J, Loubeau JM (1985) Acquired immune deficiency syndrome--related lymphadenopathies presenting in the salivary gland lymph nodes. Arch Otolaryngol 111(8): 554-556.

Safrin S, Grunfeld C (1999) Fat distribution and metabolic changes in patients with HIV infection. Aids 13(18): 2493-2505.

Schiodt M, Greenspan D, Daniels TE, Nelson J, Leggott PJ et al. (1989) Parotid gland enlargement and xerostomia associated with labial sialadenitis in HIV-infected patients. J Autoimmun 2(4): 415-425.

Schiodt M, Dodd CL, Greenspan D, Daniels TE, Chernoff D et al. (1992) Natural history of HIV-associated salivary gland disease. Oral Surg Oral Med Oral Pathol 74(3): 326-331.

Shanti RM, Aziz SR (2009) HIV-associated salivary gland disease. Oral Maxillofac Surg Clin North Am 21(3): 339-343.

Shugar JM, Som PM, Jacobson AL, Ryan JR, Bernard PJ et al. (1988) Multicentric parotid cysts and cervical adenopathy in AIDS patients. A newly recognized entity: CT and MR manifestations. Laryngoscope 98(7): 772-775.

Som PM, Brandwein MS, Silvers A (1995) Nodal inclusion cysts of the parotid gland and parapharyngeal space: a discussion of lymphoepithelial, AIDS-related parotid, and branchial cysts, cystic Warthin's tumors, and cysts in Sjogren's syndrome. Laryngoscope 105(10): 1122-1128.

Sooy CD (1987) The Impact of AIDS on Otolaryngology - Head and Neck Surgery. In: Meyers EM, editor. Advances in Otolaryngology - Head and Neck Surgery. Chicago: Year Book Medical Publishers, Inc. pp. 1-28.

Steel JL, Landsittel D, Calhoun B, Wieand S, Kingsley LA (2006) Effects of lipodystrophy on quality of life and depression in HIV-infected men on HAART. AIDS Patient Care STDS 20(8): 565-575.

Taiwo B, Hicks C, Eron J (2010) Unmet therapeutic needs in the new era of combination antiretroviral therapy for HIV-1. J Antimicrob Chemother 65(6): 1100-1107.

Tall AR, Krumholz S, Olivecrona T, Deckelbaum RJ (1985) Plasma phospholipid transfer protein enhances transfer and exchange of phospholipids between very low density lipoproteins and high density lipoproteins during lipolysis. J Lipid Res 26(7): 842-851.

Tao LC, Gullane PJ (1991) HIV infection-associated lymphoepithelial lesions of the parotid gland: aspiration biopsy cytology, histology, and pathogenesis. Diagn Cytopathol 7(2): 158-162.

Tien PC, Grunfeld C (2004) What is HIV-associated lipodystrophy? Defining fat distribution changes in HIV infection. Curr Opin Infect Dis 17(1): 27-32.

Wotherspoon AC, Isaacson PG (1996) Letter. Histopathology 29: 196.

4

Lipoplasty of the Back

Francisco Agullo, Sadri O. Sozer and Humberto Palladino
Texas Tech University Health Sciences Center El Paso,
Paul L. Foster School of Medicine, and El Paso Cosmetic Surgery
United States

1. Introduction

Suction lipectomy is among the most common invasive surgical procedures performed. The most common target area is the abdomen although other body parts such as flanks, thighs, arms and breast are also subject to lipoplasty in the hands of the most experienced practitioners.

In recent years and with the increase in body contouring demand as a result of the popularity of the bariatric procedures the back has presented as a challenging area to treat. Although there are few publications available addressing this important anatomic area, a broad spectrum of techniques has been utilized to address this problem, and following the usual trend a most conservative approach is preferred.

Geometrically speaking, the waist and back area form an "hourglass figure". [1, 2] This ideal shape provides much insight into how any lipodystrophy should be treated.

2. Indications

Ideal candidates for lipoplasty of the back present with excess subcutaneous fat in the flank and back which often create "rolls". There are many techniques available to treat excess skin and fat in the trunk area. Liposuction is an excellent treatment method for the back and flanks in most circumstances. Excess skin with laxity, stretch markss, or a lack of excess subcutaneous fat are clear contraindications.

As with any surgical procedure, a strict preoperative workup is essential to determine risk factors and optimize postoperative results.

3. Technique

Suction assisted lipectomy (SAL) and most recently, ultrasound assisted lipectomy (UAL) and laser assisted lipaedtomy (LAL), play an essential role in the management of this problem. While direct excision is the method of choice for those cases where a significant amount of excess tissue is present, liposuction is the alternative for patients in the obese and overweight group with mild to moderate excess tissue. This technique has the benefit of being significantly less invasive and morbid than direct excision avoiding incisional complications and the presence of scars across the back.

The back should be addressed as a three dimensional structure and different considerations apply to male and females. Female's back has a lateral contour with widening at the level of the ribs and hips. The center portion is narrow and this creates a more appealing lateral contour. From the lateral view, the midline shows a superior kyphosis and lumbar lordosis accentuating the shape of the buttocks. In males this is different, with narrower hips translating into a V shape type due to the difference in the fat deposits and more muscular structure. [3]

There are many fibrous connections between the superficial fat of the back and the underlying fascia that often form into rolls. There is a lack of medical literature on treatment through liposuction of fat rolls. Some authors have described a direction for suctioning that is parallel to the fat roll axis. Other authors have described the release of folds in a transverse manner. Some have even advocated a cranio-caudal axis of liposuction.

We individualize the treatment per patient. Different cannulas and type of liposuction are selected for different patients. Body habitus, quality of skin, sex, age, race and amount and distribution of subcutaneous tissue are taken in consideration when making the decision. In our practice we utilize tumescent technique with SAL and UAL. We have not personally used the LAL and although we are aware of its advantages, there has not been consistent scientific proof that LAL is better than SAL or the combination of SAL and UAL. The cannulas are usually of large diameter and multiple access points are utilized using a crisscross technique to cover the large back surface including paraspinal, bra line, infrascapular, flanks, and lumbar regions.

In males we always combined the UAL with SAL since the tissues are denser with greater amount of fibrous connections between the superficial fat and underlying fascia. Some females with lax tissues have been treated with SAL alone although the tissues of the flanks and back often times are denser and require UAL to obtain and optimal result. [4]

Most of the time, four incisions are utilized to perform adequate liposuction of the back. One incision is placed at the midline of the bra strap area, one incision above the buttock cleft at the level of the sacrum, and two incisions at the waistline, one for each side. In certain cases, two to three incisions per side are required to be able to perform the multiplane liposuction appropriately.

In our series of patients treated with this modality we routinely achieve a significant improvement in the contour of the back, flanks, lumbar and gluteal area. By combining liposuction with fat grafting techniques we broaden the possibilities of improvement addressing not only the back but also the surrounding areas thus, providing an optimal result for the patient. Fat grafting of the buttocks along with suction lipectomy of the lumbar, flanks and upper back significantly impact the over all result by emphasizing the projection of the buttocks and reshaping the lumbar contour at the same time. The suction lipectomy of the upper back and flanks allows for the harvest of the adipose tissue to be transplanted removing the usual creases on the lateral upper back and flank regions.

As a side note, besides the aesthetic improvement of the back and lumbosacral area there could be an added benefit in cases of back pain, with improvement and strengthening of the paraspinal muscles. [5]

4. Complications

In our experience, complications of lipoplasty in the back are rare when performed by experienced surgeons. The back and flanks are very "forgiving" areas for lipoplasty, making deformities due to superfluous liposuction extremely rare. The most common complication is under-correction of the deformities and need for a secondary "revision" procedure.

Hyperpigmentation of the liposuction port scars is common, specially in Hispanic and black patients. This pigmentation is often post-inflamatory hyperpigmentation and resolves over a period of four to six months.

Although other complications are rare, they are still possible and thus described at length in the "Complications of Liposuction" chapter.

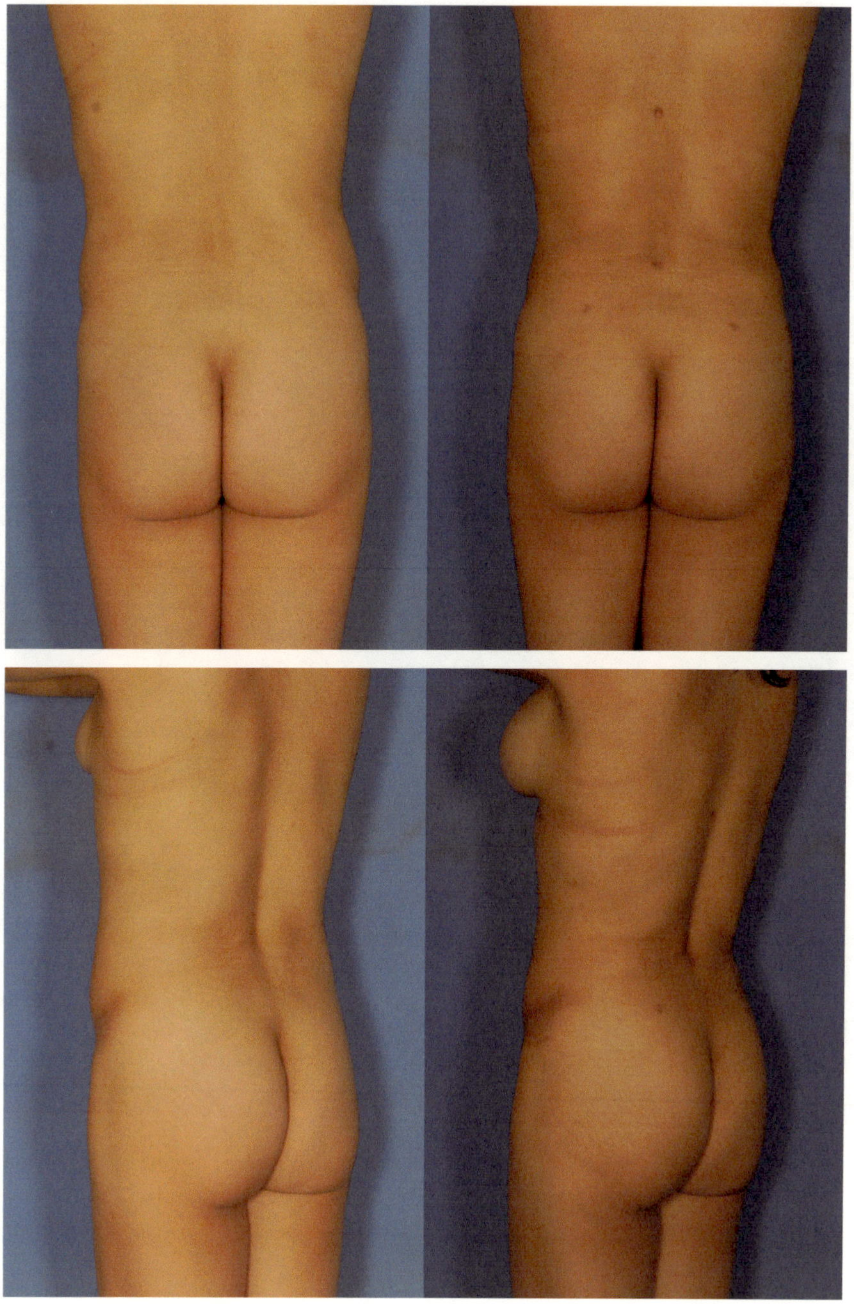

Fig. 1. Liposuction of the back and fat injections to the buttocks.

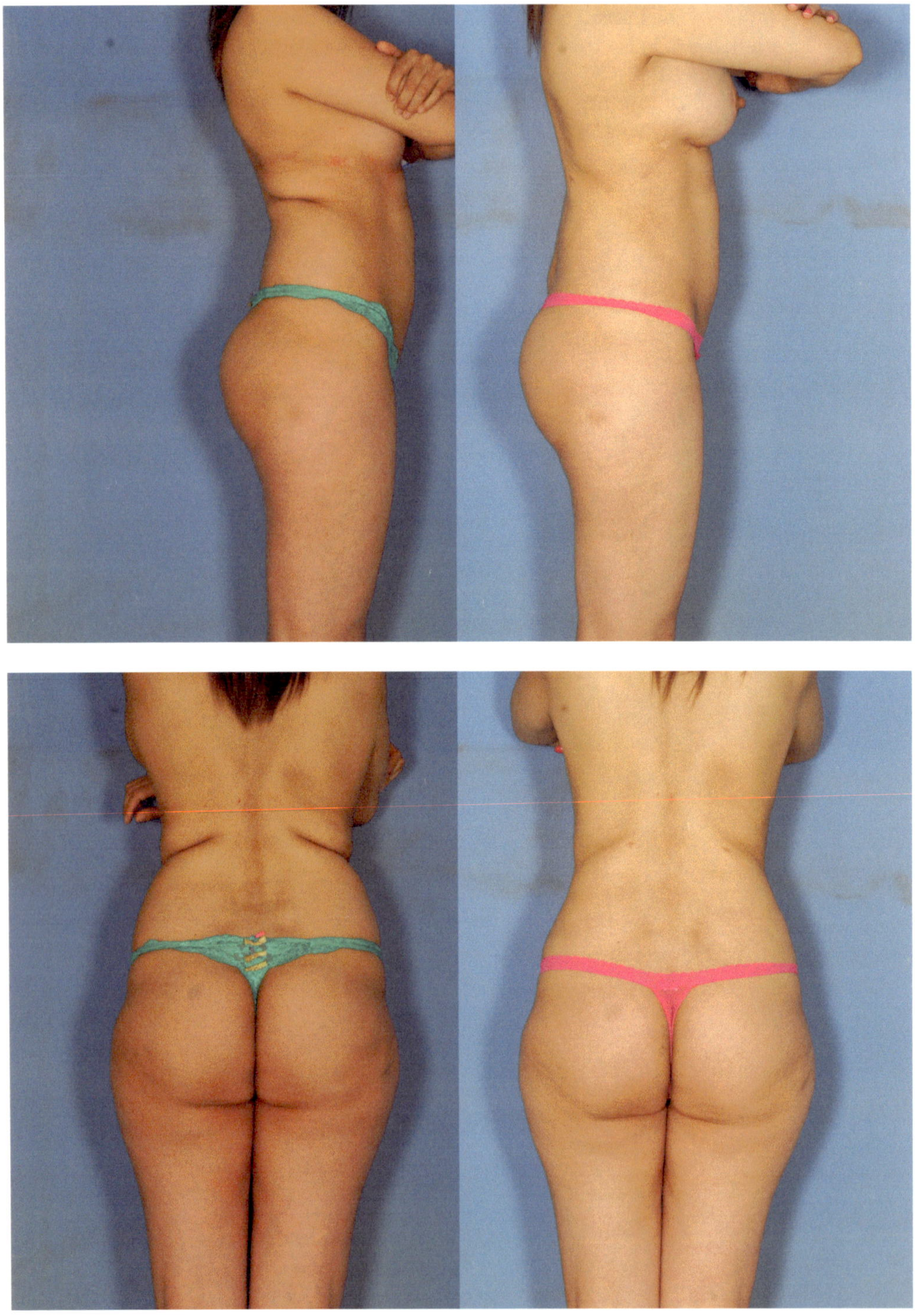

Fig. 2. Ultrasound assisted liposuction of the back.

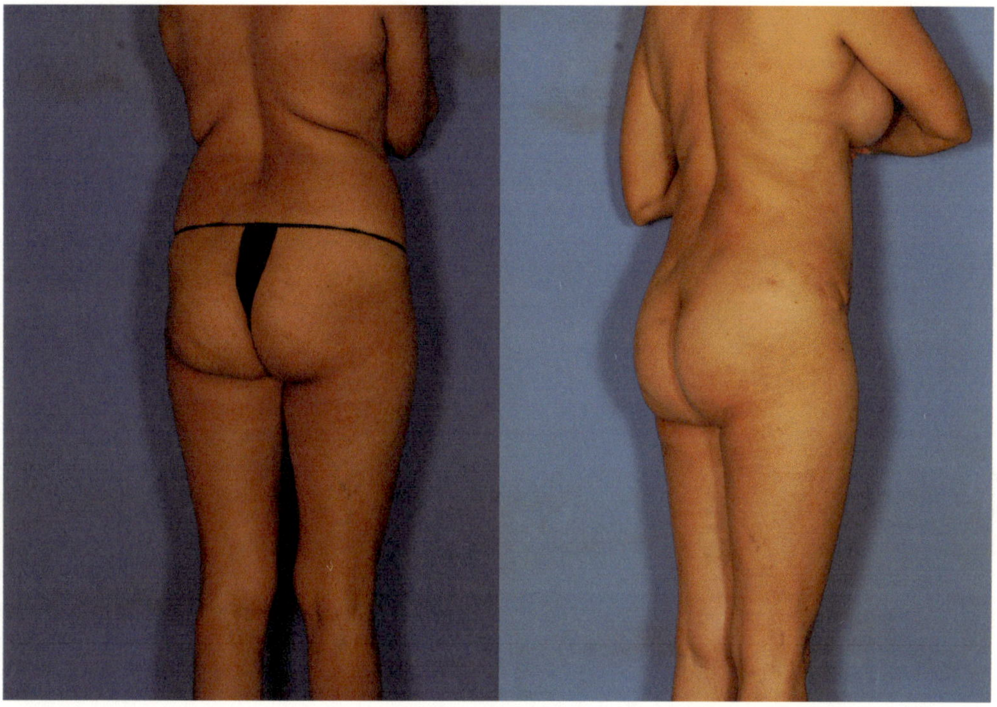

Fig. 3. Suction assisted liposuction of the back and fat injections to the buttocks.

5. Conclusion

Suction lipectomy of the back has become an essential tool in body contouring. The combination of these techniques with fat grafting allows simultaneous improvement of many areas in the back resulting in a significant over all enhancement of the body contour.

6. References

[1] Pawlowski B, Grabarczyk M: Center of body mass and the evolution of female body shape. Am J Hum Biol 2003, 15(2):144-150.

[2] Apfelberg DB: The vast "waistland": a rediscovered area in liposuction. Ann Plast Surg 1994, 33(3):237-240.

[3] Matarasso SL: Liposuction of the chest and back. Dermatol Clin 1999, 17(4):799-804, vi.

[4] Zocchi ML: Ultrasonic assisted lipoplasty. Technical refinements and clinical evaluations. Clin Plast Surg 1996, 23(4):575-598.

[5] Theron J, Guimaraens L, Casasco A, Coellar H, Sola T: Lumbosacral liposuction. A new tool for the treatment of low back pain. Interv Neuroradiol 2007, 13(2):153-160.

5

Power-Assisted Liposuction (PAL) vs. Traditional Liposuction: Quantification and Comparison of Tissue Shrinkage and Tightening

Gordon H. Sasaki[1], Ana Tevez[2] and Erica Lopez Ulloa[2]
[1]*Loma Linda University, Medical University Center, Private Practice, Pasadena*
[2]*Sasaki Advanced Aesthetic Medical Center*
USA

1. Introduction

Traditional liposuction with blunt-tip fenestrated cannulas remains the most commonly performed surgery for localized fat deposits. Refinements in the use of tumescent solutions, improvements in technique/instrumentation and selection of optimal candidates are critical to maintain its safety profile and effectiveness[1]. Since the introduction of power-assisted liposuction (PAL) by MicroAire Surgical Instruments (FDA 510(K) December 1998, the device has undergone developmental changes to improve mechanical disruption of normal and fibrotic fatty areas, in gynecomastia and within firmer tissues after secondary surgery for superior fat extraction[2-8]. To date, however, there have been no studies that objectively determine whether the effects of mechanical injury, produced by a PAL device with potential increased surgical trauma, result in increased tissue shrinkage and tightening, after extraction of fat which is not apt to occur with traditional manual liposuction (TL).
The purposes of this chapter were to review a 12-year clinical experience with powered-assisted liposuction and, in a limited study, obtain additional quantitative data on tissue shrinkage (accommodation or retraction) and tightening (elasticity) comparing PAL liposuction vs. traditional manual liposuction alone.

1.1 Device

The current upgraded MicroAire™ PAL device was an electrically powered and ergonomically re-designed model that was lighter and transmitted less vibrations, allowing easier penetration, removal of fatty tissue and reduced surgeon fatigue. A multi-fenestrated 4.0mm helix triport 3 cannula reciprocated at 2000 to 4000 cpm at a 2-3mm stroke. Although the speed of cannula movement could be adjusted by surgeon-preference, the instrument was operated either at full power (4000 cpm) or without power (manual) for this study.

1.2 Clinical protocol

From 1998 to 2011, ASA 1 patients presented for body contouring with PAL. Treatments were indicated for patients with moderate collections of adiposity and mild to moderate amount of tissue laxity. Patient exclusion criteria included pregnancy, uncontrolled diabetes mellitus, collagen disorders, cardiovascular diseases, and bleeding disorders. Standardized digital photography was obtained before surgery, along with data about each patient's weight, height, percentage body fat, and body mass index. Patients were marked in the standing and sitting positions to the localized zones of treatment. Patients were offered preoperative oral medication for pain and sedation. An intravenous line and urinary catheter were inserted for access before surgery and removed upon discharge

All surgeries were performed in an office setting under tumescent local anesthesia (500mg lidocaine, 1mg epinephrine, 20ml 8.4% sodium bicarbonate, 1000 ml 1 normal saline), utilizing superwet technique (1:1 ratio of tumescent fluid infiltration:lipoaspiration). Multiport blunt cannulas (2.4-4.0mm openings) removed fat, tissue debris, and tumescent fluid under a vacuum pressure between 450-500mm Hg for small-to-moderate volume cases for safe and effective fat removal in one session. The maximum amount of lipoaspirate did not exceed 5000ml in any one patient, respecting the safe maximum 35mg/kg of lidocaine dosage, while monitoring fluid replacement, hemodynamic stability, blood loss, and urinary output during surgery and in the post-operative recovery period. Temporary 0.25-inch (0.635-cm) Penrose drains were inserted into dependent sites and removed within 1-2 days. Compression garments with sponge inserts were applied for 2-3 weeks, after which a series of weekly external ultrasound treatments were given to reduce irregularities and swelling.

1.3 Study design for quantitative tissue shrinkage and tightening

A randomized, controlled study was designed to measure tissue shrinkage and tightening in 3 female volunteers who presented with localized lower abdominal adiposity, minimal-moderate skin laxity, and absence of rectus abdominis diastasis. Conditions for exclusion included abdominal surgeries, current weight reduction programs, diabetes mellitus, collagen disorders, cardiovascular diseases, local infections and bleeding disorders. Biopsies from treated sites were obtained at baseline and 6 months later to correlate histologic observations with tissue shrinkage changes. At the completion of the study, a complete abdominal liposuction was offered to achieve an aesthetic result in each patient. Informed consents were obtained with IRB and HIPPA-approved protocols.

In the upright position, patients' skin-fat folds were measured across by a caliper (Harpenden Skinfold Caliper, Baty International, West Sussex, UK). Two 10cmx10cm square templates were marked on the lower half of each abdomen and were separated by a 5cmx10cm rectangular zone at the midline of the abdomen. The corners of each treated site were tattooed with India ink deposited through a 21 gauge multipronged needle. The Vectra 3D System software (Canfield Scientific, Fairfield, New Jersey) would capture the permanent markers around each targeted site and calculate quantitative changes in tissue shrinkage by measuring the horizontal, vertical, diagonal and perimeter distances at baseline compared to findings at 3 and 6 month follow up visits (Figure 1).

Tissue elasticity was evaluated by three repetitive measurements a tattooed site at the center of each targeted zone with the Reviscometer® RVM 900 (Courage-Khazaka, Colone, Germany) at baseline and 3 months after manual or power-driven liposuction. Measurements were calculated on the principle of stress-strain relationships when the skin was drawn up with negative pressure of 400mbar within 3 seconds and then released and moves back to its original position for another 3 seconds. The pressure differential between measurements, determined optically during suction and relaxation, is expressed as a percentage: tissue resistance during negative pressure = A; tissue's ability to return to original position=B

$$\frac{A\text{-}B}{A} \times 100 = E\ (\text{elasticity in }\%)$$

Internal subdermal temperatures were recorded with a thermal sensing device at baseline and during the end of the procedures along with simultaneous surface skin temperatures with a handheld infrared noncontact thermometer (MiniTemp® MT6, Raytek Corp, Santa Cruz, CA, USA).

One subject consented to tissue punch biopsies within the target zones at baseline, 3 and 6 months after completion of the study. Samples were fixed in 10% formaldehyde-buffered solution, paraffin embedded, sectioned at 4-5 µm, and interpreted with hematoxyline-eosin and trichome stains. The pathologist interpreted the microscopic findings in each specimen without knowledge of the given treatments.

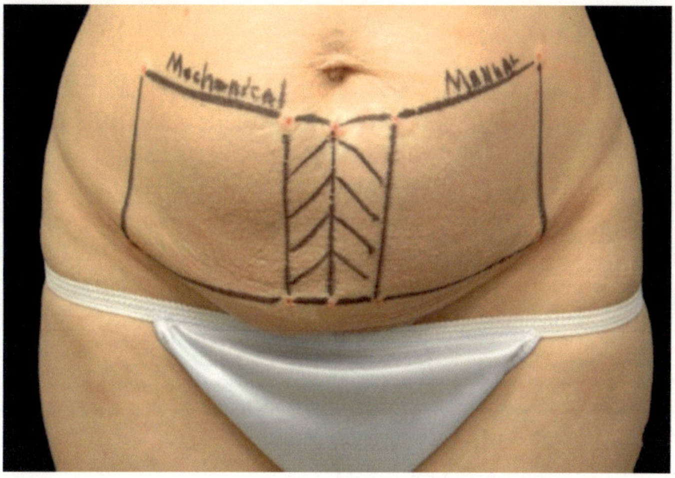

Fig. 1. Two 10cmx10cm target zones are identified by 8 tattoos whose surface areas are assessed by Vectra 3D Analyses between manual and powered-driven procedures.

1.4 Study protocol

Upon completion of their markings, measurements and photographs, patients were offered preoperative medications and prescribed a postoperative antibiotic. A 2mm incision below each of the square target zones permitted access for treatment. In a random fashion amongst the three subjects, once each of the 10cmx10cm areas received one of the following assignments, that zone remained as either a manual or power-driven site through baseline, three months and 6 months treatments regimens (Table1). During passages of the cannula in the **non-suction mode** within panels A & B at baseline treatments, simultaneous recording of temperatures were determined in the deep subcutaneous fat and surface of the skin. Identical temperature recordings were obtained during passages of the cannula in the suction mode within panels A & B at the 3rd month study period. Final Vectra 3D quantitative evaluations, elasticity measurements, and punch biopsies were obtained at the 6th month evaluation period, 3 months after the liposuctioning phases were completed. After each surgical procedure, access incisions were closed with a single suture. Subjects were dressed with sponge inserts and compression garments. Postoperative antibiotic and pain medications were prescribed.

Time	Panel Zone	Treatment
Baseline Vectra 3D & Intraop Temp. Monitoring	A	200ml tumescent solution (500mg plain Lidocaine, 1 mg epinephrine, 20ml of 8.4% sodium bicarbonate in 1000ml normal saline); 500 **manual** passes of a 4.0mm helixed triport 3 cannula in the **non-suction mode*** throughout the superficial and deep layers of subcutaneous fat.
Baseline Vectra 3D & Intraop Temp. Monitoring	B	200ml tumescent solution; 500 **power-driven** passes of a 4.0mm helixed triport 3 cannula in the **non-suction mode*** throughout the superficial and deep layers of subcutaneous fat.
3 Months Vectra 3D & Intraop Temp. Monitoring	A	200ml tumescent solution (500mg plain Lidocaine, 1 mg epinephrine, 20ml of 8.4% sodium bicarbonate in 1000ml normal saline); 500 **manual** passes of a 4.0mm helixed triport 3 cannula in the **suction mode*** throughout the superficial and deep layers of subcutaneous fat (250 ml aspirate).
3 Months Vectra 3D & Intraop Temp. Monitoring	B	200ml tumescent solution; 500 **power-driven** passes of a 4.0mm helixed triport 3 cannula in the **suction mode*** throughout the superficial and deep layers of subcutaneous fat. (250ml aspirate)
6 months	A & B	Vectra 3D & Elasticity Measurements, Biopsies

*MicroAire Surgical Instruments, Inc. Charlottesville, VA, USA

Table 1. Assignment and Treatment per Target Zone

2. Results

2.1 Clinical patient demographic data

Beginning in February 1998 to April 2011, 547 patients (498 women, 49 men) received PAL treatments in the author's private practice were able to be evaluated. Patients had a mean age of 48.3 years (range, 19 to 67 years), mean height of 162.7 cm (range, 146 to 192 cm), a mean weight of 69.2 (range, 53.6 to 115 kg), a mean body fat of 28.6% (range, 25.4.2% to 36.5%), and a mean body mass index of 24.6 (range, 18.2 to 32.2). Among the 547 patients, liposuction was performed in 13 anatomical sites (face, neck, brachia, axillae, brassiere/lumbar/hip rolls, breasts, abdomen, saddlebags, banana rolls, thighs and calves). Four hundred sixty-eight patients (85.6%) elected to undergo liposuction more than one site at the same session (average 4.2 sites; range, two to eight sites).

The average volume of tumescent infiltration was 2700 ml (range 1250ml to 3500ml), while the average aspiration volume was 2500ml (range 1750ml to 3200ml). The average infiltration:aspiration ratio was 1.08:1.0 (range, 0.9:1.0 to 1.2:1.0). The average volume of fat was 1785ml (range 1500ml to 2700ml). The average lidocaine dosage was 3.5mg/kg (range, 1.7-4.7mg/kg), below the recommended safe level of 7mg/kg in the *Physicians Desk Reference*[10].

In general, patients reported 85% satisfaction with the changes in their bodies after PAL liposuction at the six-month postoperative visit (Figures 2-3). Ten patients (1.8%) requested excision of redundant skin after liposuction to the brachia, upper inner thighs and lower abdomens. The majority of patients experienced skin accommodation or retraction after volume reduction of the fat. Nineteen patients (3.5%) requested surgical revisions because of incomplete fat removal of at selected sites or asymmetries. Each patient was asked to record his or her impression of the degree of intraoperative pain on a visual analog scale from 0 to 10. Patient responses indicated an average intraoperative pain level between 1 to 4 and a postoperative pain level of 1 to 3 on the second or third day after surgery. Almost all patients were able to resume their presurgical routines by the tenth postoperative day, depending on the extent and number of treatment sites.

During surgery, and the first forty-eight hours after surgery, none of the patients demonstrated any hemodynamic instability due to larger infiltration and aspiration volumes. Patients did not observed or exhibit lidocaine side effects such as prolonged lightheadedness, euphoria, digital or circumoral paresthesias, tremors, blurred vision, tinnitus or severe nausea and vomiting. Total blood loss was negligible, as determined by lipocrit measurements of less than 1.0% in lipoaspirates in over 50 patients.

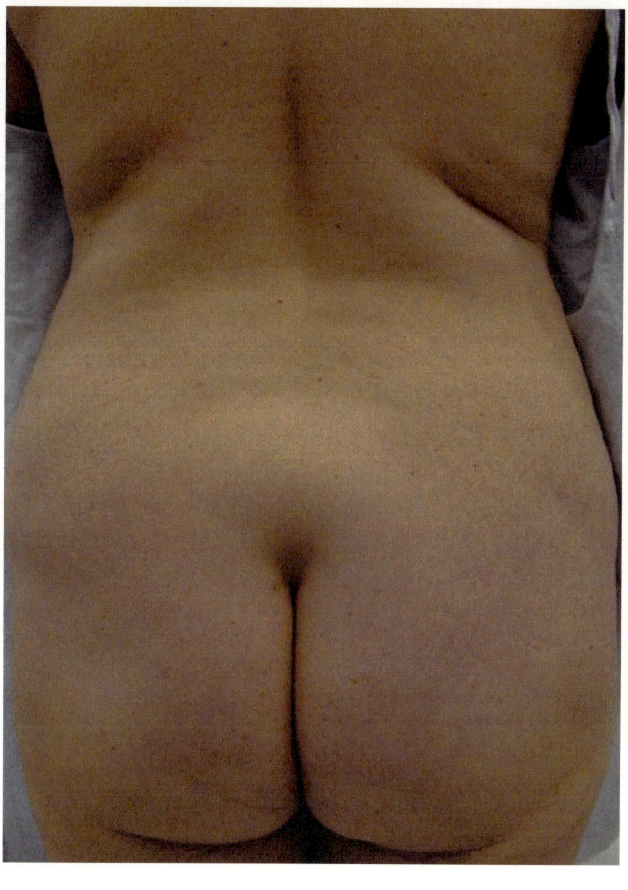

Fig. 2. 43 Year old female with lipodystrophy to the brassiere, lumbar, and hip rolls

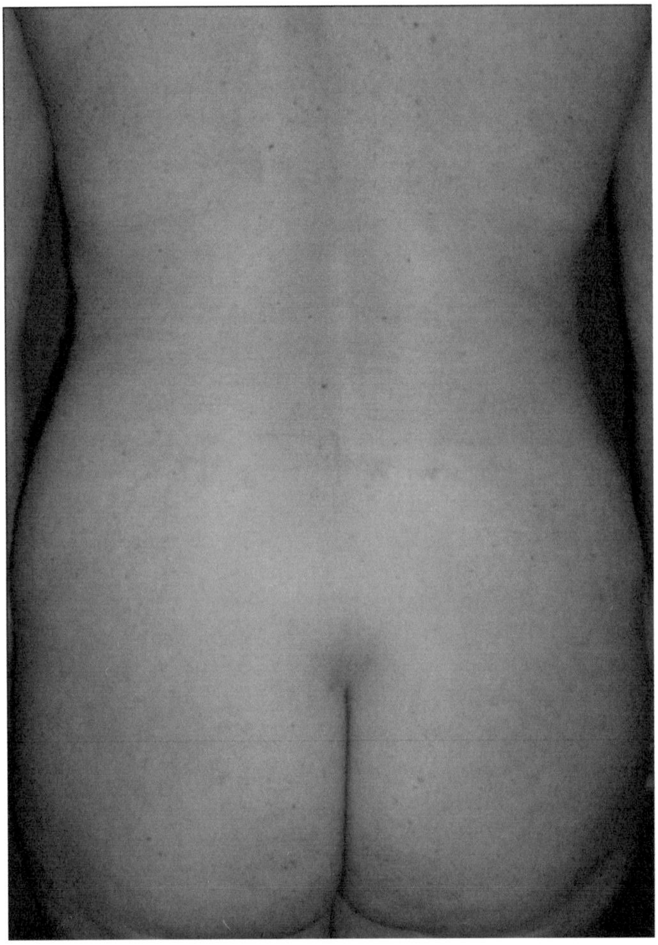

Fig. 3. Tissue accommodation after PAL procedure provided contour improvement

Patients developed fibrotic nodules (5.0%), prolonged indurations (3.0%), and seromas (less than 1.0%) but did not experience cellulitis, skin necrosis, blisters or prolonged edema. Nodules resolved spontaneously or were successfully managed by intralesional steroid injections along with a series of external ultrasound treatments. Prolong indurations took longer to resolve by 3 months with ultrasound treatments and lymphatic massages. Seromas resolved spontaneously without aspiration. Surgeon fatigue was negligible during surgery, while the learning curve was not steep.

2.2 Study patient demographic data

The mean age of the three female patients was 46.7± 2.2 years. The average pretreatment weight (57.7 kg), percent body (fat 33%), BMI (25 kg/m$^{2)}$, waist diameter (85.3 cm), and hip diameter (95cm) varied during the post-treatment measurements at 3 and 6 months (Table 2). Abdominal skin-fat fold thickness, measured by calipers, varied between 1.7-2.3 cm. Subjects experience no complications from surgery and returned to their normal activity levels within 1 to 3 days.

Subject	Weight (kg)			Body Fat %*			BMI (kg/m2)*			Waist (cm)			Hips (cm)		
	0 Months	3	6	0	3	6	0	3	6	0	3	6	0	3	6
Pt. #1 (48y)	58	56	59	33.5	34.4	36	23.6	22.6	23.9	81	81	85	95.5	91	93
Pt. #2 (45y)	61	64	67	34.6	37.6	38.7	24.7	25.8	27.1	86	88.5	92.5	95	94	96
Pt. #3 (47y)	54	54	54	31.2	32.9	32.9	21.7	21.9	22.1	89	88.5	85	95	93	92

*Body Fat Analysis Futrex-5500

Table 2. Patient Demographic Data

2.3 Vectra 3D skin shrinkage surface area changes

Results of surface area changes from baseline measurement, as determined by Vectra 3D Analyses at 3 months after **non-suction** manual or power-driven cannulations and at 6 months after manual or power-driven **liposuctions**, are shown in Table 3. A positive change in percentage surface area within the tattooed square reflected an increase of target site compared to baseline value. In contrast, a negative percentage value in surface area indicated a smaller area after treatment compared to baseline measurement. Outcomes were tested for significance with a paired *t* test, using $p<0.05$ as the cutoff value.

	Zone A Manual/ Non-Suction 3 Mos	Zone B Power-Driven/ Non-Suction 3 Mos	Zone A Manual/Suction 6 Mos	Zone B Power-Driven/ Suction 6 Mos
Subject 1	0.0%	-2.40%	-1.70%	-5.20%
Subject 2	3.30%	6.10%	-10.10%	-3.80%
Subject 3	0.70%	-2.90%	-0.90%	-7.50%
Average	1.3%	0.27%	-4.2%	-5.50%

Table 3. Zonal Surface Area Changes after Manual or Motor-Driven Procedures over Time

As depicted in Figure 4, manual cannulations without suctioning demonstrated an small increase in the area measurement from its baseline value (average 1.4%), while power-driven cannulations without suctioning resulted in no appreciable surface area change from its baseline value (average 0.2%) at the 3 month evaluation period. At 6 months, the surface area after power-driven suctioning exhibited a greater reduced surface area (average -5.8%) than after manual suctioning (average -4.2%) from their baseline values.

2.4 Skin elasticity changes

Calculations of biomechanical measurement for skin elasticity at 6 months (3 months after completion of liposuction) and expressed as mean percent changes over baseline. No statistically significant elasticity changes were observed in zones treated by either manual or power-driven suctioning from their adjacent control sites.

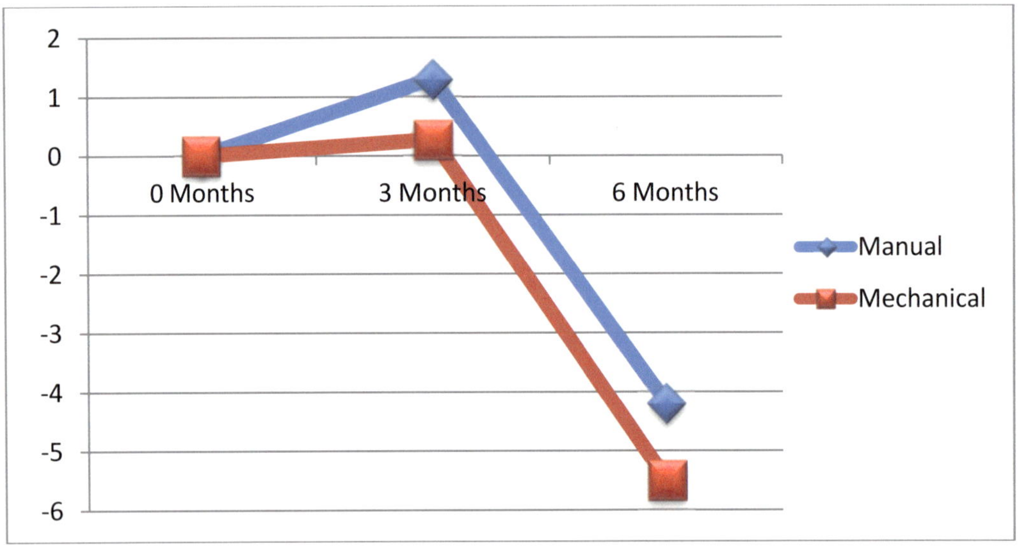

Percent Time

Fig. 4. Vectra 3D Analyses of reductions in surface changes at 3 and 6 months compared to baseline measurements after manual or power-driven procedures.

2.5 Subdermal and surface skin temperatures

The average oral temperature for the three subjects at baseline was recorded at 36°C (range 36.4-37.2°C). Throughout each of the assigned treatments, as listed in Table 4, the deep subdermal temperatures did not significantly differ from the simultaneously measured surface skin temperatures in each patient. Since manual/motor-driven cannulations or active suctioning did not result in any elevation of the subdermal or skin temperatures, the area changes observed during treatments, as tabulated in Table 3, is unlikely to be attributed to localized tissue trauma or thermal denaturation of collagen/elastin fibers and their secondary remodeling/contraction.

Pt	Zone A (3 Mos) Manual/Non-suction	Zone A (3 Mos) Power-driven/Non-suction	Zone A (6 Mos) Manual/Suction	Zone A (6 Mos) Power-driven/Suction
1	T_D* 30°C	31°C	29°C	30°C
	T_S** 27°C	28°C	27°C	29°C
2	T_D* 29°C	29°C	30°C	29°C
	T_S** 25°C	26°C	26°C	27°C
3	T_D* 31°C	31°C	30°C	31°C
	T_S** 29°C	28°C	27°C	28°C

* Temperature in deep subcutaneous fat (1-2cm below dermis)
** Temperature of surface skin

Table 4. Deep and Surface skin Temperature during Assigned Treatments

3. Histology

Microscopic examination of punch tissue biopsies of in panels A & B after the 6th month procedures did not demonstrate any significant epidermal, dermal or subdermal changes by hematoxyline-eosine and trichome staining (Figure 5). The use of manual suctioning or motor-driven suctioning did not produce any visible damage within the epithelial cell layers, dermal collagen or elastin fibers, and subdermal septae.

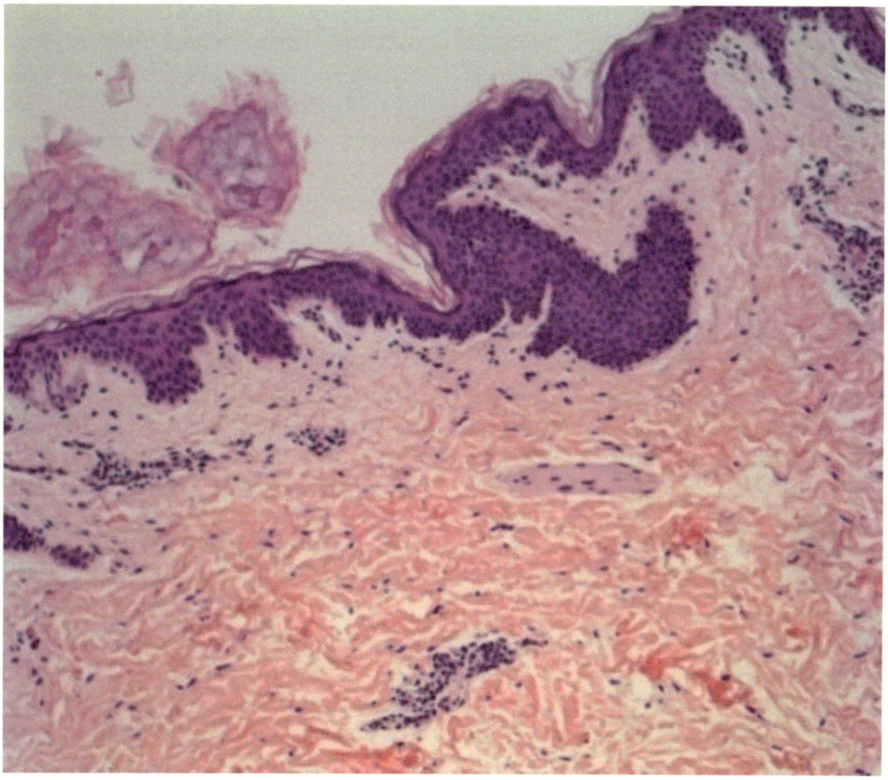

Fig. 5. Histologic changes in Panel B at three months after motor-driven suctioning in subject 3 demonstrating no observable damage to the epidermal, dermal or subdermal structures.

4. Discussion

Power-assisted liposuction has been shown to be effective and safe for small-to-large volume liposuction cases. Studies[2-3,9] that compared power-assisted to traditional liposuction found that power-assisted liposuction was superior in the ease and speed of fat extraction, faster healing and recovery time for patients, shorter procedure times with less surgeon fatigue, and lower incidence of touch-up secondary procedures. However, neither technique demonstrated a distinct advantage over the other in the post-operative evaluations for ecchymosis, edema, results, recovery times and complications.

Our extensive experience confirms previous findings that PAL represents a safe and efficient method for small-to-moderate volume cases with superwet tumescent technique. About 85%

of the aspirate volume was composed of fat, while blood loss was minimal with lipocrits less than 1.0% of the lipoaspirates. The average lidocaine dosage was calculated at a safe level of 3.5mg/kg, which resulted in no overt signs or symptoms of lidocaine toxicity. All patients experienced stable hemodynamics during surgery and in the 48 hour recovery period.

Over 85% of patients were satisfied with their surgical results with an acceptable revision rate of about 3.5%. A secondary procedure for removal of excess skin after liposuction occurred only in 1.8% of patients in areas of primary skin laxity (brachii, upper inner thighs, and lower abdomen). In the vast majority of cases, the overlying skin accommodated or contracted to its new environment after fat debulking. Patients rated their intraoperative and postoperative pain at relatively low levels and returned to presurgical activity levels by the tenth day. Postoperative complications, such as nodularity, induration and seromas, were low and resolved spontaneously or with postop massaging and external ultrasound treatments.

The limited clinical study for quantitative tissue shrinkage and tightening determined that the mechanical injury produced by the power-assisted device resulted in no significant difference in abdominal tissue shrinkage (accommodation and/or retraction) 3 months after powered mechanical cannulations compared to manual identical manual cannulations by 3D Vectra Analyses after the passage of the same number of strokes with a 4.0mm helixed triport 3 cannula without liposuction. Patients served as their own controls in a paired comparison analysis of powered cannulations and traditional manual cannulations within adjacent 10cmx10cm target zones. When powered mechanical liposuction was compared to manual liposuction, utilizing the same diameter and designed cannula, identical negative aspiration pressures, and similar lipoaspirated volumes, an increase in abdominal tissue shrinkage was observed with PAL over TL. Since power-assisted liposuction did not generate any temperature changes to the skin or subdermal tissues compared to manual liposuction, as determined in this study, there were no thermal effects on tissue elasticity or histology detected at the 6th month evaluation period. Since PAL did not elicit any significant thermal injury to the collagen fibers in the septae and dermis, no active tissue contraction was observed clinically or determined in the elasticity study. Although the number of patients in this limited study was small for statistical significance, the observed results indicated a trend in greater tissue accommodation after PAL treatments. However, the study did not provide an explanation for power-assisted liposuction's ability to result in a small increase in the amount of tissue shrinkage (accommodation and retraction) over manual liposuction, after fat extraction and in the absence of temperature effects. Further studies will be necessary to examine this salutary tissue response from powered mechanical liposuction over traditional liposuction that, if confirmed, may provide an additional advantage, resulting in safer, more effective and precise surgery.

5. Conclusions

Power-assisted liposuction represents a safe and effective method to remove small-to moderate collections of fat for body contouring purposes. With super-wet tumescent technique, the average infiltration to aspiration volumes approaches a ratio of 1.08:1.0 in most surgeries. PAL appears to be an efficient method because the average percent of fat within the lipoaspirate approaches 85% in the majority of cases. Over 85% of patients were satisfied with the body contouring procedure with only 3.5% of patient requesting revisional surgeries for incomplete fat removal. Appropriate tissue accommodation or retraction occurred after liposuction in most treated sites, except in areas that exhibited preoperatively a significant degree of tissue laxity (brachii, upper inner thighs, and lower abdomen) that required tissue excision after surgery in 1.8% of cases. All patients were hemodynamically stable during and after surgery, and did not exhibit any signs or symptoms of lidocaine side effects. Complication rates were low and involved temporary tissue fibrous nodularity, induration and seromas.

The study for quantitative tissue shrinkage and elasticity indirectly confirmed the postoperative findings among the 547 patients. The limited clinical study obtained quantitative measurements of non-significant differences in shrinkage of tissue surfaces in zones treated by either manual cannulations without suctioning or by power-driven liposuction without suctioning under other identical assignments (blunt cannula, tumescent volumes, number of stroke passages). Greater differences in surface area reductions were observed, however, in the same zones that were treated by power-driven liposuction than by manual liposuction only, under the same identical treatment conditions (blunt cannula, tumescent volumes, number of stroke passages, and volumes of aspiration). Since skin surface and deep subcutaneous temperatures did not approach threshold levels for collagen denaturation of 40-42°C with these non-thermal treatments, the observed shrinkage of surface areas may be due to tissue accommodation and retraction from volume reductions rather than to active skin contraction from denatured collagen fibers and their subsequent reorganization. These conclusions are substantiated by the normal microscopic findings after manual or power-driven liposuction at the 6th month evaluation period within the skin and subdermal layers. Further objective studies will be required to validate these observations.

6. Acknowledgement

The author wishes to thank Dennis DaSilva, Canfield Scientific, Fairfield, CT for Vectra 3D Analysis and Margaret Gaston, BS for statistics and computer assistance.

7. References

Coleman W, Katz B, Bruck M, et al. The efficacy of powered liposuction. Dermatol Surg 2001; 27:735- 738.

Flynn TC. Powered liposuction. Clin Plast Surg 2006; 33:91-105.

Fodor PB, Vogt PA. Power-assisted lipoplasty (PAL): A clinical pilot study comparing PAL to traditional lipoplasty (TL). Aesth Plast Surg 1999; 23:379-385.

Hunstad JP. Power-assisted liposuction. Semin Plast Surg 2002; 16:175-182.

Katz BE, Bruck MC, Felsenfeld L, et al. Power Liposuction: A report of complications. Dermatol Surg 2003; 29:925-927.

Katz BE, Bruck MC, Coleman WP III. The benefits of power liposuction versus traditional liposuction: A paired comparison analysis. Dermatol Surg 2001; 27:863-867.

Mann MW, Palm MD, Sengelmann RD. New advances in liposuction technology. Semin Cutan Med Surg 2008; 27:72-82.

Rebelo A. Power-assisted liposuction. Clin Plast Surg 2006; 33:91-105.

Young VL. Power-assisted lipoplasty. Plast Reconstr Surg 2001; 108:1429-1432.

Private Practice, Pasadena, CA. Clinical Professor, Department of Plastic Surgery, Loma Linda University School of Medicine, Loma Linda, CA.

6

Larger Infiltration/Aspiration Volumes, Plasma/ Subcutaneous Fluid Lidocaine Levels and Quantitative Abdominal Tissue Accommodation After Water-Assisted Liposuction (WAL): Comparative Safety and Efficacy to Traditional Liposuction (TL)

Gordon H. Sasaki and Ana Tevez
Loma Linda University Medical Center Private Practice
Pasadena, CA RN Pasadena, CA
USA

1. Introduction

Traditional liposuction[1] remains a standard procedure for removal of unwanted fat. In contrast, water-assisted liposuction[34-39](WAL), introduced in the United States less than three years ago, utilizes larger volumes of superwet tumescent anesthesia in small-moderate volume liposuction than that commonly employed by traditional liposuction (TL) in comparable cases. In larger infiltration-volume WAL cases, therefore, potential fluid overloading and lidocaine side-effects can occur as a consequence of technique. Thus, the first purpose of this preliminary report is to compare the infiltration and aspiration volumes, operating and recovery times, urine output rates in surgery and in the recovery period in larger infiltration-volume WAL cases to similar volume cases treated by traditional liposuction. The second purpose is to determine lidocaine levels in plasma and fluids within the subcutaneous space over 24 hours in a separate cohort of two patients undergoing larger-volume WAL procedures. The third purpose is to determine quantitatively by 3D Vector Analysis the significance of the WAL technique on percentages of tissue area reduction within panels on the lower abdomen in three separate patients.

2. Patient and methods

2.1 Study designs

All consented participants underwent either WAL or traditional liposuction procedures under local anesthesia by superwet tumescent infiltration and were offered preoperative oral sedation. An intravenous catheter was inserted in the arm as an access for drugs and intravenous fluid support during the entire surgical procedure and recovery period. The following demographic measurements were obtained prior to surgery: age, weight (kg), height (m), BMI, body fat analysis (Futrex 5500, Futrex Inc., Hagerstown, MD), hematocrit/hemoglobin and blood chemistries Prior to surgery, patients were encouraged to drink electrolyte-containing fluids *ad libitum* and have a light protein breakfast.

In the first study, patients underwent larger volumes of infiltration by either WAL or traditional liposuction to their abdomens, back rolls, thighs, axillae and brachii to obtain data on 1) total infiltration/aspiration volumes, 2) total lidocaine dose (mg), total lidocaine dosage (mg/kg), and 3) hemodynamic stability and urine output. WAL uses a two-chambered cannula that can independently either channel pulsations of tumescent solution (to loosen the fat and provide anesthesia) or spray pulses of tumescent fluid and simultaneously suction the rinsed, mobilized fatty tissue. Each WAL patient was treated in the three sequential stages. In Phase 1, pulses of tumescent solution [0.05% lidocaine (50ml of 1% lidocaine), 1:1,000,000 epinephrine (1ml of 1:1000 epinephrine), and 20ml 8.4% sodium bicarbonate per liter of 0.9% normal saline] were infused at the lowest rate of 90 ml/minute to provide localized anesthesia, vasoconstriction and tissue rinsing in a non-turgid manner to the planned site(s). During Phase 2, simultaneous suctioning (750mm Hg) and continuous pulsed infiltration, using a tumescent solution containing a reduced 0.025% lidocaine dose, evacuates the fatty tissue and a significant portion of the infusate. In Phase 3, a finishing cannula removes remnants of fatty tissue beneath the dermis with concurrent suctioning and lower rates of pulsed infiltration with 0.025% lidocaine solution. On the other hand, traditional liposuction patients were treated by superwet technique with the same tumescent solution, used in Phase 1 of WAL, prior to liposuction. Volumes (ml) and ratios of infiltration/aspiration/fat, lipocrits and urine output were calculated during and after surgery in the recovery room with each type of liposuction method.

In the second IRB study, two patients participated in the investigation of plasma and subcutaneous fluid lidocaine concentration levels, obtained over twenty-four hours during and after WAL abdominal liposuction, to determine the time and magnitude of peak values. In addition, total infiltration/aspiration volumes, total lidocaine dosage (mg), total lidocaine dosage (mg/kg), and urine output were recorded. Lidocaine concentration levels of plasma and fluid within the subcutaneous space were measured by the Emit 2000 Lidocaine Assay (Dade Behring, Inc., Cupertino, CA), a homogeneous enzyme immunoassay technique, based on competition between drug in the sample and drug labeled with recombinant glucose-6-phosphate dehydrogenase for antibody binding sites. Active enzyme converts oxidized nicotinamide adenine dinucleotide (NAD) to NADH, resulting in an absorbance change measured by spectrophotometric analysis.

In the third study (IRB, controlled, randomized), three patients received randomly assigned treatments of three cumulative phases of a WAL procedure within 4 x 10cm rectangles on their abdomens, with an additional control panel, listed in Table 1. Standardized photography, weight, body fat analyses, waist and hip circumferences were obtained at baseline and three months after treatment. Tissue reduction was assessed by using the Vectra 3D Software System (Canfield Scientific, Fairfield, NJ), that identified the permanent India ink markers around corners of each targeted site and calculated changes in horizontal, diagonal and perimeter baseline measurements compared to findings at three months. At the completion of the study, total abdominal liposuction was performed on each subject to achieve a final aesthetic result.

Results

Study 1. As shown in Table 2, twelve WAL patients (8 females; 4 males) with an ASA I classification underwent large infiltration volume and fat aspiration. Participants averaged a mean age of 49.0 years (range 29-61 years), mean weight of 71.1kg (range 51.7-98.9 kg), mean height of 1.7 meters (range 1.3-1.9 meters), mean body mass index of 25.2 (range 21.0 -30.2), and mean body fat of 31.9% (range 23.0-35.0%). As summarized in Table 3, thirteen TL patients (10 females; 3 males) with an ASA I classification underwent large infiltration volume and fat aspiration. This group of patients averaged a mean age of 53.3 years (range 32-63 years), mean weight of 77.5kg (range 67.1-94.3kg), mean height of 1.7 meters (range 1.5-1.9 meters), mean body mass index of 27.4 (range 24.0-30.3), and mean body fat of 33.7% (range 27.8-36.4%).

Panel	Treatment Assignment
1	Control
2	Phase 1: Infiltration Solution (25ml) (25 cannula passes)
3	Phase 1: Infiltration Solution (25ml) (25 cannula passes) Phase 2: Simultaneous Suctioning (100ml) and Infiltration (225ml) (25 cannula passes)
4	Phase 1: 25ml Infiltration Solution (25 cannula passes) Phase 2: Simultaneous Suctioning (100ml) and Infiltration (225ml) (25 cannula passes) Phase 3: Simultaneous Suctioning (25ml) and Infiltration (50ml) (10 cannula passes)

Table 1. Target Zones and Treatments

WAL patients received almost all their total fluid support from infiltration solutions which served as their anesthetic solution, maintenance fluid, and volume replacement fluid (Table 2). The average total subcutaneous infiltration volume was measured at 6239ml (range 4920-7500ml), while the average aspiration volume was calculated at 5460ml (range 4350-6900ml). The average infiltration-to-aspiration ratio was 1.2:1 (range 1.1:1-1.3:1). The average volume of aspirated fat was 2456ml (range 1716-3105ml), which calculated to an average infiltration-to-fat ratio of 2.6:1 (range 2.2:1-3.0:1) and an average fat-to-aspirate percentage of 44.9% (range 37.6-56.2%). During surgery, patients received an average total lidocaine dose of 1702mgs (range 1423-2095mgs) and an average lidocaine dosage of 24.2mg/kg (range 18.9-33.6mg/kg)

In contrast, TL patients received their total fluid support both from the infiltration tumescent solution and intravenous saline fluid resuscitation (Table 3). The average total subcutaneous infiltration volume was measured as 5350ml (range 4500-6500ml), while the average aspiration volume was calculated at 5042ml (range 4000-6000ml). The average infiltration-to-aspiration ratio was 1.1:1 (range 1.0:1-1.1:1). The average volume of aspirated fat was 4036ml (range 3280-4800ml), which calculated to an average infiltration-to-fat ratio of 1.3:1 (range 1.2-1.6) and an average fat-to-aspirate percentage of 80.2% (range 70.0-86.0%). During surgery, patients received an average total lidocaine dose of 2675mg (range 2450-3100mg) and an average lidocaine dosage of 34.8mg/kg (range 27.0-40.9mg/kg).

Pt #	Age	Wt (kg)	Ht (m)	BMI	Total Lido (mg)	Lido Dosage (mg/kg)	Total Infiltration (ml)	Total Aspiration(ml)	I/A Ratio*	Total Fat (ml)	I/F Ratio**	F/A (%)
1	29	97.5	1.8	30.2	1690	17.3	5760	4900	1.2:1	2500	2.3:1	51.0
2	44	51.7	1.7	23.0	1735	33.6	5940	4700	1.3:1	2021	2.9:1	43.0
3	61	54.0	1.5	21.8	1480	27.4	4920	4400	1.1:1	1716	2.9:1	39.0
4	57	56.2	1.3	23.4	1550	27.6	5200	4812	1.1:1	2117	2.4:1	44.0
5	42	92.5	1.7	28.0	2095	22.6	7375	6900	1.1:1	3105	2.4:1	45.0
6	60	98.9	1.9	28.0	1600	16.2	5400	4350	1.2:1	1783	3.0:1	41.0
7	55	70.3	1.7	23.5	1767	25.1	7000	6885	1.0:1	2592	2.7:1	37.6
8	45	67.0	1.6	27.1	1833	27.5	7500	6550	1.1:1	3050	2.4:1	46.5
9	44	63.5	1.6	25.8	1684	26.5	6550	5575	1.2:1	2174	3.0:1	39.0
10	46	52.0	1.6	21.0	1423	18.9	6050	5550	1.1:1	2775	2.2:1	50.0
11	56	82.5	1.8	27.0	1767	21.4	6600	5375	1.2:1	3020	2.2:1	56.2
12	49	66.8	1.7	23.3	1800	26.9	6575	5525	1.2:1	2630	2.5:1	47.6
Avg.	49	**71.1**	1.7	25.2	1702	24.2	6239	5460	1.2:1	2456	2.6:1	44.9

* Infiltration-to-Aspiration Ratio ** Infiltration-to-Fat-Ratio

Table 2. Demographic and Clinical Data in Twelve Patients for Larger Volume Water-Assisted Liposuction

Pt #	Age	Wt (kg)	Ht (m)	BMI	Total Lido (mg)	Lido Dosage (mg/kg)	Total Infiltration (ml)	Total Aspiration (ml)	I/A Ratio*	Total Fat (ml)	I/F Ratio**	F/A (%)
1	61	74.8	1.7	26.0	2750	36.8	5500	5200	1.1:1	4108	1.3:1	79.0
2	53	73.4	1.5	26.0	3000	40.8	6000	5500	1.1:1	3850	1.6:1	70.0
3	37	81.6	1.7	28.2	2625	32.4	5250	5000	1.1:1	4050	1.3:1	81.0
4	68	92.9	1.9	26.5	2600	27.9	5200	4990	1.0:1	4142	1.2:1	83.0
5	63	79.3	1.6	28.0	3250	40.9	6500	6000	1.1:1	4740	1.4:1	79.0
6	62	78.4	1.6	29.2	3100	39.5	6200	6000	1.0:1	4800	1.3:1	80.0
7	49	72.5	1.6	25.2	2500	34.4	5000	4950	1.0:1	3811	1.3:1	76.9
8	32	74.8	1.6	30.3	2250	30.1	4500	4000	1.1:1	3280	1.4:1	82.0
9	53	67.1	1.5	28.0	2650	39.5	5300	5000	1.1:1	4150	1.3:1	83.0
10	62	94.3	1.8	29.0	2550	27.0	5100	5000	1.0:1	3900	1.3:1	78.0
11	49	74.8	1.7	26.0	2500	33.4	5000	4900	1.0:1	4214	1.2:1	86.0
12	49	70.4	1.5	29.0	2450	35.1	4900	4500	1.1:1	3645	1.3:1	81.0
13	55	72.7	1.6	24.0	2550	34.8	5100	4500	1.1:1	3780	1.3:1	84.0
Avg	53.3	77.5	1.7	27.4	2675	34.8	5350	5042	1.1:1	4036	1.3:1	80.2

*Infiltration-to-Aspiration Ratio **Infiltration-to-Fat Ratio

Table 3. Demographic and Clinical Data in Thirteen Patients for Larger Volume Traditional Liposuction

The average operating time for the larger volume WAL group was 4.0 hours (range 3.0-5.0 hours), while the average time in the recovery room was 1.4 hours (Table 4). The average tumescent infiltration fluid rate was 24.8ml/kg/hr (range 13.1-38.8 ml/kg/hr). The average urine output in surgery was 1.8 ml/kg/hr (range 1.3-2.5 ml/kg/hr), while the average urine output in the recovery room was 2.2ml/kg/hr (range 1.5-2.7ml/kg/hr). As cited in Table 5, similar data was obtained from the larger volume TL patients who demonstrated an average operating time of 3.5 hours (range 3.0-4.0 hours) and an average recovery time of 1.3 hours (range 1.0-1.5 hours). The average tumescent infiltration fluid rate during surgery was 20.4ml/kg/hr (range 15.5-27.0ml/kg/hr). The average urine output in surgery was 2.0ml/kg/hr (range 1.3-2.7ml/kg/hr), while the average urine output in the recovery room was 2.1mlkg/hr (range 1.7-2.4ml/kg/hr). The majority of patients were monitored for over 12 hours after surgery.

Pt #	OR Time (hrs)	Recovery Time OR (hrs)	Infiltration Fluid Rate (ml/kg/hr) During Surgery	Urine Output Rate (ml/kg/hr) During Surgery	Recovery Room Urine Output (ml/kg/hr)
1	4.5	1.5	13.1	1.3	1.2
2	3.0	1.5	18.4	1.8	1.7
3	3.0	1.25	16.8	1.7	1.5
4	4.0	1.5	11.9	1.3	1.2
5	3.0	1.5	11.7	2.0	1.2
6	3.5	1.5	15.2	1.3	1.3
7	5.0	1.5	19.9	2.1	2.5
8	4.0	1.0	28.0	1.7	2.0
9	3.5	1.2	29.5	1.5	2.2
10	3.0	1.5	38.8	1.8	2.3
11	5.0	1.5	16.0	2.5	2.7
12	5.0	1.0	19.7	2.2	2.4
Avg.	4.0	1.4	24.8	1.8	2.2

Table 4. Operating/Recovery Times, Infiltration Fluid Rates and Urine Output Rates in Larger Volume Water-Assisted Liposuction

In both WAL and TL groups, lipocrits of less than 1.0% were estimated from millimeters of red blood cell presence and millimeters of non-red blood cell containing fluid from aspirates measured within centrifuged capillary tubes from final aspirates in each patient. Preoperative hematocrit, hemoglobin, electrolytes, blood urea nitrogen/creatinine and liver function test levels demonstrated no significant changes from their 3-month postoperative values. During surgery and the perioperative period, episodes of tachycardia, hypotension, excessive bleeding, dyspnea/wheezing, significant detectable fluid shifts, pulmonary edema, congestive heart failure, or low urine output were not observed. Each patient was assessed to be stable hemodynamically throughout the entire procedure and in the recovery period.

None of the TL or WAL patients developed in the immediate postoperative period or after 6-month follow-ups infections, deep venous thrombosis or skin loss. Subjective assessments of postoperative pain suggest that WAL patients on an individual basis experienced less pain and discomfort and were able to resume normal pre-surgical activities more rapidly than TL patients. There were no significant differences in the low incidences of ecchymoses, surface irregularities and nodular fibroses between the two treatment groups.

Pt. #	OR Time (Hrs)	Recovery Time OR (Hrs)	Parenteral and Infiltration Rate (ml/kg/hr) During Surgery	Fluid Urine Output Rate (ml/kg/hr) During Surgery	Recovery Room Output (ml/kg/hr)
1	3.5	1.5	20.9	2.3	2.2
2	3.0	1.5	27.0	2.0	2.4
3	3.0	1.0	21.3	2.5	2.1
4	2.5	1.5	22.4	2.6	2.3
5	4.0	1.0	20.6	2.7	2.0
6	3.5	1.0	22.0	1.9	2.0
7	4.0	1.0	17.2	1.5	1.7
8	4.0	1.5	15.0	1.3	1.5
9	4.0	1.5	19.8	2.1	2.4
10	3.5	1.0	15.5	2.0	2.2
11	3.0	1.0	22.3	1.7	1.9
12	3.0	1.5	23.2	1.5	2.0
13	4.0	1.5	17.5	1.9	2.2
Avg	3.5	1.3	20.4	2.0	2.1

Table 5. Operating/Recovery Time, Infiltration Fluid, Rates and Urine Output Rates in Larger Volume Traditional Liposuction

Study 2. Two female subjects with an ASA I classification volunteered for lidocaine levels in plasma and fluid within the subcutaneous space during and after liposuction of their abdomens. The following demographic measurements from subject 1 and subject 2 were obtained, respectfully: age (33yr, 47yr), height (1.7m, 1.6m), weight (78.6Kg, 59.0Kg), body fat (38.3%, 36.0%), and BMI (27.2, 23.9). For each respective subject, the total tumescent infiltration volumes (5900ml, 3050ml), final aspiration volumes (5500ml= 750ml fat + 4750ml infranate); 3050ml = 575ml fat + 1875ml infranate), total lidocaine doses (1700mg, 975mg), and lidocaine dosages (29.5mg/kg, 12.5mg/kg$_2$) were tabulated. In subject 1, the average tumescent infiltration fluid rate was 25.0ml/kg/hr, while the average urine output during surgery and in the recovery room was 1.5ml/kg/hr. In subject 2, the average tumescent infiltration fluid rate was 17.2ml/kg/hr, while the total urine output was 2.1ml/kg/hr. Serial lipocrits were calculated less than 1.0% of infranates collected from each subject. Preoperative blood work demonstrated no significant changes from 3 month post-operative values. During surgery and postoperative recovery period (average 3 hours), subjects did not exhibit any deleterious signs or symptoms that could be attributed to lidocaine toxicity or fluid overload. Patients received no parenteral fluid support other than tumescent infiltration and were observed to be hemodynamically stable throughout the office procedure and continued recovery at home.

Lidocaine concentrations in plasma and fluids with the subcutaneous space were measured by enzyme immunoassay technique and plotted by connecting the sequential levels for a continuous curve over 24 hours (Figure 1). The peak occurrence of the peak plasma lidocaine concentration, were observed at about 9 hours in both subjects. At 30 minutes, elevated plasma levels were measured at 0.5-0.1μg/ml, gradually rising to peak levels between 0.80-0.95μg/ml, and falling to 0.30μg/ml at 24 hours. All recorded plasma levels were lower than elevated levels from subcutaneous fluids within the tumescent-treated abdomens measured between 1-1 ½ hours (95-130ug/ml) and after 6-8 hours (66-95μg/ml) from the start of lidocaine infiltration.

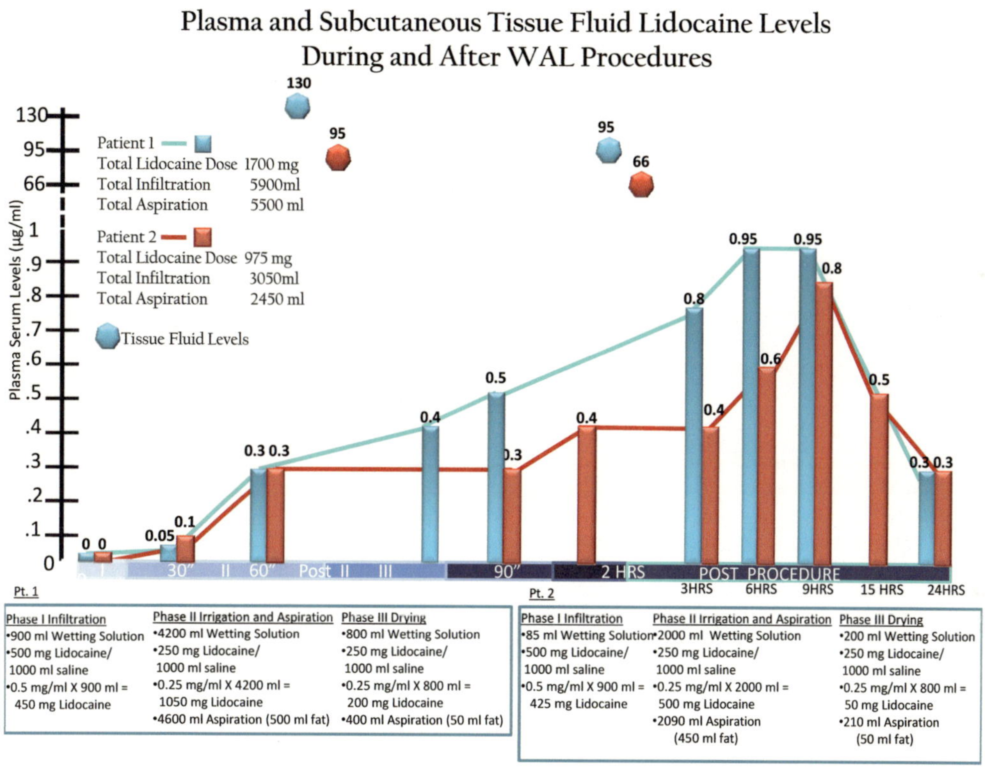

Fig. 1. Serial lidocaine levels in plasma and fluid within subcutaneous space during and after WAL procedures.

Study 3. Three female patients with ASA I classifications had an average age of 46 years (range 26-66 years). Each patient's pretreatment weight, percent body fat, BMI, and hip circumference did not vary significantly from the measurements 3 months after surgery. In each subject, a reduction in waist circumference from baseline to 3 months was observed (Table 6).

Results of surface area changes from baseline to 3 months within the four isolated rectangles, as determined by Vectra 3D analysis, are shown in Figure 2. Each target panel received cumulative components of the standard treatment protocol for a WAL procedure. At the three month evaluation period, the difference in mean percent area of tissue reduction between panel 1 (control) and panel 2 (subcutaneous infiltration) was negligible.

However, the increases in mean percent area of tissue reduction, observed in panel 3 (6.8%) and in panel 4 (6.7%) over control (0.0%) and panel 1 (1.2%), indicate that the removal of fat facilitates increased the accommodation, retraction or contraction of the overlying skin.

Pt #	Weight (kg)		% Body Fat		Body Mass Index		Waist Circum.(cm)		Hip Circum. (cm)	
	0 mos	3 mos	0 mos	3 mos	0 mos	3 mos	0 mos	3 mos	0 mos	3 mos
1	67.3	68.6	40.8	42.6	26.2	26.8	94.5	92.0	106.0	106.0
2	79.5	79.1	38.1	37.5	25.9	25.8	109.5	105.0	108.0	107.5
3	83.6	83.2	39.6	40.5	30.7	30.5	105.0	101.0	107.0	106.0

Table 6. Patient Demographics in Abdominal Tissue Tightening Study

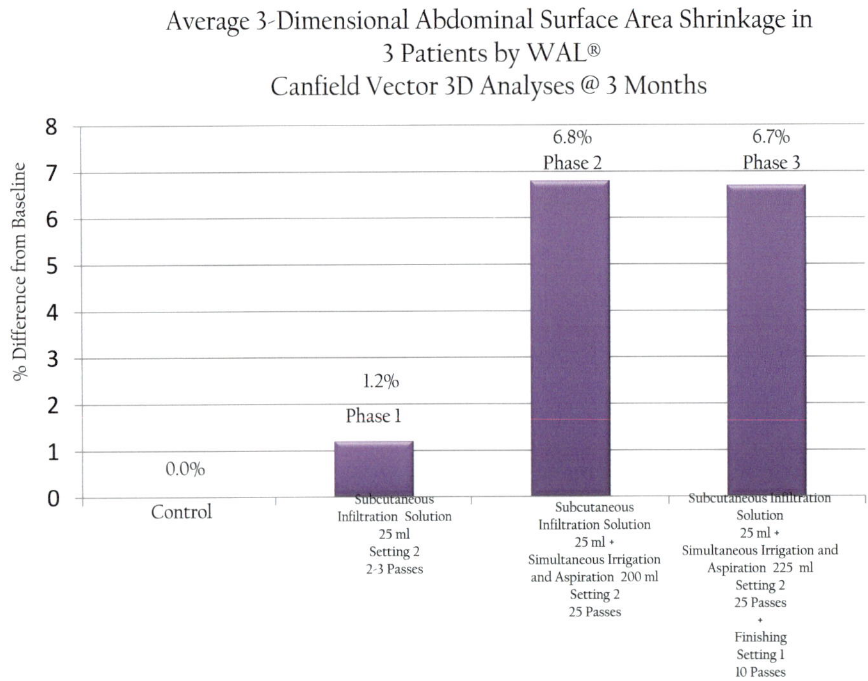

Fig. 2. Average 3-Dimensional Abdominal Surface Area Reduction in 3 Patients by Treatment Phases of WAL by Canfield Vector 3D Analyses at 3 Months.

3. Discussion

Traditional liposuction continues to be the gold standard to remove fat and contour body shapes. Since 1986, advocates preferred either a superwet[9,15-17,28-31] or a tumescent technique[2-8,10,], each of which have established proven safety and efficacy profiles using similar anesthetic solutions, but with significantly differing ratios of infiltration volume to total aspiration volumes. Each technique appears to be safe when strict clinical criteria[11-14] are observed such as selecting ASA I patients, using less than 5 liters of dilute volumes of lidocaine and epinephrine for average cases, limiting total lipoaspirates to less than 5 liters in the outpatient setting, respecting the safe maximum 35mg/kg of lidocaine, and prolonging patient discharge for large volume cases because of various factors delaying peak lidocaine levels as late as 10 to 15 hours. In particular, safer outcomes have been reported when the physiologic impact of larger volume liposuction is understood in cases that are associated with significant fluid shifts, third space losses, and potential epinephrine and lidocaine side-effects and toxicities.

In larger cases, superwet technique[28-31] is usually associated with the use of parenteral fluid maintenance and replacement with total intravenous or general anesthesia, while Klein's tumescent technique[6-7, 10] recommends the elimination for parenteral fluid support or total intravenous/general anesthesia in large volume cases. With either technique, however, the issue of absorption of the tumescent fluid infiltrate is complicated by the removal of the infiltrate along with fat and blood during suctioning. Since most of the infiltrate, ranging from 22-29 percent, is not removed by suctioning, at least 70 percent of the infiltrate is believed to remain after the procedure[20, 49]. Fluid overload[28, 33, 41, 51-53] becomes possible whenever substantial amounts of tumescent infiltrative fluids or parenteral fluids are used in high volume cases with the tumescent (3-4:1 ratio) and superwet (1- 1.5:1) techniques. Since WAL's variable force infusion pump pulses fan-shaped jets of tumescent solution into the subcutaneous fatty tissue during its three procedural phases, but only suctions simultaneously the loosened fat and fluid during the latter two phases, the final physiological and pharmacological impact is expected to reflect more closely the infiltration-to-aspiration ratios (between 3-4:1) observed with the tumescent technique. The author's recent WAL publication[39] provided, however, evidence to the contrary by recording an average 1.1:1 infiltration to aspiration ratio in fifty small-moderate infiltration volume cases.

Although the present study 1 data was underpowered for statistical significance, the observed results indicated that WAL and TL exhibited a comparative safety margin in similar types of cases for larger volumes of infiltrated tumescent solution, lipoaspiration, and fat removal, respectfully: average total infiltration (WAL, 6239ml; TL, 5350ml); total aspiration (WAL, 5460ml; TL, 5042ml, and total fat (WAL, 2456ml; TL, 4036ml). In these cases, the average calculated infiltration-to-aspiration ratios were similar (WAL, 1.2:1; TL, 1.1:1), approaching that observed in typical cases using superwet technique (1-1.5:1) rather than that experienced with the Klein tumescent technique (3-4:1). Although explanations for WAL's findings as a superwet technique are unclear, the data suggest that simultaneous infiltration- aspiration for the greater part of the procedure in phases 2 and 3 may account for the observed balanced I/A ratio, as found with TL procedures. In this study, the use of WAL, however, resulted in a lower average fat-to-aspiration ratio (44.9%) than that observed with TL (80.2%) or with other devices[17, 19-21, 42, 46, 54] that commonly experience 70-90% fat-to-aspiration ratios in comparable volume cases. These findings suggest that WAL may be more inefficient in removing more fibrous fat from the back rolls and upper abdomen than TL.

In this study, the average total lidocaine dose was larger in TL patients (2675mg) than in WAL patients(1702mg) because of higher concentrations delivered during the entire procedure in TL patients (0.05% lidocaine, average 5350ml total tumescent infiltration) than in WAL patients (phase 1, 0.05%; phases 2-3, 0.025% lidocaine, average 6239ml total tumescent infiltration). For similar reasons, the lidocaine dosage exposure was greater in the TL patients (34.8mg/kg) than in WAL patients (24.2mg/kg).

Although the average tumescent fluid infiltration volume (24.8ml/kg/hr) in the WAL patients provided the only fluid replacement, urine output safely averaged about 1.8 ml/kg/hr during surgery and 2.2ml/kg/hr in the postoperative recovery period. In the TL patients, the average tumescent fluid infiltration volume (5350ml) was augmented by parenteral intravenous fluid support (average 1000ml ringer's lactate) for a total infiltration fluid rate of 20.4ml/kg/hr during surgery to maintain an average urine output rate of 2.0ml/kg/hr in surgery and 2.1ml/kg/hr in the recovery room. In both procedures, clinical parameters of fluid overload (pulmonary edema, dyspnea, wheezing, congestive heart failure), low maintenance fluid replacement (tachycardia, hypotension, low urine output), and significant blood loss attributable to the procedure were not observed. In larger infiltration volume WAL or TL cases, however, patients must be provided with an available intravenous access site, be the recipient of prewarmed tumescent fluids, supported by a warming blanket and an anti-embolic calf/ankle pumps, and monitored fluid outputs with a urinary catheter. The information from this limited comparison of techniques does not significantly add to previously published data[4, 6,10,15,50], but confirms the safety profile during larger infiltration and liposuction cases under local anesthesia. Along with sound clinical judgment, both techniques may be performed safely under strict preoperative criteria, intraoperative fluid monitoring, and postoperative assessments for at least 12 hours. Overnight stays are recommended for monitoring of vital signs and fluid resuscitation in larger volume cases.

The pharmacokinetics of dilute amounts of lidocaine[4, 6, 21], approaching 35mg/kg, and epinephrine into subcutaneous fat with relatively large volumes of fluid have been found to be safe with the tumescent technique because of slow absorption of lidocaine in the presence of epinephrine, poor vascularity of fatty tissue, and the removal of a variable amount of much of the infused lidocaine by suction before systemic absorption. In studies[21-27, 55] associated with high dosages, peak serum levels below toxic levels of 5µg/ml were measured about 10-12 hours after infiltration. In the second part of this study, the lidocaine dosages used in the two patients were calculated at 12.5mg/kg and 29.5mg/kg, exceeding the recommended the safe limit of lidocaine dosage of 7mg/kg with epinephrine in normal healthy adults[31,40], but below the estimated maximal safe dosage of 35mg/kg, as recommended in the Klein tumescent technique[12]. The low plasma peak levels between 0.80-0.95µg/ml at 9 hours and the elevated subcutaneous fluid levels from lipoaspirates at 1-1 ½ hours (95-130µg/ml) and after 6-8 hours (66-95µg/ml) from the start of lidocaine infiltration were consistent and similar with those observed in previous cited publications. These results confirm the relative safeness of using larger infiltration volumes with simultaneous liposuction during the WAL technique. Because of costs, the study was limited to few patients and used an enzyme immunoassay technique that was unable to measure the variability in protein binding and active metabolites of lidocaine (monoethylglycinexylide and glycinexylidide)[32], which can be over 80% active and contribute to lidocaine toxicity. Although no significant side effects have been reported with higher lidocaine dosages[33, 55], further expanded clinical and laboratory studies need to be performed to determine the optimal lidocaine dose for WAL to provide complete local anesthesia.

Although the number of patients in third part of the study is small for statistical significance, the observed results indicated tissue accommodation after WAL treatments. In younger patients who present with minimal laxity to the overlying skin, the removal of fat can be expected to result in normal skin retraction, as observed in panels 3 and 4. There exists no evidence from this study that this beneficial finding was due to the preservation of the septal architecture. In the future, one of the challenges for WAL, as with other energized liposuction devices[42-47], is to investigate the contribution of energy in the form of mechanical or thermal injury to improve tissue reduction/contraction in the skin-challenged patient. Their limited clinical benefit brings into perspective the cost-benefit value of thermally-equipped devices for tissue tightening and emphasizes the need for further clinical research and applications[48].

In conclusion, we believe that larger-volume liposuction is safe and efficacious by WAL compared to TL, provided attention is directed to tumescent anesthesia, fluid replacement and overload, blood loss and postoperative monitoring for potential lidocaine side-effects.

4. Conclusions

On the basis of our limited and preliminary study, patients undergoing WAL procedures, as well as TL procedures, are safe for cases involving larger infiltration/aspiration volumes that introduce the possibility of lidocaine side-effects and toxicities and fluid imbalance. Patients did not experience significant adverse events in this study. Specifically, this brief study demonstrated that current algorithm with WAL treatments results in peak plasma lidocaine levels between 0.80-0.95ug/ml around 9 hours when subcutaneous fluid levels were elevated around 95-130ug/ml at 1-1½ into surgery and 66-95µg/ml at 6-8 hour after lidocaine infiltration. Although the correlation between total plasma lidocaine concentration (<5µg/ml) and the predictability of specific toxicity is tenuous at best and can lead to false sense of security, the surgeon must always be mindful of careful clinical monitoring during and at least 24 hours after completion of the procedure. In addition, preliminary results, indicating a small but positive trend for skin reduction by Vectra 3D analysis, remain underpowered for significance and will require larger number of patients for statistical validation.

5. Acknowledgements

The authors thank Dennis DaSilva, Canfield Scientific (Fairfield, New Jersey) for Vectra 3D analysis, Erica Lopez Ulloa and Margaret Gaston, BS for clinical and statistical assistance.

5. References

[1] Illouz Y. Body contouring by lipolysis: A 5-year experience with over 3000 cases. Plast Reconstr Surg 72:591-597, 1983.
[2] Klein J. Tumescent technique. Am J Cosm Surg 1987; 4:263-267.
[3] Klein JA. Anesthesia for liposuction in dermatologic surgery. J Derm Surg Oncol 1988; 14:1124- 1132.
[4] Lillis PJ. Liposuction surgery under local anesthesia: Limited blood loss and minimal lidocaineabsorption. J Derm Surg Oncol 1988; 14:1145-1148.
[5] Bernstein G, Hanke CW. Safety of liposuction: A review of 9478 cases performed by dermatologists. J Dermatol Surg Oncol 1988; 14:1112-1114.
[6] Klein JA. The tumescent technique: Anesthesia and modified liposuction technique. Dermatol Clin 1990; 8:425-437.

[7] Lillis PJ. The tumescent technique for liposuction surgery. Dermatol Clin 1990; 8:439-450.

[8] Hanke CW, Berstein G, Bullock S. Safety of tumescent liposuction in 15,336 patients. Dermatol Surg 1995; 21:459-461.

[9] Fodor PB, Watson JP. Wetting solutions in ultrasound-assisted lipoplasty. Clin in Plast Surg 1999; 26:289-293.

[10] Habbema L. Safety of liposuction using exclusively tumescent local anesthesia in 3,240 consecutive cases. Dermatol Surg 2009; 35:1728-1735.

[11] Morello D, Colon G, Fredricks S, et al. Patient safety in accredited office surgical facilities.Plast Reconstr Surg 1997; 99:1496-1500.

[12] Haeck PC, Swanson JA, Iverson RE, et al. Evidence-based patient safety advisory: Patient selection and procedures in ambulatory surgery. Plast Reconstr Surg 2009; 124:6S-27S.

[13] Haeck PC, Swanson JA, Gutowski KA, et al. Evidence-based patient safety advisory: Liposuction. Plast Reconstr Surg 2009; 124:28S-44S.

[14] Lipschitz AH, Kenkel JM, Luby M, et al. Electrolyte and plasma enzyme analyses during large volume liposuction. Plast Reconstr Surg 2004; 114:766-775; discussion 776-777.

[15] Rohrich RJ, Kenkel JM, Janis JE, et al. An update on the role of subcutaneous infiltration in suction-assisted lipoplasty. Plast Reconstr Surg 2003; 111:926.

[16] Basile AR, Fernandes F, Basile V, et al. Fluid resuscitation in liposuction: A prospective analysis of infiltration-to-total aspirate ratios lower than used for the superwet technique. Aesth Plast Surg 2006; 30:659-665.

[17] Pitman GH, Aker JS, Tripp ZD. Tumescent liposuction: A surgeon's perspective. Clin Plast Surg 1996; 23:633-641; discussion 642-645.

[18] Meister F. Possible association between tumescent technique and life-threatening pulmonary complications. Clin Plast Surg 996; 23:642-645.

[19] Karmo FR, Milan MF, Silbergleit A. Blood loss in major liposuction procedures: A comparison study using suction-assisted versus ultrasonically assisted lipoplasty. Plast Reconstr Surg 2001; 108; 241.

[20] Samdal F, Amland PF, Bugge JF. Blood loss during suction-assisted lipectomy with largevolumes of dilute adrenaline. Scand J Plast Reconstr Surg Hand Surg 1995; 29:161-165.

[21] Klein JA. Tumescent technique for regional anesthesia permits lidocaine doses of 35mg/kg for. liposuction. J Dermatol Surg Oncol 1990; 16:248.

[22] Samdal F, Amland PF, Bugge JF. Plasma lidocaine levels during suction-assisted lipectomy using large doses of dilute lidocaine with epinephrine. Plast Reconstr Surg 1994; 93:1217.

[23] Klein JA, Kassarjdian N. Lidocaine toxicity with tumescent liposuction: A case report of drug interactions. Dermatol Surg 1997; 23:1169.

[24] Hagerty T. Klein P. Fat partitioning of lidocaine in tumescent liposuction. Ann Plast Surg 1999; 42:372-375.

[25] Burk RW III, Guzman-Steiin G, Vasconez LO. Lidocaine and epinephrine levels in tumescent technique liposuction. Plast Reconstr Surg 1996; 97:1379-1384.

[26] Brown Sa, Lipschitz AH, Kenkel J, et al. Pharmacokinetics and safety of epinephrine use in liposuction. Plast Reconstr Surg 2004; 114:756.

[27] Nordstrom H, Stange K. Plasma lidocaine levels and risks after liposuction with tumescent anesthesia. Acta Anaesthesiol Scand 2005; 49:1487-1490.

[28] Trott, S, Beran S, Rohrich RJ, et al. Safety considerations and fluid resuscitation in liposuction; An analysis of 53 consecutive patients. Plast Reconstr Surg 1998; 102:2220-2229.

[29] Kenkle JM, Lipschitz AH, Luby M, et al. Hemodynamic physiology and thermoregulation in liposuction. Plast Reconstr Surg 2004; 114:503.

[30] Rohrich RJ, Leedy JE, Swamy R, et al. Fluid resuscitation in liposuction: A retrospective reviewof 89 consecutive patients. Plast Reconstr Surg 2006; 117:431-435.

[31] Commons GW, Halperin B, Chang CC. Large volume liposuction: A review of 631 consecutive cases over 12 years. Plast Reconstr Surg 2001; 108:1753-1763; discussion 1764-1767.

[32] Naguib M, Magboul MM, Samarkandi A, et al. Adverse effects and drug interactions associated with local and regional anesthesia. Drug Saf. 1998; 18:221-225.

[33] Lehnhardt M, Homann HH, Daigeler A, et al. Major and lethal complications of liposuction: A review of 72 cases in Germany between 1998 and 2002. Plast Reconstr Surg 2008; 121:396e- 403e.

[34] Heymans O, Castus P, Grandjean FX, Van Zele D. Liposuction: Review of the techniques, innovations and applications. Acta chir belg 2006; 106:647-653.

[35] Mann MW, Palm MD, Sengelmann RD. New Advances in Liposuction Technology. Semin Cutan Med Surg 2008; 27:72-82.

[36] Taufiz AZ. Water-jet-assisted liposuction. In: Shiffman MA, Di Giuseppe A, editors. Liposuction: Principles and Practice. New York: Springer-Verlag; 2006; Chapter 49, pages 326-330.

[37] Stutz J, Krahl D. Water jet-assisted liposuction for patients with lipoedema: Histologic andimmunologic analysis of the aspirates of 30 lipoedema patients. Aesth Plast Surg 2008; June.

[38] Wanner M, Jacob S, Schwarzl F, Honigmann K, Oberholzer M, Pierer G. Wasser-jet dissection im fettgewebe. Swiss Surg 2001; 7:173-179.

[39] Sasaki GH. Preliminary Report: Part 1. Water-Assisted Liposuction (WAL) for body contouring and lipo-harvesting: Safety and Efficacy with 50 consecutive patients. Aesthetic Plastic Surgery Journal. Spring Issue, 2011.

[40] Gilman AG, Goodman LS, Rall TW, et al. Goodman and Gilman's The Pharmacologic Basis ofTherapeutics, 7th Ed. New York: Macmillan, 1985:310.

[41] Grazer FM, Meister FL. Factors contributing to adverse effects of the tumescent technique.Aesth Surg J 1997; 17:411-413.

[42] Scheflan M, Tazi H. Ultrasonically assisted body contouring. Aesth Surg J 1996; 16:117-122.

[43] Prado A, Andrades P, Danilla S, et al. A prospective, randomized, double-blind, controlled Clinical trial comparing laser-assisted lipoplasty with suction-assisted lipoplasty. Plast Reconstr2006; 118:1032-1045.

[44] DiBernardo BE, Reyes J, Chien B. Evaluation of tissue thermal effects from 1064/1320-nm laser-assisted lipolysis and its clinical implications. J Cosm Laser Ther 2009; 11:62-69.

[45] DiBernardo BE, Reyes J. Preliminary report: evaluation of skin tightening after laser-assistedliposuction. Aesth Surg J 2009; 29:400-408.

[46] Sasaki GH, Tevez A. Laser-assisted liposuction for facial and body contouring and skin tightening: A 2-year experience with 75 consecutive patients. Sem Cut Med Surg 2009; 8:226-235.
[47] Sasaki GH. Preliminary report: Quantification of human abdominal tissue tightening and contraction after component treatments with 1064nm/1320nm laser-assisted lipolysis: Clinical implications. Aesth Surg J 2010; 30:239-245. Commentary: Jewell M, 246-248.
[48] Goldman A, Gotkin RH, Sarnoff DS, et al. Cellulite: A new treatment approach combining subdermal Nd:YAG laser lipolysis and autologous fat transplantation. Aesth Surg J 2008; 28:656-662.
[49] Pitman GH, Aker JS, Tripp ZD. Tumescent liposuction. Clin Plast Surg 1996; 23:633.
[50] Rohrich RJ, Beran SJ, Fodor PB. The role of subcutaneous infiltration in suction-assistedlipoplasty: A review. Plast Reconstr Surg 1997; 99:514.
[51] Gilliland MD, Coates N. Tumescent liposuction complicated by pulmonary edema. Plast Reconstr Surg 1989; 99:215.
[52] Pitman GH. Tumescent technique for local anesthesia improves safety in large-volume liposuction (Discussion). Plast Reconstr Surg 1993; 92:1099.
[53] Fodor PB. Wetting solutions in aspirate lipoplasty: A plea for safety in liposuction (Editorial). Aesth Plast Surg 1995; 19:379.
[54] Maxwell GP, Gingrass MK. Ultrasound-assisted lipoplasty: A clinical study of 250 consecutivepatients. Plast Reconstr Surg 1998; 101:189.
[55] Klein JA. Tumescent technique for regional anesthesia permits lidocaine doses of 35 mg/kg for liposuction. Dermatol Surg Oncol 1990; 16:248.

7

Gynoid Lipodystrophy Treatment and Other Advances on Laser-Assisted Liposuction

Alberto Goldman[1], Sufan Wu[2], Yi Sun[2],
Diego Schavelzon[3] and Guillermo Blugerman[3]
[1]*Clinica Goldman of Plastic Surgery, Porto Alegre, RS*
[2]*Department of Plastic and Reconstructive Surgery*
Zhejiang Provincial People's Hospital, Hangzhou, Zhejiang
[3]*Centro B&S de Excelencia en Cirugía Plástica, Buenos Aires*
[1]*Brazil*
[2]*China*
[3]*Argentina*

1. Introduction

Localized adiposis invariably disturbs the natural contours of the face and body, and can further cause the inferiority of the patients. Moreover, excessive obesity could be harmful for the health. Therefore, removal of the excess adipose tissue to keep the perfect shape and maintain a healthy physical state is now a common pursuit. Many methods have been used to treat the local adiposis and general obesity, including diet, medication, exercise and liposuction. For the purpose of improving the body contour, liposuction is the most widely used due to its long lasting result and positive effect. Over the past 30 years, liposuction has become an increasingly popular procedure and one of the most frequent aesthetic surgical operations.

At the earlier stage of the liposuction in the 1980s, the operation was usually performed as a hospital in-patient procedure, under general anesthesia and often required blood transfusion due to the blood lost during the operation. The procedure was usually related to a lot of potential complications. In 1988, Klein [1] published his important scientific contribution on the tumescent technique, administering large quantities of very dilute buffered lidocaine and epinephrine which could significantly reduce intra-operative bleeding and post-operative ecchymoses [2]. Although Klein's tumescent technique dramatically improved the safety and recovery of patients, it has some shortages and the complications after liposuction, including bleeding, pain, operative trauma, slow recovery with weeks down time to the patients, and hard work for the surgeons.

On the other hand, Liposuction can work well for treating large areas of adiposis with thicker layers and looser texture, but it is less effective for the compact adipose tissues found in some localized positions such as the neck, in secondary procedures or in cases of gynecomastia. The adiposis in these locations consists of firm fibrous connective tissue and compact adipose tissues, which makes conventional liposuction more difficult to perform. It is difficult to insert and move the suction cannula within the compact tissues, and the compact adipose tissues are not easily aspirated. If force is exerted repeatedly, it causes great damage to the tissues. For these reasons, surgeons are continuing to refine the procedures and seek more advanced procedures with less injury, shorter down time, and more effective, such as interventional ultrasound-assisted liposuction [3-5], external ultrasound-assisted lipoplasty [6] and power-assisted lipoplasty [7]. In the search for a better solution, laser lipolysis was used to treat localized adiposis instead of conventional liposuction.

Laser is an important innovation and has become a popular device in surgery, which is mainly used to treat hemangioma, tattoo, pigmentation, scars and so on. By its thermal effects on the tissue, laser was also studied on the liposlysis. From the 1990s, several papers have discussed the effects and results of different types of lasers on adipose tissues. Apfelberg [8-10] was beginning to study laser-assisted liposuction; this preliminary investigation utilized a YAG optical fiber contained within a liposuction cannula. The investigators concluded that no clear benefit was demonstrated with the laser. Since FDA did not approve the technique, the researchers did not pursue the study. In the late 1990s, Neira and colleagues began studying the effects of low-level laser on adipose tissue [11-14]. At the same time, Blugerman [15] /, Schavelzon [16] and Goldman [17-18] were studying 1064 nm neodymium:yttrium-aluminum-garnet (Nd:YAG) laser on the lipolysis. They found that the laser could cause adipocytes lysis effectively and had less side-effect. The characteristics of laser lipolysis are less intra-operative blood loss, less post-operative ecchymoses and improved skin tightening and skin re-draping during the recovery process [19, 20]. The procedures of lipolysis made small tunnels in the adipose tissue, resulted in small blood vessels coagulation and coagulation of reticular dermis [21-24].

The accumulated experience and scientific publications of the senior author and colleagues during the last 10 years enhance the knowledge about laser and tissue interactions, as well as the possibility of obtaining not only fat-cell disruption but also tissue tightening, supports the efficacy and safety of subdermal laser-assisted use in the body and facial treatments. Current laser-assisted liposuction is designed to provide more selective adipose damage, facilitate fat removal, enhance hemostasis, and increase tissue tightening. Recent advances demonstrating the use of the laser in direct contact with targets like the fat, sweat glands, vessels and dermis layers opened up new applications on different conditions. Although some negative or neutral views have been reported, most of the results have shown that laser lipolysis has the advantages of less bleeding, pain, and edema, a quicker recovery and better comfort. Most of the patients obtained satisfactory results, with significant reduction of their adiposes. The clinical results have proved that laser lipolysis is an effective therapy for these patients. In subsequent histologic studies, the findings showed that the adipose cells had been damaged and "melted." Their cell membranes had shrunk, curled, or ruptured, leading to loss of integrity and shape of the cells, with consequent loss of cellular content.

The purpose of the chapter is to demonstrate the evolution and new indications of laser lipolysis as well as new concepts and trends related to this technique. Treatment of localized fat, skin and tissue flaccidity, cellulite, lipomas, hyperhidrosis and osmidrosis, vascular alterations, treatment of complications related to permanent fillers, combine treatments with traditional surgeries and new indications will be described in the chapter.

2. Laser biology

A laser (light amplification by stimulated emission of radiation) is a device which generates a coherent beam of stimulated emission light resulted from a quantum mechanical effect. The first working laser was a ruby laser with a wavelength of 694nm, invented by Maiman in 1969, who later received the Albert Einstein Award. There are several properties of laser beams: 1) monochromatic: all of the waves of a laser having the same wavelength; 2) collimated: a laser generally emits photons in a narrow direction, and the waves parallel and have minimal variation in convergence or divergence; 3) coherent: describes the property of having waves that are in phase with on another in both space and time; 4) high brightness: a laser light can be highly intense, and to be focused to very high intensities and used for cutting, burning or even vaporizing materials.

The tissue interactions produced by lasers are 1) photothermal effect: converting light energy into heat energy, which then heat tissue up to be coagulated and even be vaporized; 2) photochemical effect: the light of laser making target cells to produce chemical reactions, such as photodynamic reactions; 3) photobiological effect, 4) electromechanical effect: dielectric breakdown in tissue caused by shock wave plasma expansion resulting in localized mechanical rupture. The processes of laser after arrival on the tissue are transmission, absorption, reflection, and scatter. There are several important parameters determining the action level of laser on the tissue: 1) wavelength: it is the primary parameter of the laser, which affects the absorption of laser by tissues; 2) power density: related to the power and spot size, and plays a critical role in determining tissue interaction; 3) exposure time: the more exposure time, the more energy acted on the tissue; 4) laser types: Q-switched, pulsed and continuous wave (CW), which was used for different purposes clinically. Laser is an important innovation and has become a popular device in surgery. Nd:YAG laser produces a beam in the near-infrared region, with a wavelength of 1064nm. Its main effect on the tissue is coagulation, which could be used to destroy tumors or to coagulate vascular vessels, for the treatment of hemangioma, tattoo, pigmentation, scars and so on. The Nd:YAG laser could be transmitted through flexible quartz fiber optics, making its use in endoscopy possible.

The Nd:YAG laser beam scatters in tissue to create the coagulation and can also produce retrograde scatter. The YAG lasers using in the lipolysis usually have high output power of 6 to 30 watts, which are highly dangerous of safety classes IV. Because of its danger, special eye protection is necessary. All personnel should wear glasses with side panels or goggles that are appropriated for the laser in use, since the eye is the most delicate organ commonly exposed to laser injury. Green filter glass is needed for the Nd: YAG laser. Moreover, during tissue vaporization, smoke is produced, which contains nonviable particles, and so should be avoided to be breathed in.

3. Histological study of laser lipolysis

Observed by the optical microscope and SEM, lipocytes were separated into fat lobules in normal adipose tissue (Fig. 1-3). They were spherical, surrounded by vessels and connective tissues. Small nucleus was located at the edges of cells. After irradiated by the laser, the adipose tissues became loose and messy, blank areas were observed that the closer to the blank areas the more serious destruction appeared. Fibers were broken. Some crater-like depressions were seen. Lipocytes shrunk, broke and melted, and a large number of lipid droplets leaked. Connective tissues melted, twisted and adhered.

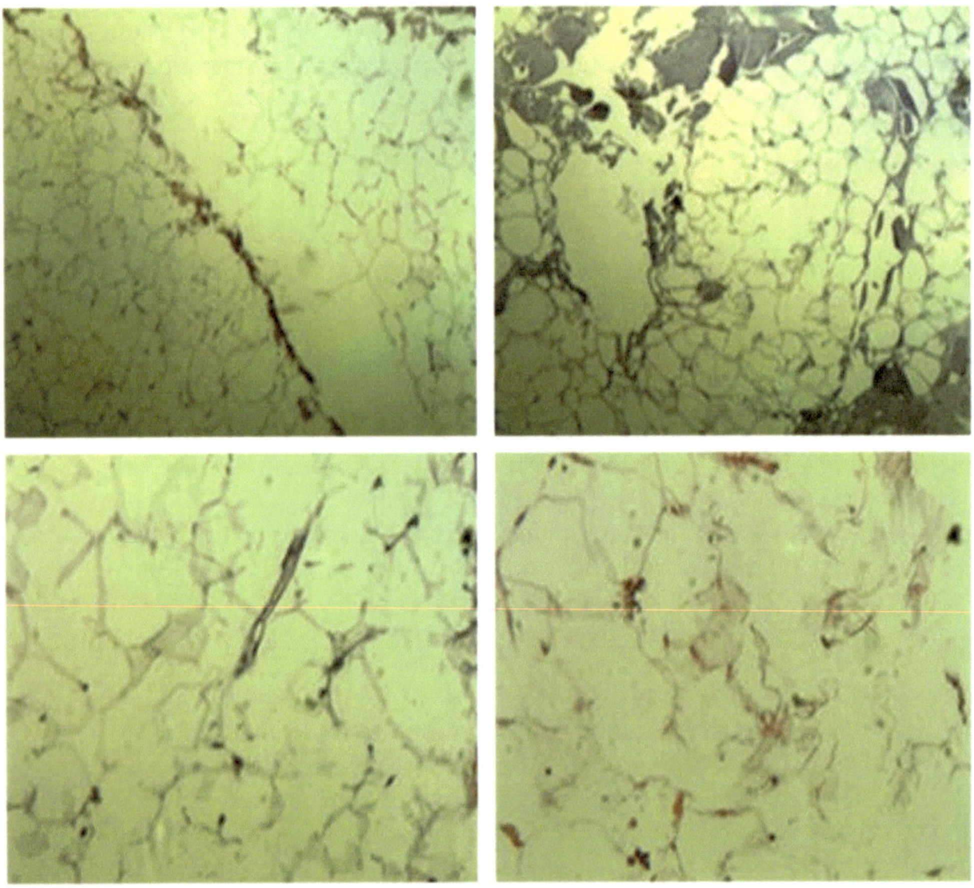

Fig. 1. Adipose tissues irradiated by the laser (optical microscope). The adipose tissues became loose and messy, blank areas were observed that the closer to the blank areas the more serious destruction appeared. Fibers were broken. Some crater-like depressions were seen. Lipocytes shrunk, broke and melted.

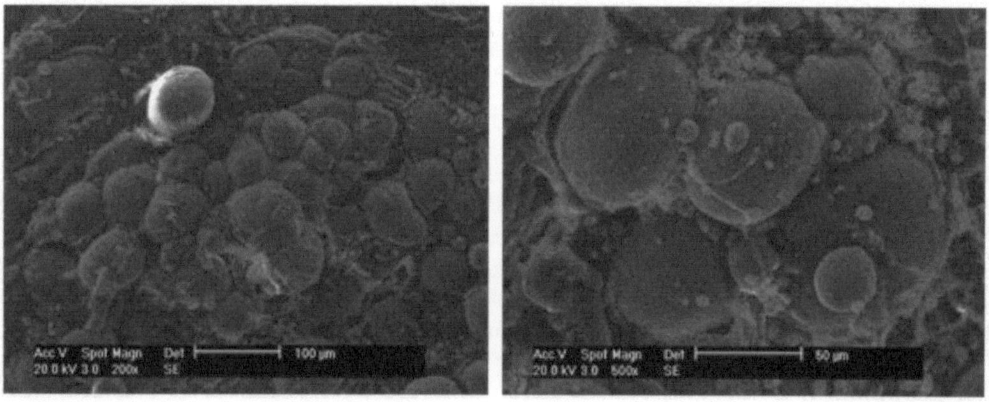

Fig. 2. Normal adipose tissues (SEM). Lipocytes were separated into fat lobules in normal adipose tissue. They were spherical, surrounded by vessels and connective tissues.

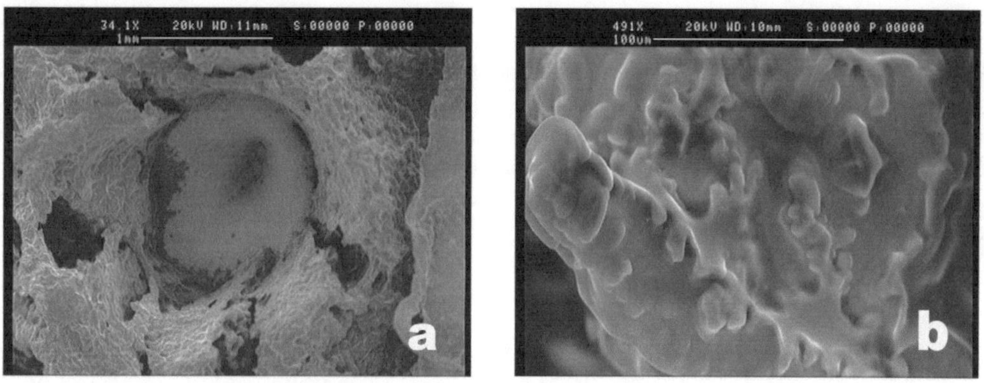

Fig. 3. a. The adipose tissue after laser treatment is examined by the scanning electron microscope. Adiposis is melted, and a channel is made. The arrow indicates that the diameter of the channel is approximately 1 mm (bar = 1 mm). b. Adipose cells are damaged and melted by the laser treatment, with the cell membrane shrunken, curled, and ruptured (asterisks). The shape of the cells is not intact (bar = 0.1 mm)

3. Fundaments of laser lipolysis

As the laser has the biothermal effect on tissues, it is expected can overcome the shortage of traditional surgical method, disrupt adipose tissues selectively, shorten surgery and recovery time, enhance hemostasis, promote tissue retraction, and reduce complications. From the 1990s, several papers have discussed the effects and results of different types of lasers on adipose tissues. The accumulated experience and scientific publications of the authors and colleagues enhance the knowledge about laser and tissue interactions, as well as the possibility of obtaining not only fat-cell disruption but also tissue tightening, supports the efficacy and safety of subdermal laser-assisted use in the body and facial treatments. Current laser-assisted liposuction is designed to provide more selective adipose damage, facilitate fat removal, enhance hemostasis, and increase tissue tightening. Recent advances demonstrating the use of the laser in direct contact with targets like the fat, sweat glands, vessels and dermis layers opened up new applications on different conditions.

Adipose tissue distribution is dependent on genetic and environmental factors. The total and regional masses of adipose tissue are dependent on the number of adipocytes as well as their degree of filling with depot fat. [25] The subcutaneous tissue consists of a superficial and deep adipose layer. The superficial adipose layer is contained within organized, compact fascial septa. The deep adipose layer demonstrates regional variations, but is contained within a relatively loose, less organized, and more widely spaced fascial septa. Energy substrate, storage of lipids and vitamins, protection of vital organs, physical support and insulation, maintenance of serum lipids, source of hormones and generation of heat are some of important functions related to the adipose tissue. The adipocyte represents one of the most important targets in laser lipolysis process. These adipose cells store lipids and are normal constituents of connective tissue. Adipose tissue is composed mostly of fat cells organized into lobules. Lobules of fat are separated and supported by loose connective tissue called septa.

Dermis represents another important target to be treated in the laser-assisted liposuction (laser lipolysis). The primary function of the dermis is to sustain and support the epidermis. Dermis is a complex structure and is composed of two layers, the more superficial papillary dermis and the deeper reticular dermis. The papillary dermis is thinner, consisting of loose connective tissue and some collagen. The reticular dermis consists of a thicker layer of dense connective tissue containing larger blood vessels, closely interlaced elastic fibers, fibroblasts and coarse bundles of collagen fibers arranged in layers parallel to the surface. Other targets related to this surgical procedure are represented by small blood vessels, eccrine and apocrine glands, fibrous tissue presented in cellulite and body regions previously submitted to surgical procedures like liposuction.The mechanism of action on a cellular level is due to a specific laser-tissue interaction that is defined by the process of selective photothermolysis [26]; some features of this interaction are wavelength-dependent and some are independent of wavelength used.

The progresses of laser lipolysis are: 1. melting adipose tissue into liquid state by heating adipocytes; 2. heating adipocytes to disrupt their membrane and allow extracellular drainage and facilitated suctioning; 3. heating collagenous fibrous septae and reticular dermis for enhanced tissue tightening; 4. coagulating microvasculature to improve hemostasis and to reduce postoperative bleeding. 5. minimal intervention of the procedure improving rapid recovery.

4. Instruments of laser lipolysis

The instrument of laser lipolysis consists of 3 main parts: laser machine, transfer system, and control system.

4.1 Laser machine

The effects of laser-assisted lipolysis are caused by photothermal energy as well as photomechanic effect. The various wavelengths for laser-assisted liposuction have been selected based on the theory of selective photothermolysis. There are several wavelengths (1032nm, 1064nm) that have recently been studied, in which the Nd:YAG laser is the main option. The laser machine is usually a pulsed (40-80 Hz) Nd:YAG laser, with a wavelength of 1064nm and an output power ranging from 6 to 18 watts.

4.2 Transfer system

The transfer system basically includes optical fiber, handpiece, and cannula. The laser is conducted via an optical fiber, covered by a 1 mm introducer cannula, which could inserted into the body and directly treat the adipose tissue. The fiber extends beyond the end of the cannula by 2-3 mm (Fig. 4). This 2-3 mm extension enables the direct reaction of laser energy within the adipose tissue. The laser is conducted through a very fine (small diameter around 300um) optical fiber. Lipolysis and tissue coagulation occur during the laser irradiation. The transillumination of the 3mW diode laser beam associated with the system allows for precise localization of the fiber tip so that the surgeon is constantly aware of the location of laser activity.

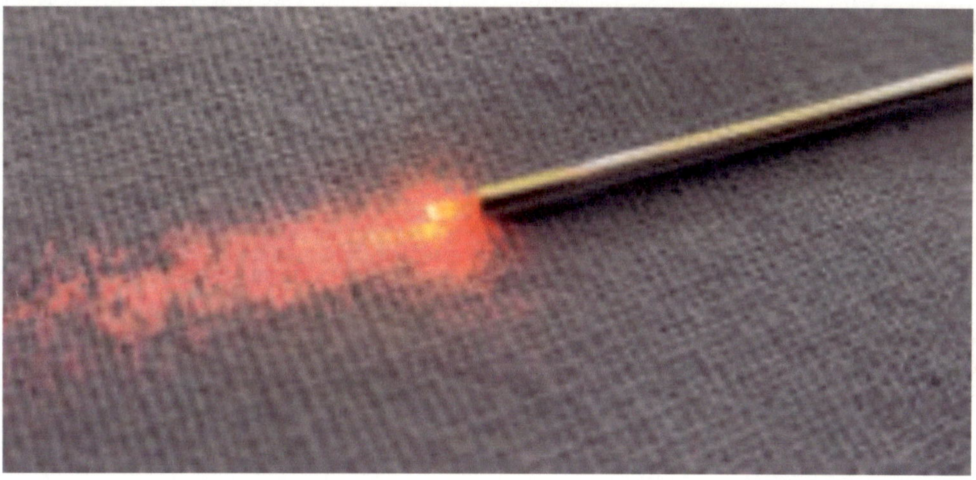

Fig. 4. One-millimeter cannula containing fiber optic extended approximately 2mm from the distal end and emitting laser energy.

4.3 Control system

The total energy of laser acted on the tissue depends on power and time. The lipolyses laser machine can display and record total irradiation energy automatically (accumulated energy). The moving speed of handpiece is also important for the clinical effect: too high speed will decrease the photothermal effect on the tissue, whereas to lower speed will damage the tissue due to the thermal effect remained in small part. The authors experience of the speed is about 3-5 cm/second [31]. The laser emission is usually controlled by a foot switch. During the laser irradiation, the handpiece should be kept moving within the tissues, otherwise the tissue will be injured by the laser heating. In some modified system, the laser emission could be shut off automatically once the handpiece stopped.

5. Techniques of operation

5.1 Pre-operative preparation

Medical and psychosocial evaluation plays a fundamental role in safe and successful laser-assisted liposuction treatment. Physical evaluation includes assessment of the general medical health of the patient. A well documented medical history, physical examination, and appropriate laboratory analysis based upon the patient's general health and age must be performed on all candidates. Special attention must be paid to the skin quality, laxity and texture, presence and distribution of fat, and previous scars and treatments. Considering that body sculpturing is primarily an aesthetic procedure, patients should be of good general health. Laser-assisted liposuction is contraindicated in patients who are pregnant or lactating; patients with severe cardiovascular disease or with coagulation disorders including thrombophilia. The medical history must be evaluated in any history of bleeding disorders, emboli, thrombophlebitis, infectious diseases, previous surgical procedures and complications, poor wound healing and metabolic diseases. Psychosocial evaluation and patient's expectations are also important factors to consider. Laboratory studies must be performed (blood count with quantitative platelet assessment, prothrombin time, partial thromboplastin time and chemistry profile including liver function tests and hepatitis screen) prior to any elective surgery. Clinical examination should include planning and evaluation of all regions being treated, including the presence of hernias, scars, asymmetries, cellulite, sweat gland disease and stretch marks. The quality and texture of the skin and, particularly, its elasticity or the presence of flaccidity must also be carefully evaluated. Finally, digital photographic documentation is required for all patients.

5.2 Operative procedures

Laser-assisted liposuction may be performed under local anesthesia alone, or supplemented with intravenous sedation, epidural block or general anesthesia. The patient is marked in the standing position. The sites of laser lipolysis are marked by contour lines in ring form, and the central point of the localized adiposis is emphasized. If treatment is for cellulite, it is helpful to use various markers of different colors in order to mark areas of elevation and depression [27]. The patients were placed in appropriate positions according to the lipolysis sites. External pneumatic compression devices are placed on the legs and the patient is sedated if desired. The operation areas are cleaned and draped in the usual fashion. Subcutaneous infiltration of warmed Klein's tumescent solution, or some similar solution combining buffered lidocaine and epinephrine, precedes laser application to the areas of unwanted fat. The total volume of subcutaneous infiltration depends upon the surgeon preference and the overall size of the treatment area. The solution is warmed to minimize any discomfort associated with a temperature difference between the tissue and the fluid. Warming also helps to maintain core body temperature. The solution is injected into the subcutaneous adipose layer, and should be well distributed until the target areas are turgid. The procedure is initiated following a 10 to 20 minute delay to allow for appropriate diffusion of the fluid and adequate vasoconstriction. According to the location of the adiposis, appropriate entry points are chosen for insertion of the cannula, such as the corner of the mouth, the preauricular, or nasolabial fold for face access, or beneath the chin for neck access. More incisions are made if the treatment area is large. Direct laser application into the adipose tissue occurs via an optical fiber. This fiber (200 - 600 μm in diameter) is conducted within a stainless steel microcannula of 1-1.5 mm external diameter using a pulsed 1064nm Nd-YAG laser (Smartlipo, Deka, Italy). Lasers have biologic effects on living tissues in the form of thermal, mechanical, electromagnetic, and photochemical reactions. Laser lipolysis melts and liquefies the adipose cells mostly by its thermal effect. The wavelength of the Nd:YAG laser is 1,064 nm, which has great penetration in soft tissue of about 8 mm and can be transmitted through an optic fiber. It frequently is used in tissue vaporization, vessel coagulation, and dissection, which enable it to be used effectively for melting adipose tissues.

Based on the photothermal effect of the laser, the localized adiposis is melted and liquefied, resulting in multiple fan-shaped channels in the adipose tissue. Various insertion routes are used, allowing the fan-shaped delivery of laser heat (irradiation) to overlap, resulting in a three-dimensional lipolysis. The movement of the cannula in the adipose tissue should be gentle and slow to avoid penetrating the skin and breaking the optic fiber. When encountering compact adipose tissues, the movement of the cannula should be slowed down until the compact fat has been broken up. It is important to keep the coordination between the moving of the handle and the control of the footswitch. The laser fiber optic should be kept moving as long as the laser emission is switched on to prevent energy accumulation at any one spot that might burn the skin. The duration of laser activity in the tissues is highly variable and depends upon the overall size of the treatment area, the thickness and volume of fat being removed, the degree of skin laxity and the presence of previous internal scarring. The surgeon senses a diminishing resistance to cannula movement as the procedure progresses. This indicates lipolysis and the presence of more liquefied fat (lysate) and less normal, untreated fat. The "pinch test" is another important method in determining the clinical endpoint of treatment.

The laser energy was related to the treatment region. The larger the region was, the greater the laser energy was needed. In different parts of the body, parts with more fibrous tissues required more laser energy. When the local adipose thickness is reduced to the expected grade, the laser irradiation is stopped. The resultant product of laser-assisted lipolysis is an oily lysate which contains ruptured adipocytes and cellular debris mixed with tumescent solution. Aspiration of this lysate is the surgeon's choice. If the surgeon chooses to remove the mixture, it is removed by gentle aspiration using a 2 mm or 3 mm external diameter cannula and a negative pressure of 0.3 to 0.5 atm (<50 kPa or 350 mm Hg). It is the authors' experience that very small areas of treatment with low volumes of lysate do well without aspiration. In larger areas such as the upper arms or abdomen, a vacuum liposuction machine could be used to remove the liquid adipose mixture. This may be the case, for example, in the treatment of the anterior cervical area or in the improvement of prominent malar fat pad. In situations when minimal lipolysis is desired, and the laser is being used mainly for the photostimulatory effect of collagen contraction, here, too, it may not be necessary to aspirate. This latter example often applies to the treatment of cellulite.

5.3 Post-operative care

Following surgery, tight garments are usually helpful in reducing edema and improving skin re-draping. During the first week following the procedure, the patient may be started on a post-operative physiotherapeutic routine to hasten the resolution of edema. Antibiotics should be used for 1 week.

6. Indications of laser lipolysis

Based on the senior authors' experience using the subdermal laser treatment with a 1064nm Nd-YAG laser, the most frequent conditions could be treated with this technique are:

6.1 Local fat deposits

Localized fat deposits in the body and face is the most frequent condition treated with this technique. The procedure is usually performed under local tumescent anesthesia. Combining laser-assisted liposuction with traditional techniques can improve the result and decrease the surgical trauma and complications. The technique is not indicated for treatment in obese subjects and severe skin flaccidity. Mild to moderate cases of skin and tissue laxity can be adequately treated and attenuated with the use of the subdermal laser-assisted application. The laser can be used even in cases without localized fat, with the intention of inducing neo-collagenesis production and a consequent tightening effect.

Cellulite, also known as gynoid lipodystrophy and edematous fibrosclerotic panniculopathy, is an alteration in the surface contour of the skin in which areas of lumpy bumpiness seem to alternate with areas of skin dimpling. This uneven skin texture is most prevalent in the abdomen, hips, thighs, and buttocks. It is estimated that 85% of postpubertal women have some degree of cellulite. The anatomic basis of cellulite has been determined through histology and, more recently, by magnetic resonance imaging studies that further revealed the ultrastructure of the subcutaneous tissue in women and men. In men, the septa are arranged in a criss-cross pattern, dividing the fat cell chambers into small, polygonal units. In women, fat cell chambers, or papillae adiposae, are sequestered by septa of connective tissue, positioned in a radial or diagonal manner, anchoring the dermis to the muscle fascia via the subcutaneous fat. The papillae adiposae of the subcutis bulge up into the dermis (sometimes close to the dermoepidermal junction), changing the gross appearance of the skin surface [31]. This condition (cellulite) can also be treated with laser lipolysis. In this latter indication, the use of the laser with other techniques such as physiotherapy, external ultrasound and autologous fat injections can lead to a greater improvement.

6.2 Laser-assisted lipoabdominoplasty

The lipoabdominoplasty is a relatively new surgical procedure based on the selective undermining of the abdominal flap in the superior medium line, preserving the perforating and lymph vessels almost completely, reducing the complications. The use of the internal laser represents another useful tool in this technique. The laser builds tunnels in the tissue facilitating the flap mobilization; disrupts the fat cells, and induces new collagen production with a consequent tissue retraction.

6.3 Lipomas and flaps

Large and giant lipomas can be effectively treated with the laser. Two effects are especially improved in these cases: cellular lysis and skin tightening. This is an alternative and less invasive option for the treatment of lipomas. Non-esthetic use of the internal Nd-YAG laser includes the treatment of fat flaps (it refines and contours flaps according to specific anatomical characteristics). This indication can be applied to breast reconstruction using the rectus abdominal technique or in the improvement of tumoral and traumatic lesions previously reconstructed with cutaneous and adipose flaps to thin or to contour these flaps.

6.4 Sweat gland diseases

The subdermal approach for axillary hyperhidrosis, osmidrosis and bromidrosis treatment using a 1064 nm Nd-YAG laser results in significant clinical improvement. It is an alternative treatment option for these sweat gland disorders. Patients suffering from this condition indicate that their sweating is difficult to tolerate and frequently interferes in their daily activities or is intolerable and always interferes in their daily activities. Axillary hyperhidrosis, osmidrosis and bromidrosis has a strong negative impact on different domains of quality of life. It often interferes with patient's daily activities with occupational, emotional, social, and physical implications. Numerous treatments have been described to improve this condition. Topical antiperspirants such as acids, aldehydes, and metal salts; iontophoresis; botulinum toxin injections; anticholinergic and other drugs; surgeries; curettage; liposuction; and open or endoscopic sympathectomy represent some of the main treatment options. Each treatment presents advantages and limitations and, so far, there is no ideal option. Among the surgical methods, minimal skin excision combined with subcutaneous curettage is the gold standard in many countries, yet a major disadvantage of this method is the formation of operative scar and hematoma. Suction curettage in tumescent anesthesia is a less invasive method although the number of recurrences is higher. Sympathectomy has been reported to cause compensatory hyperhidrosis in up to 90% of patients. This highlights the need for further improvement of surgical treatments for the more severe cases. The laser energy acts directly on the anatomical location of the sweat glands. Subdermal action of laser is better than transcutaneous action, since the laser could reach its target directly and by only one small hole on the skin.

6.5 Gynecomastia

This is another interesting indication for the use of the subdermal Nd-YAG laser. The laser facilitates cannula penetration (very important mainly in glandular and fibrous tissue treatment). There is effective cellular disruption (lipolysis), and the small tunnels in the male breast tissue as well as the new collagen stimulation, help tissue retraction and attenuation of small breast ptosis or skin laxity. Also, in the case of glandular tissue (mixed gynecomastia), the laser can be applied with traditional glandular excision with limited scarring.

6.6 Wrinkles

The same principle - new collagen stimulation - can be applied to the improvement of wrinkles (subdermal application).

6.7 Treatment of permanent filler injections

Polymethylmethacrylate and other products have been used as synthetic permanent fillers for soft-tissue augmentation in the face and body. Complications related to these injections include tissue necrosis, local infections, granulomas, chronic inflammatory reactions, etc. Preliminary studies have shown excellent results using the intralesional application of the 1064 nm Nd-YAG laser in the treatment of these granulomas related to permanent fillers.

7. Typical cases of laser lipolysis

Case 1. Congenital localized adiposis.

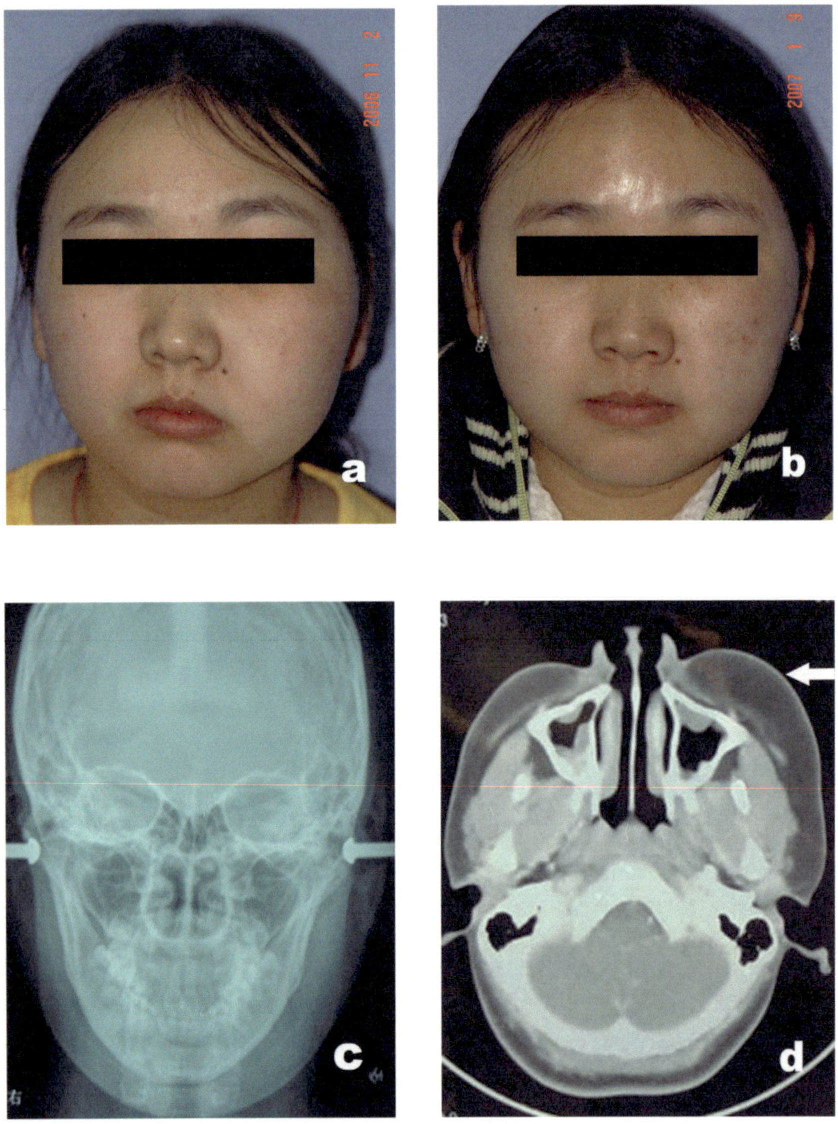

Fig. 5. a. The facial contour is asymmetric due to the congenital localized adiposis in the left face. Note that the left corner of the mouth is moved down. b. At 2 months after laser lipolysis, the enlarged adipose tissue has been removed; the asymmetry is significantly improved; and the corners of the mouth are symmetric. c. Anteroposterior x-ray of the skull before the operation. The bilateral maxilla and mandible are symmetric (arrows), whereas the soft tissues of the left face (asterisk) are obviously thicker than those of the right side. d. Magnetic resonance imaging (MRI) indicates the enlarged soft tissue on the left side of the face (asterisk), which basically consists of adipose tissue

Case 2. Congenital subcutaneous fat pad in the neck.

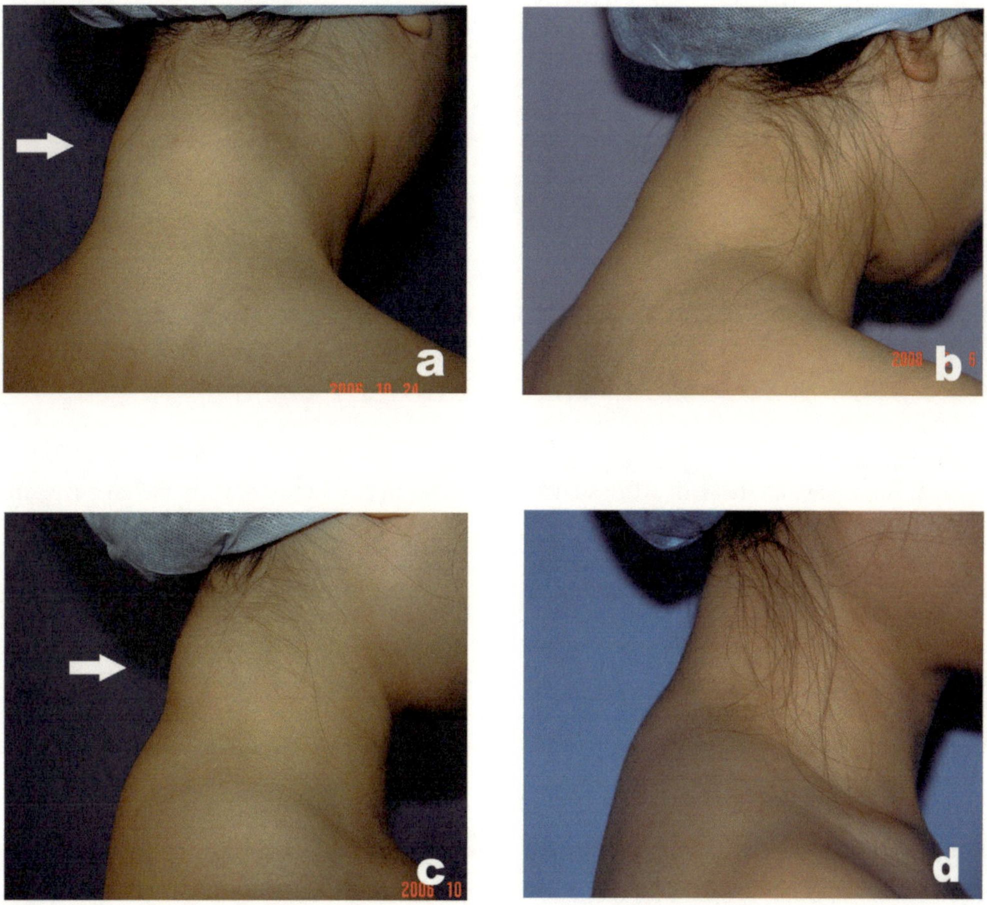

Fig. 6. a Oblique view of the congenital subcutaneous fat pad in the neck (arrow). There is a prominent swelling in the middle part of the neck from the inferior border of the hairline to the superior border of the seventh cervical vertebrae. The swelling is hemispheric in shape. b Oblique view 20 months after laser lipolysis showing that the prominence of the fat pad is eliminated and that the overall contour is normal. c Lateral view of the congenital subcutaneous fat pad in the neck (arrow). d Lateral view of the patient 20 months after laser lipolysis

Case 3. Submental adipose deposit.

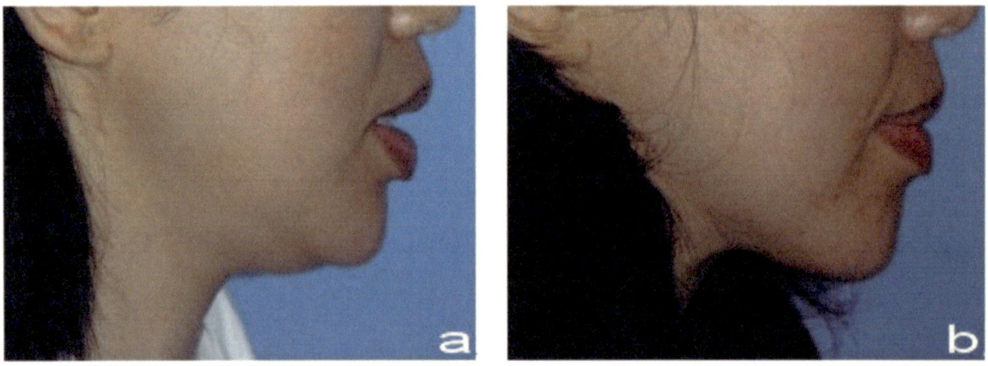

Fig. 7. a. A female patient with adipose tissues deposit in her submental. b. Seven days after laser lipolysis shows great appearance.

Case 4. Facial adipose deposit

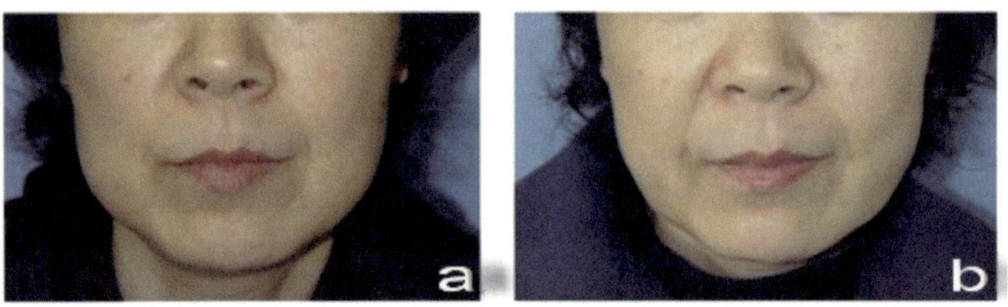

Fig. 8. a. A female patient with adipose tissues deposit in her cheeks. b. The face contour of hers is tighten up after laser lipolysis.

Case 5. Adipose deposit in neck

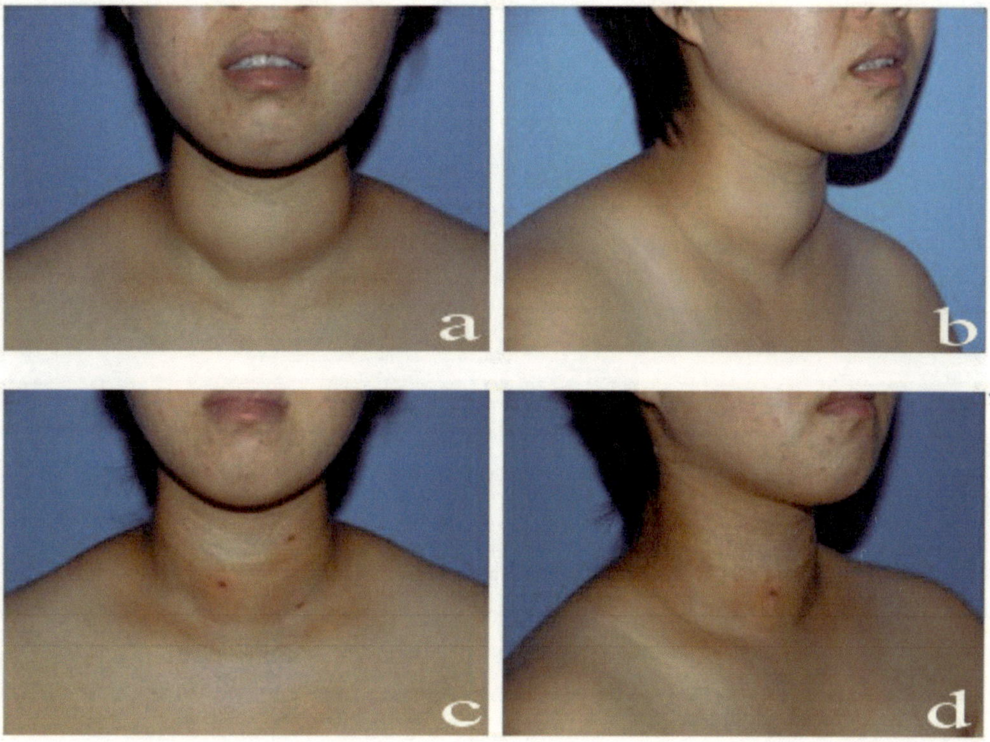

Fig. 9. a.b. A female patient with adipose tissues deposit in her front neck. c.d. One day after laser lipolysis.

Case 6. Adipose deposit in the arms

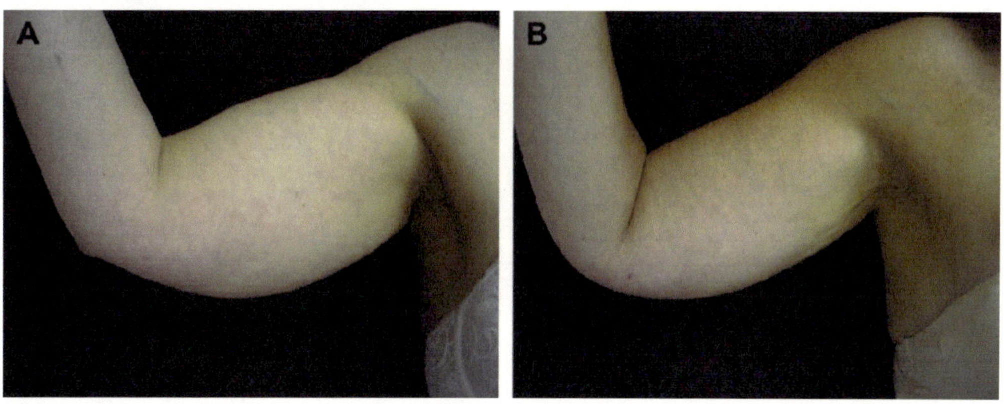

Fig. 10. 54-year-old woman is shown before (A) and 8 months after (B) laser-assisted liposuction of the arms.

Case 7. Adipose deposit in the abdomen and flanks.

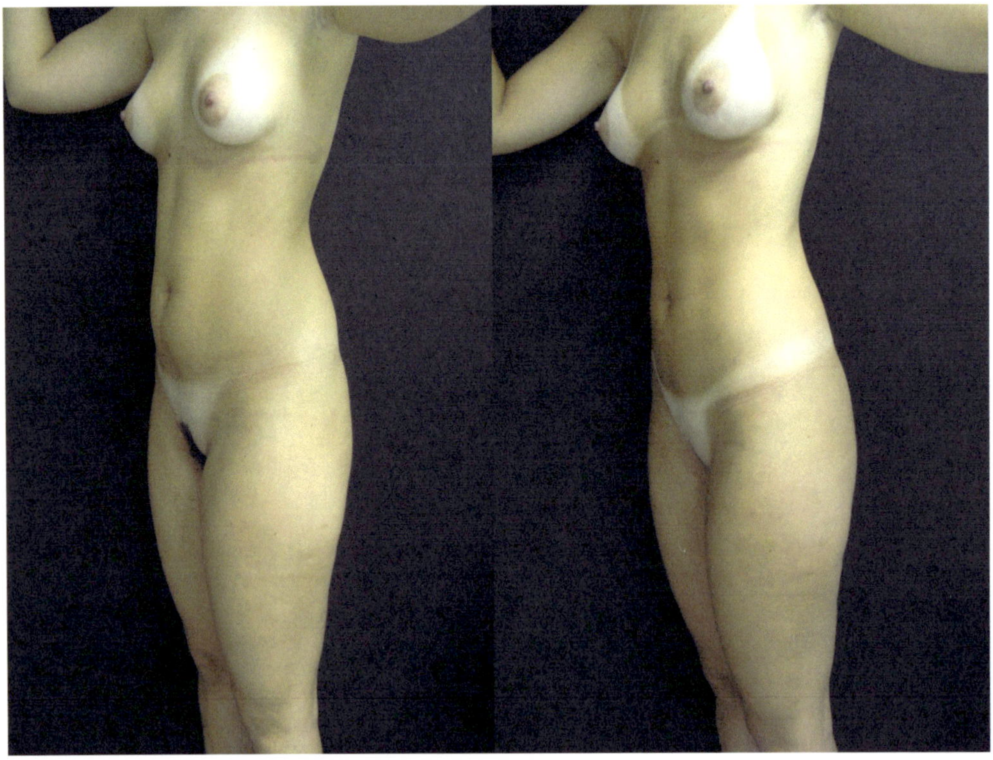

Fig. 11. 29-year-old woman is shown before (A, C) and 6 months after (B, D) laser-assisted liposuction of the abdomen and flanks.

Case 8. Adipose deposit in the abdomen, hips, and flanks.

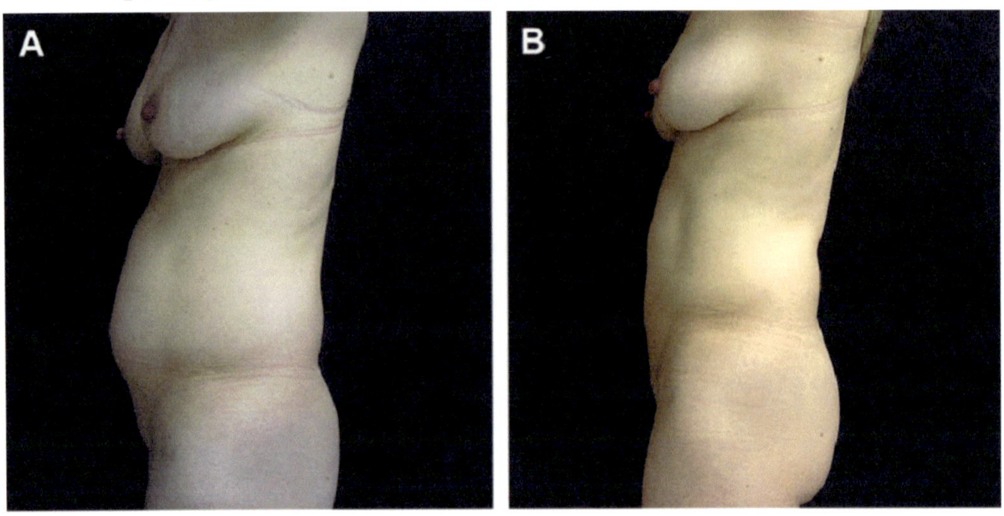

Fig. 12. 38-year-old woman is shown before (A, C) and 6 months after (B, D) laser-assisted liposuction of the abdomen, hips, and flanks.

Case 9. Adipose deposit in the hips.

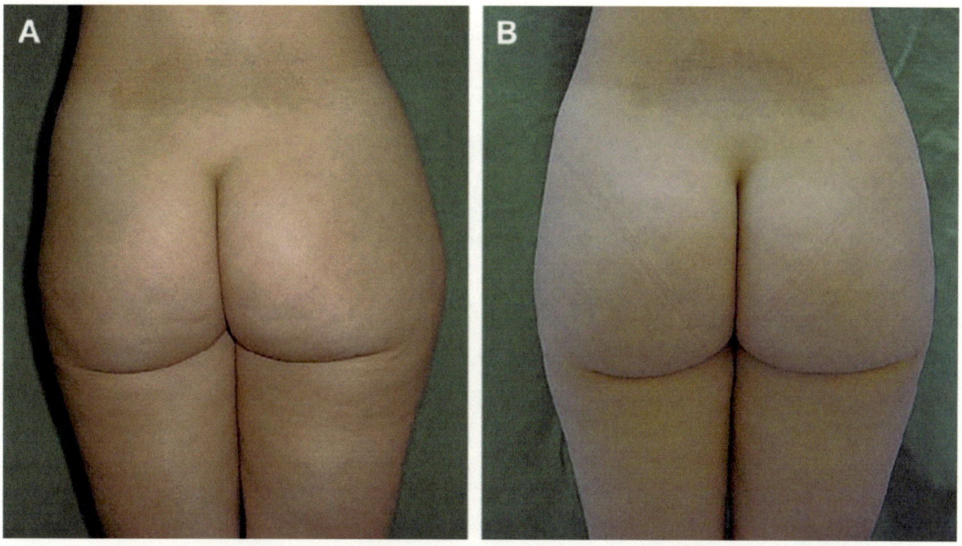

Fig. 13. 32-year-old woman is shown before (A) and 6 months after (B) laser-assisted liposuction of hips and thighs.

Case 10. Lipoma on the back.

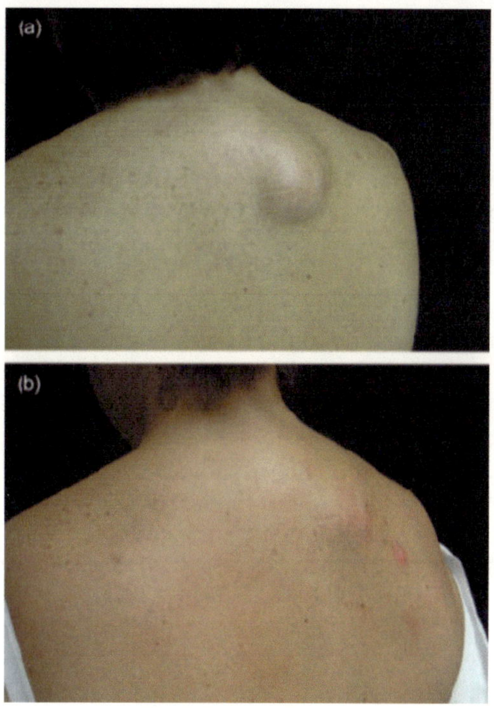

Fig. 14. (a) Lipoma on the back. Observe the scar produced by a previous surgical excision. (b) Five days after subdermal treatment with an Nd:YAGlaser. Edema and small scar.

Case 11. Axillary Hyperhidrosis.

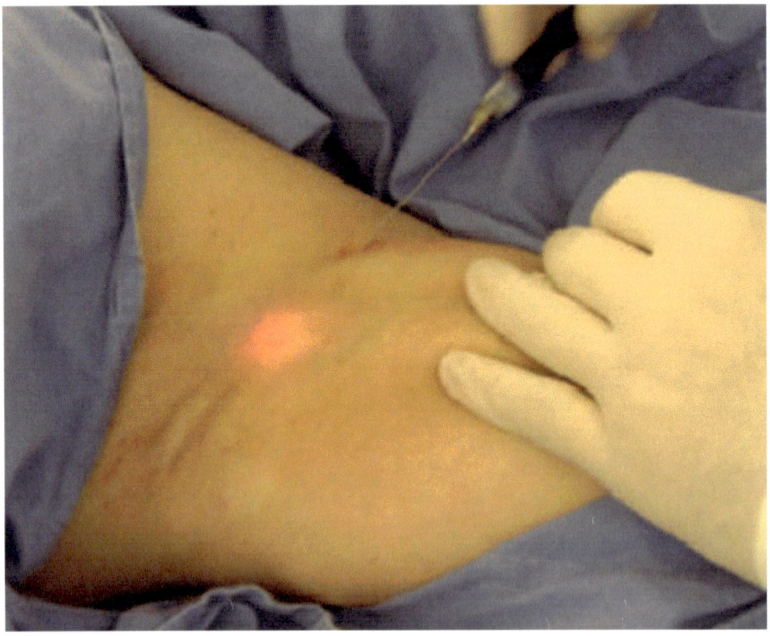

Fig. 15. Subdermal laser acting on the axillary region and the transillumination effect due to the red helium-neon laser. The incision was placed in a natural axillary fold.

8. Discussion

Lipolysis depends on the thermal effect of the laser. The laser can vaporize and melt tissues that it irradiates. Adipose tissues are located under the skin and above the deeper tissues, which include nerves and large vessels. It is very important to avoid excess tissue injury except for the target adipose tissue, especially in facial lipolysis. To achieve satisfactory therapeutic effects, the optimal energy of the laser should be set according to the regions of the treatment. The more fibrous and compact the tissues contained in the adiposis, the higher the laser energy density was needed. However, it was found that a long operation time was needed when laser lipolysis was applied in larger regions such as the abdominal wall. Therefore, laser lipolysis is more suitable for treating small regions and compact locations such as the face and cheeks, the mental region, the nuchal region, the upper arm, and the legs. Furthermore, it can also be used to improve local unevenness after conventional liposuction. Compared with the conventional liposuction technique, laser lipolysis has the following characteristics. The laser coagulates the small vessels and reduces the bleeding during the operation. Laser lipolysis has a well-distributed effect, and the skin surface is less uneven after the operation. Laser stimulates the formation of collagen in the region, which enhances the elasticity of the skin and facilitates the skin contraction in the operative regions. The laser breaks down the compact fibrous tissues of the localized adiposis, reduces the resistance of the suction cannula, and makes the operation easier. Finally, the trauma is mild, which brings a rapid recovery with fewer complications of edema, neural damage, and adipose embolism.

Laser lipolysis makes adipocytes rupture and shrink, with necrosis and carbonization. Reduction of the number of adipocytes improves the local shape, but the photothermal effect should also be controlled in a certain range. A variety of coagulation and other serious damage on lipocytes and collagen fibers must be taken into account. This method is suitable for small-scale, high-density area, and also unsatisfied areas after liposuction.
Although some negative or neutral views have been reported, most of the results have shown that laser lipolysis has the characteristics of less bleeding, pain, and edema; a quicker recovery; and better comfort. Most of the patients obtained satisfactory results, with significant reduction of localized fat. The clinical results have proved that laser lipolysis is an effective therapy for these patients. In subsequent histologic studies, the findings showed that the adipose cells had been damaged and "melted." Their cell membranes had shrunk, curled, or ruptured, leading to loss of integrity and shape of the cells, with consequent loss of cellular content.

9. Conclusion

Laser lipolysis is a new approach in the treatment of localized adiposis, which has satisfactory effects and potential clinical applications of other diseases. The approach is still in its initial stage, and the operation indications and criteria are not complete. Further studies and researches are needed to optimize the operation routes and methods.

10. References

[1] Klein JA. Anesthesia for liposuction in dermatologic surgery. J Dermatol Surg Oncol. 1988 Oct; 14(10):1124-1132.
[2] Klein JA. Tumescent technique for local anesthesia improves safety in large volume liposuction. Plast Reconstr Surg. 1993 Nov; 92(6):1085-1098.
[3] Zocchi ML. Ultrasonic liposculpturing. Aesthetic Plast Surg. 1992; 16:287-298.
[4] Maxwell GP, Gingrass MK. Ultrasound-assisted lipoplasty: A clinical study of 250 consecutive patients. Plast Reconstr Surg. 1998 Jan; 101(1):189-202.
[5] Zocchi ML. Ultrasonic-assisted lipectomy. Adv Plast Reconstr Surg. 1995; 11:197.
[6] Silberg BN. The technique of external ultrasound-assisted lipoplasty. Plast Reconstr Surg. 1998 Feb; 101(2):552.
[7] Fodor PB, Vogt PA. Power-assisted lipoplasty (PAL): A clinical pilot study comparing PAL to traditional lipoplasty (TL). Aesthetic Plast Surg. 1999 Nov-Dec; 23(6):379-385.
[8] Apfelberg DB. Laser-assisted liposuction may benefit surgeons, patients. Clin Laser Mon. 1992 Dec; 10(12):193-194.
[9] Apfelberg DB, Rosenthal S, Hunsted JP, et al. Progress report on multicenter study of laser-assisted liposuction. Aesthetic Plast Surg. 1994 Summer; 18(3):259-264.
[10] Apfelberg DB. Results of multicenter study of laser-assisted liposuction. Clin Plast Surg. 1996 Oct; 23(4):713-719.
[11] Neira R, Solarte E, Reyes MA, et al. Low-level laser-assisted lipoplasty: A new technique. In: Proceedings of the World Congress on Liposuction. Dearborn, MI: 2000.
[12] Neira R, Arroyave J, Ramirez H, et al. Fat Liquefaction: effect of low-level laser energy on adipose tissue. Plast Reconstr Surg. 2002 Sept; 110(3):912-922.

[13] Neira R, Ortiz-Neira C. Low-level laser-assisted liposculpture: Clinical report of 700 cases. Aesthetic Plast Surg. 2002 Sept-Oct; 22(5):451-455.
[14] Neira R, Toledo L, Arroyave J, et al. Low-level laser-assisted liposuction: the Neira 4L technique. Clin Plast Surg. 2006 Jan; 33(1):117-127.
[15] Blugerman, G. Laser lipolysis for the treatment of localized adiposity and "cellulite." In: Abstracts of the World Congress on Liposuction. Dearborn, MI: 2000.
[16] Schavelzon D, Blugerman G, Goldman A, et al. Laser lipolysis. In: Abstracts of the 10th International Symposium of Cosmetic Laser Surgery. Las Vegas, NV: 2001.
[17] Goldman A, Schavelzon DE, Blugerman GS. Laser lipolysis: liposuction using Nd:YAG laser. Rev Soc Bras Cir Plast. 2002 Jan-Apr; 17(1):17-21.
[18] Goldman, A. Lipoaspiração a laser - laserlipólise no contorno corporal. Revista Brasileira de Cirurgia. 92, 2002.
[19] Goldman, A., Schavelzon, D., Blugerman, G. Laserlipólise - lipoaspiração com Nd:YAG laser. Revista da Sociedade Brasileira de Laser em Medicina e Cirurgia. 2(5), 2002.
[20] Goldman A, Schavelzon D, Blugerman G. Liposuction using neodymium:yttrium-aluminum-garnet laser. International Abs. Plast Reconstr Surg. 2003 June; 111(7):2497.
[21] Badin AZD, Moraes LM, Gondek LB, et al. Laser lipolysis: Flaccidity under control. Aesthetic Plast Surg. 2002 Sept-Oct; 26(5):335-339.
[22] Goldman, A., Submentale Laserassistierte Liposuktion: Klinishe Erfahrungen und Histologische Ergebnisse, Kosmetische Medizin 3:5 4-11, 2005
[23] Badin AZD, Gondek LB, Garcia MJ, et al. Analysis of laser lipolysis effects on human tissue samples obtained from liposuction. Aesthetic Plast Surg. 2005 Jul-Aug; 29(4):281-286.
[24] Goldman A. Submental Nd:YAG laser-assisted liposuction. Lasers Surg Med. 2006 Mar; 38(3):181-184.
[25] Wollina U, Goldman A, Berger U, et al. Esthetic and cosmetic dermatology. Dermatol Ther. 2008; 21:118-130.
[26] Goldman A, Wollina U. Subdermal Nd-YAG laser for axillary hyperhidrosis. Dermatol Surg 2008; 34:756-762.
[27] Goldman A, Gotkin RH, Sarnoff DS, et al. Cellulite: A new treatment approach combining sub-dermal Nd:YAG laser lipolysis and autologous fat transplantation. Aesthetic Surg J. 2008 (in press).
[28] Björntorp P. Adipose tissue distribution and function. Int J Obes. 1991 Sep;15 Suppl 2:67-81.
[29] Anderson RR, Parrish JA. Selective photothermolysis: precise microsurgery by selective absorption of pulsed radiation. Science. 1983 April 29; 220:524-527.
[30] Goldman A, Gotkin RH, Sarnoff DS, et al. Cellulite: A new treatment approach combining sub-dermal Nd:YAG laser lipolysis and autologous fat transplantation. Aesthetic Surg J. J 2008;28:656–662.
[31] Sun Y, Wu SF, Yan S, et al. Laser lipolysis used to treat localized adiposis: a preliminary report on experience with Asian patients. Aesthetic Plast Surg. 2009;33:701-705.

8

Radio-Frequency Assisted Liposuction (RFAL)

Guillermo Blugerman et al.*,
[1,3]*Argentina*

1. Introduction

The increased prevalence of obesity worldwide has grown the body contouring market, as patients demand more solutions. One of the most popular body contouring methods is liposuction. Pioneered in Europe in the early 1980's as a simple fat aspirating technique, liposuction has quickly expanded its breadth to incorporate a variety of energy sources and modus operandi.

Many types of energies have been combined with standard liposuction techniques in an attempt to improve and optimize treatment outcomes. The current chapter is dedicated to the authors' experience with the most recent addition to the liposuction family, Radio-Frequency Assisted Liposuction (RFAL). RFAL delivers RF energy for a thermal effect to the adipose tissue, skin and sub-dermal matrix in a minimally invasive manner.

Enhancing the standard lipoplasty experience with a safe and consistent thermal influence provides the following key benefits:

- Blood vessel coagulation to reduce patient downtime through less bleeding and bruising.
- Tissue tightening to expand the range of patients to now include individuals who are obese and/or have compromised skin conditions (lax skin).
- Increased patient comfort and safety will increase consumer acceptance.
- Reduced procedure time and ease of treatment will increase physician acceptance.

1.1 Earlier techniques

In previous years the liposuction procedure has stimulated the development of energy assisted lipoplasty methods, such as power-assisted lipoplasty (PAL), ultrasound-assisted lipoplasty (UAL), and laser-assisted lipoplasty (LAL).

PAL uses a reciprocating cannula that mechanically destroys the subcutaneous tissue through small rapid vibrations. This innovation was developed to accelerate the liposuction

---

*Malcolm D. Paul[2], Diego Schavelzon[3] , R. Stephen Mulholland[4], Matthias Sandhoffer[5], Peter Lisborg[6], Antonio Rusciani[7], Mark Divaris[8], Michael Kreindel[9],
[1,3]*Centros B&S de Excelencia en Cirugía Plastica, Buenos Aires, Argentina*
[2]*Aesthetic and Plastic Surgery Institute, University of California, Irvine, CA, USA*
[4]*SpaMedica Clinics, Toronto, Canada*
[5]*Astetische Dermatologie Dr. Sanhofer, Linz, Austria*
[6]*PrivatKlinik Lisborg & Parner, Klagenfurt, Austria*
[7] *Skinlaser, Roma,Italy*
[8]*Institut de Stomatologie, Chirurgie Plastique et Chirurgie Maxillo-Faciale (Université Paris VI) France*
[9]*Invasix Inc. Toronto, Canada*

process, minimize the surgeon's physical exertion and reduce patient downtime post surgery. A 15 patient study comparing PAL to standard liposuction demonstrated that PAL allowed for a faster suction removal without compromising aesthetic contour [1].
UAL has gained popularity over the past two decades especially in the niche market of male patients and as a secondary liposuction procedure. Through the cavitation of the tissue by ultrasonic energy, physicians can better treat more fibrotic tissue and perform more selective fat aspiration. However, UAL did lengthen procedure treatment time as port protectors needed to be incorporated and removed during each treatment. Port protectors increased incision size and often had to be stitched close. In addition, UAL was a two stage procedure, treatment then aspiration, which further lengthened surgeon OR time. Lastly, while treatment outcomes were satisfactory, the subsequent tightening effects of the treated area were similar to that of standard liposuction.
Laser-assisted liposuction provides a thermal experience to the skin to significantly impact dermal contraction. Dr. Barry DiBernardo's randomized blind split abdomen study, "Evaluation of shrinkage and skin tightening in laser lipolysis vs liposuction", determined that placing a laser under the skin and reaching a temperature of 42°C can result in a 17% tightening and area contraction of the skin [2].

2. Technology and procedure description

RFAL is the newest entry to the liposuction family and can be found in the BodyTite device (Invasix Ltd., Israel). RFAL deploys RF energy through a hand piece [Figure 1] to deliver a thermal effect to the adipose tissue, skin and sub-dermal matrix.

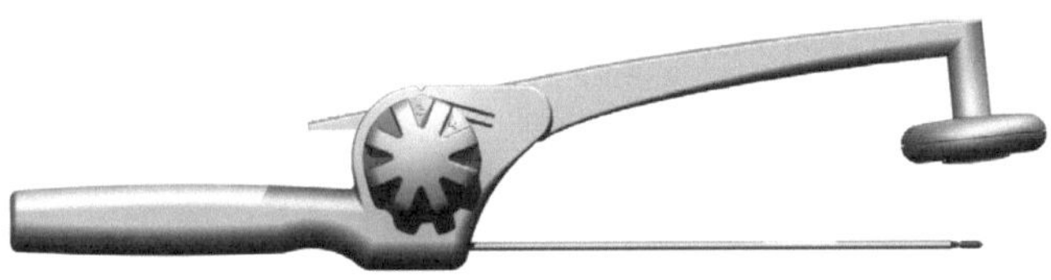

Fig. 1. Schematic presentation of the bi-polar RF hand piece.

RFAL technology uses external and internal electrode, connected by a handpiece, to create a thermal profile. During treatment the internal cannula is introduced into the adipose tissue and can be adjusted for the desired depth of treatment. This adjustment can control the distance between electrodes in the range of 5mm to 50mm that allows for targeted treatment depth and uniform treatment by layers. Contact is maintained between the external electrode and the skin by a spring-loaded pivot.
When powered, the insulated internal electrode emits RF current through a small conductive tip. The external electrode has a larger contact area and is applied to the skin surface creating a lower power density in the skin than in the adipose tissue [Figure 2]. Up to 75W of RF power can be applied between the two electrodes depending on thickness and curvature of treated area. For large and medium volume treatment, the melted fat can be aspirated; for the treatment of small areas, such as the neck and face, the fat may be dissolved naturally through phagocytosis.

The BodyTite system provides real-time monitoring of the skin temperature and a power cut-off mechanism [Figure 3]. Typical cut-off temperature is in the range of 38–42°C. When the desired temperature is reached during treatment, the system automatically turns the RF energy off to avoid overheating and ensure the maintenance of uniform temperature over the treated area. If the temperature in the zone starts to drop, or when the hand piece moves to a new zone with a lower temperature, the RF energy becomes active again. The cut-off temperature should be modified depending on the treatment area and the amount of thermal energy required for various zone and skin thicknesses. In addition, it can be adjusted to tailor to more aggressive or conservative approaches.

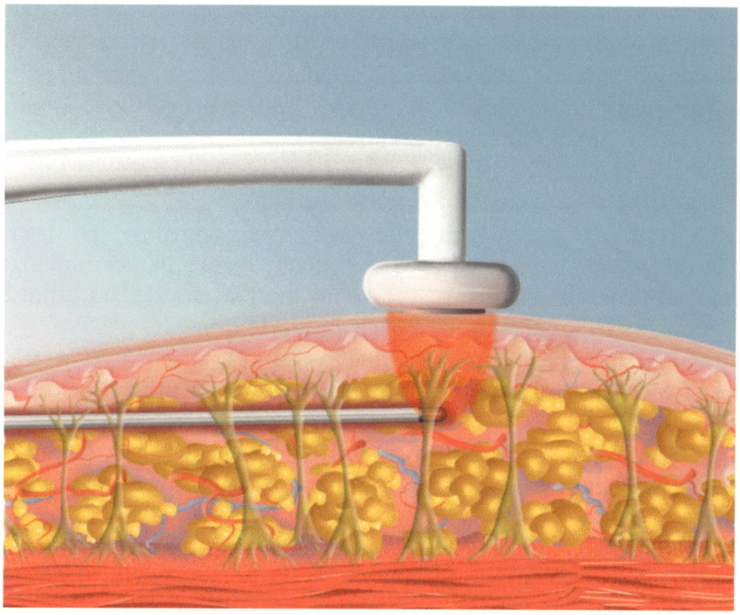

Fig. 2. RFAL hand piece inserted into the body with directional energy applied to adipose fat and septae.

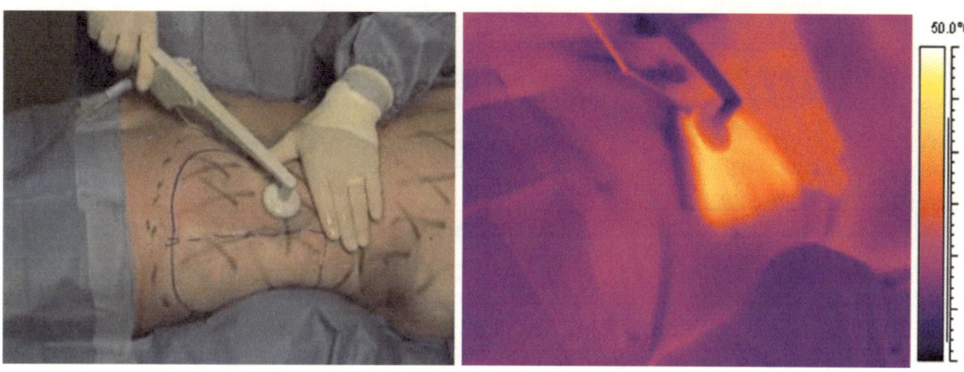

Fig. 3. RFAL uniform thermal distribution without hot spots or under-treated areas resulting from the use of a cut-off temperature control mechanism.

In addition to emitting energy, the internal electrode also serves as a cannula to provide simultaneous aspiration of the coagulated tissue. Often this coagulated tissue has less hematocrit compared to standard or power assisted liposuction, providing for less bruising post-surgery. [3] Simultaneous aspiration immediately removes treated fat from the treatment site and allows the physician to perform desired contouring, thereby reducing procedure time and associated operating costs.

To appeal to the varied areas of treatment and physician preferences, a number of RFAL hand pieces are available with multiple lengths, diameters, tip configurations, and aspiration ports allowing RFAL to be adapted to different areas and procedures.

Depending on the volume of the body, the procedure can be conducted under general anesthesia, IV sedation or local anesthesia only.

RFAL mainly comprises of the following steps:

- Patient marking of thermal zones (10 x 15cm) and planning of incision ports.
- Applying tumescent anesthesia 30-60 minutes prior the treatment. Common methods include standard Klein or Hunstad techniques.
- Applying sterile conductive gel to the skin surface to reduce friction and improve electrical contact between external electrode and skin.
- Insertion of the RFAL cannula into the tissue, after adjusting the desired treatment depth into the tissue. Treatment should start in deeper planes moving up to more superficial planes while staying in the same thermal zone. The cannula movement should be slow, with 2-3 seconds for a back and forth cycle.
- Performing RFAL treatment with simultaneous aspiration.
- Treatment of each thermal zone should end when one of the following end points are reached:
    - 6-12kJ is deposited in the treatment zone. Higher kJ can be deposited in thicker fatty layers, such as the lower abdomen, and less kJ for thinner areas such as the epigastrium or neck
    - The cut-off temperature is reached and maintained for a few minutes
    - Skin erythema
- Final contouring of the area should be done without RF, with a focus on contouring and uniformity.
- Applying drains and suturing ports, if necessary.
- Applying compressing foams and garments; considered critical for proper healing and symmetrical tightening.

2.1 Blood vessels coagulation

The coagulation of blood vessels is a process naturally associated with a thermal treatment. The coagulation of vessels may have a positive effect in reducing the bruising and blood loss, however, it may present a safety concern as the termination of blood supply to the dermis can potentially cause skin necrosis.

The macro observation of the RFAL procedure allows the authors to conclude that hematocrit in the aspirating fat is lower during RFAL procedure compared to suction assisted lipoplasty (SAL). Observation of RFAL after an abdominoplasty shows no bleeding in the adipose fatty tissue from a 5mm to 30mm depth while flowing blood vessels are observed in sub-dermal area, illustrated in Figure 4.

The histological studies and observation of tissue sections in abdominoplasty patients pretreated with RFAL concludes that small vessels such as capillaries, venules and artherioles are coagulated during the treatment [Figure 5], while the majority of larger blood vessels are not damaged and continue to supply blood to the dermis. Observations show less bleeding in the adipose fatty tissue in a 5 to 30mm depth, whereas bleeding is observed from blood vessels in the subdermal area. Bleeding of the dermis can be observed after the treatment and no skin necrosis is observed at the 6 months follow-up. [4]

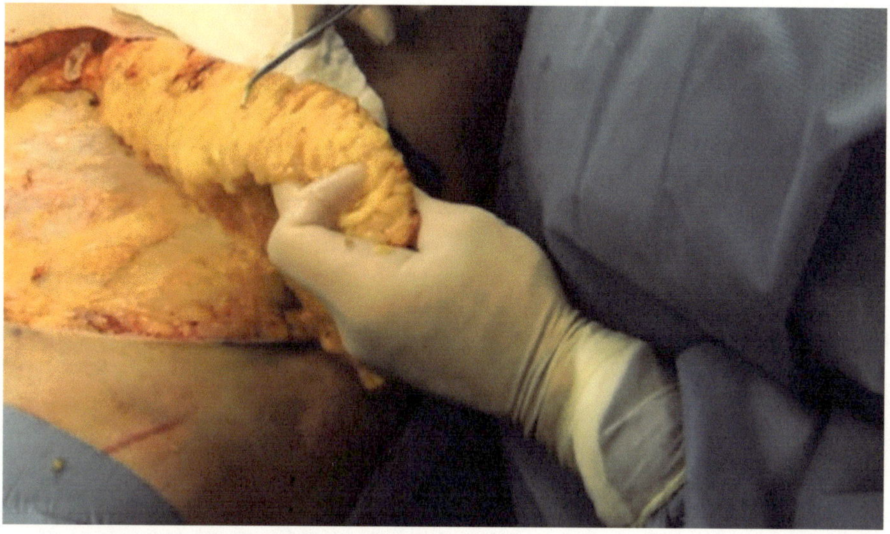

Fig. 4. Cross section of RFAL treated adipose tissue.

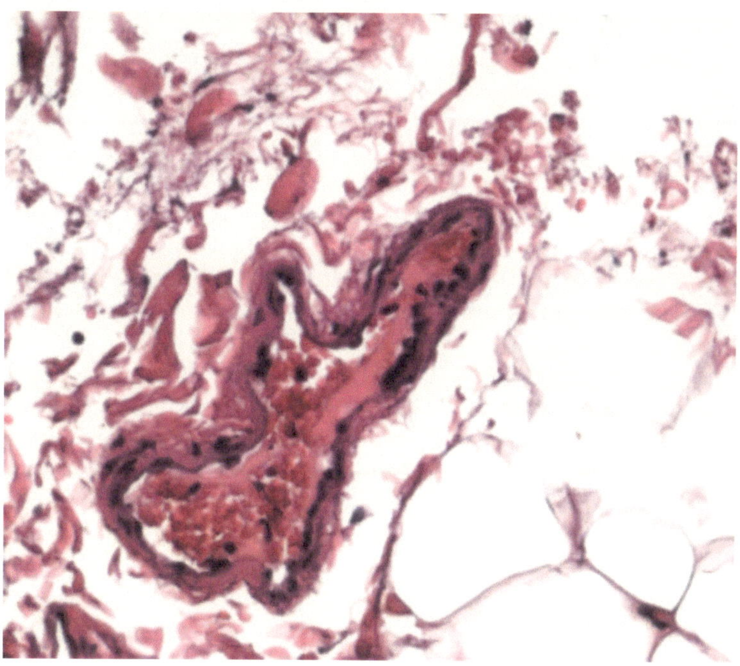

Fig. 5. Small coagulated blood vessel of the subcutaneous layer after RFAL .

2.2 Tissue tightening

Skin appearance and tightening is a common concern during one's consideration for a liposuction procedure. Patients classified as obese, or with excessive skin, or compromised skin quality are typically excluded as liposuction candidates as fat removal can often leave behind excess lax skin causing their skin and body contour to appear worse. Skin laxity post liposuction can create patient dissatisfaction with the only solution being excisional surgery. Therefore, a liposuction method that can consistently contract the skin can address these patients who were previously excluded from treatment.

RF thermal induced contraction of collagen is well documented in medicine and is used in ophthalmology, orthopedic applications and treatment of varicose veins. Each type of collagen has an optimal contraction temperature that does not cause thermal destruction of fibroblasts, but induces a restructuring effect in collagen fibers. The reported range of temperatures causing collagen shrinkage varies from 60°C to 80°C [5-9]. At this temperature tissue contraction occurs immediately after tissue reaches the threshold temperature. The shrinkage of tissue is dramatic and can reach tens of percents of the heated tissue volume. This type of contraction is well studied in cornea [5], joints [6], cartilage [7, 8] and vascular tissue [9], but its application for the skin, sub-dermal and subcutaneous tissue tightening has not been as explored.

Non-invasive RF and lasers have been used for skin tightening effects since the mid 1990's [10-15]. Due to superficial thermal safety concerns, the skin surface temperature is maintained below 45°C and in order to increase the temperature in the deep dermis the skin is heated with RF or laser energy penetrating into the tissues deeper than 1.5mm, with simultaneous skin surface cooling. This sophisticated method of trans-epidermal, non-invasive RF thermal delivery provides a variable and controversial tightening effect, which is not usually apparent, if at all, until dermal remodeling occurs, a few months after the treatment.

Recently, thermal induced tissue tightening was expanded to minimally invasive treatments [11-15]. Using laser assisted liposuction or radio-frequency assisted liposuction, physicians have attempted to achieve reduction of subcutaneous tissue with simultaneous tissue contraction. DiBernardo reported 17% skin surface shrinkage measured at three months follow-up after LAL treatment [2]. RFAL technology provides a higher power and more efficient energy transfer than laser energy systems and thus, allows the treatment of larger volumes of the subcutaneous tissue with optimal thermal profiles, facilitating the significant tightening of the tissue. Recently introduced radio-frequency assisted liposuction and soft tissue contraction technology has shown tremendous promise for thermal contouring [3, 4, 16-19].

When considering skin contraction, it is important to differentiate two-dimensional horizontal x-y tightening of the skin surface from three-dimensional x-y-z tissue tightening of the subcutaneous tissue, where the skin is also more firmly connected and adjacent to the deeper anatomical structures. If two-dimensional contraction is a function of collagen structure changes in dermis, the three-dimensional tissue tightening changes involve contraction of different types of collageneous tissue. We can separate the following types of collagen tissue in the subcutaneous space:

- Dermis - papillary and reticular.
- Fascia - relatively thick layer of connective tissue located between muscles and skin.
- Septal connective tissue - thin layers of connective tissue separating lobules of the fat and connecting dermis with fascia.

- Reticular fibers - framework of single collagen fibers encasing fat cells.

2.3 Ex-vivo tightening measurements

An ex-vivo study [16] was conducted to measure subcutaneous collageneous tissue contraction with simultaneous monitoring of local tissue temperature, to determine the threshold temperature of the collagen shrinkage on different types of ex-vivo collageneus tissue samples.
Two types of collageneus tissue were studied for thermal induced contraction:

- Fascia
- Adipose tissue with septal and reticular connective tissue

The excised post abdominoplasty tissue samples were placed between the two BodyTite RF electrodes, where the small area, internal RF active electrodes (cannula) were placed in contact with the studied tissue and the other large area electrode was applied to the opposite side, or epidermal side, of the sample [Figure 6]. Two marks were placed at a distance of 1 cm from the active internal electrode to visualize tissue displacement.

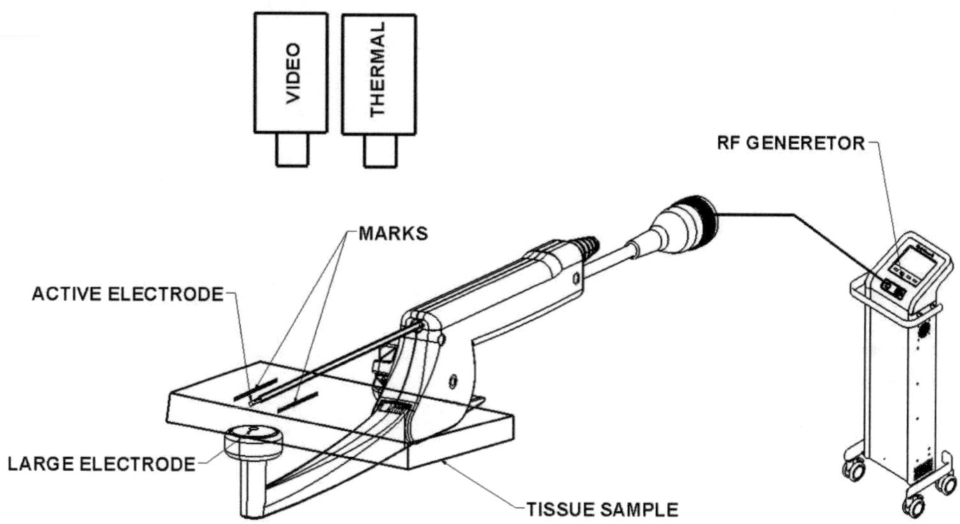

Fig. 6. Ex-vivo experiment set-up.

The delivered power was 75W, at 1MHz frequency; energy was delivered until evaporation of water from the adipocytes was observed.
Video and thermal cameras were used to monitor temperature change and tissue displacement during the treatment. The start of tissue displacement was correlated with tissue temperature to determine the contraction thermal threshold.
The adipose tissue with septal and reticular collagen behavior is shown in Figure 7.
The experiments showed that the marker movement (contraction) started within two seconds after the start of RF energy delivery. Adipose fibrous septal tissue coagulation and vaporization started to be observed at 13 seconds after initiating RF energy. Tissue contraction was not symmetrical as the displacement from one side was 8mm, and the other

side presented an average displacement of 3mm. Non-symmetrical behavior can be explained by the non-uniform structure of the connective tissue and the non-symmetrical geometry of the studied tissue sample. The average marker migration and tissue contraction for the three experiments with adipose tissue was 6.5mm.

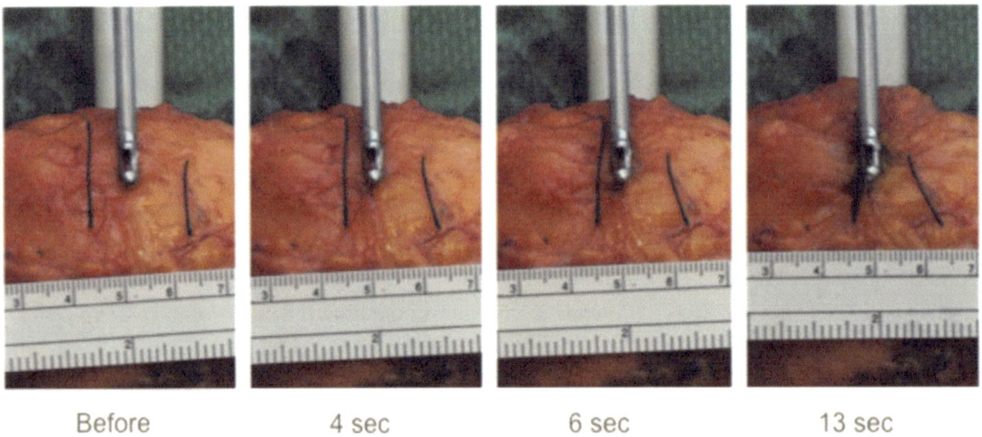

Fig. 7. Adipose-septal tissue behavior during RF energy delivery with time lapse.

Figure 8 shows thermal images of the same sample taken before the treatment, at the beginning of tissue displacement and at the end of the treatment showing the rise in thermal profile with time and onset of contraction.

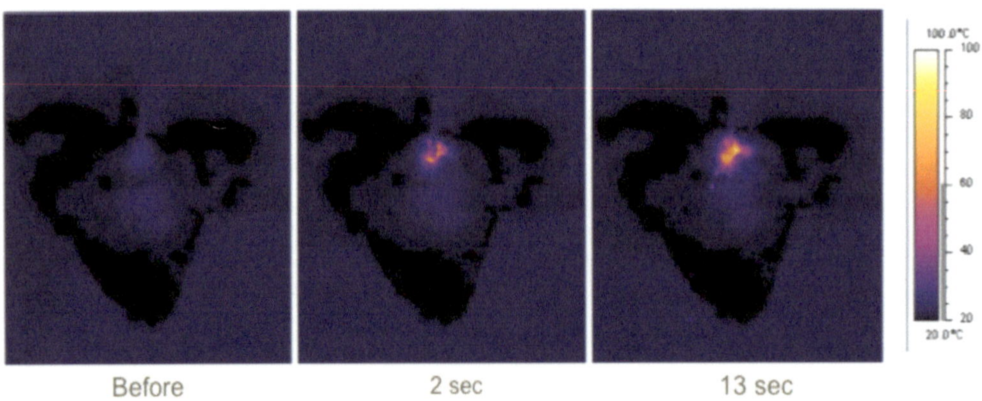

Fig. 8. Thermal images of adipose-septal tissue thermal behavior during RF energy delivery with time lapse.

For fascial tissue, contraction started when the maximal adipose tissue temperature near the active internal electrode reached 69.4^{O}C and its response is illustrated in Figure 9.
The displacement of the markers and tissue contraction in fascia were significantly less than in adipose tissue. Average movement was 2.75 mm, or approximately 2.5 times less than the mark migration and tissue contraction observed in adipose tissue.
The marker migration and medial contraction started after 3.5 sec and maximal temperature near the active electrode at this moment was 61.5°C.

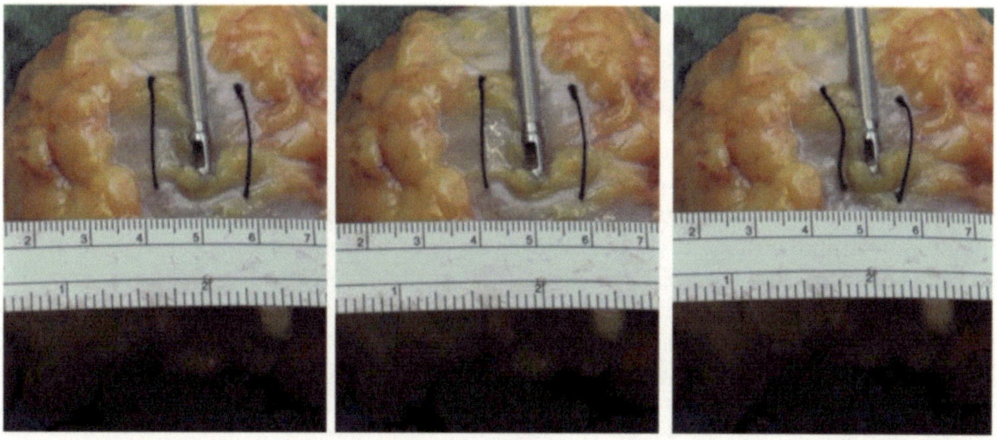

Fig. 9. Fascia contraction behavior during RF energy delivery with time lapse.

Table 1 summarizes the results on subcutaneous tissue contraction.

	Fascia	Septa/Adipose Tissue
Average Displacement, mm	2.75	6.5
Threshold Temperature, °C	61.5	69.4

Table 1. Average displacement and contraction threshold temperature.

Results show the strongest contraction response in adipose tissue containing septal connective tissue and reticular collagen fibers encasing fat cells. Fascia and septa can be heated to these high, optimal contraction temperatures, but it can be done only in an minimally invasive transcutaneous manner that deposits the thermal RF energy directly into the adipose tissue and sub-dermal space, thus avoiding heating the epidermal surfaces.

The contraction temperatures of collagen in the ex-vivo study were in the same range reported for other collageneous tissues. Tissue contraction was observed in the area with diameter of 2cm, which corresponds to a spherical contraction volume of 4.2cm^3. Knowing the tissue volume and deposited energy before the start of contraction, one can estimate the energy density required for each cubic centimeter of treated tissue to reach tissue contraction effects. It can be calculated that for 1L of adipose tissue, up to 48.3kJ is required to start to see immediate and significant collagen contraction. These tissue energy calculations for initiation of adipose contraction are consistent with empirical data obtained with LAL treatment where energy from 50kJ up to 100kJ per liter is recommended for the treatment of the abdominal area.

The ex-vivo experiments produced different degrees of contraction for septal and dermal tissues that emphasizes the balance between these processes for optimal aesthetic results. Lower two-dimensional contraction of the skin and significant three-dimensional contraction of sub-dermal adipose connective tissue may cause wrinkling of the skin surface for high volume liposuction patients.

In-vivo clinical monitoring of temperature, both in the adipose tissue and the epidermal surface, should allow the physician to more accurately predict the thermal treatment times and reduce the risk of thermal injuries.

2.4 In-vivo evaluation with radio-frequency assisted liposuction

An in-vivo study [16] enrolled 24 patients, 22 female and 2 male patients, who underwent RFAL to the abdomen and hips. The average age was 39.7 years old (range 19-52 years) with an average pre-operative weight of 71kg. The selected patients were typical candidates for a liposuction procedure. All patients were active with no significant medical diseases. 15 of 24 patients had a normal body mass index (BMI) (<25), while 9 of 24 patients were moderately overweight (BMI 25-30) and 3 patients were obese (BMI >30 but < 32).

The RF power, in the range of 40 to 75W was used for uniform heating throughout a thick subcutaneous flap. The average total energy, 72kJ, was delivered to the abdominal area. The temperature around the tip of cannula reached 70-80°C. The skin temperature was monitored and energy cut-off levels were in the range of 38-42°C, which was maintained for 1-3 minutes. The strong and sustained tissue heating during the procedure resulted in a thermal stimulation of the sub-dermal layer, the entire matrix of adipose tissue and the vertical and oblique fibrous septa, eliciting a powerful three-dimensional retraction and contraction of the entire soft tissue envelope.

All patients had their treatment area infiltrated with tumescent anesthesia prior to RFAL. Tumescent anesthesia is critical in the technique as the RF current travels through tissue most efficiently in a salinated environment.

The objective of this in-vivo study was to correlate treated soft tissue contraction results with procedure and patient variables including amount of deposed RF energy, body mass index, and amount of aspirated fat.

A zone measuring approximately 15 X 10cm (150cm^2) can be heated to a critical target temperature within 3-8 minutes, depending on the thickness of the treated fat layer and then safely maintaining uniform volumetric heating to reach uniform temperature distribution over the entire treated volume.

All patients from the study were followed at 6 weeks, 3 months and 6 months. In order to measure linear two-dimensional contraction, the distance between two fixed points was measured preoperatively and then at the 6 months postoperative visits. Distances between incision ports and natural "fixed" anatomical registration points, such as moles or the umbilicus were measured before the treatment, after the treatment and at 3 and 6 months follow-up visits. The linear contraction was measured as the relative change of distance between two points over the curved surface of the body. Distances were measured using a flexible ruler applied over the skin surface [Figure 10]. For the abdominal area, at least 3 measurements were taken between 3 different points and an average linear contraction was calculated.

All RFAL patients demonstrated some level of contraction. From 8% to 15% linear tightening was observed at the end of the surgery on the operating table, which further increased dramatically during first week when most of the swelling was reduced. The linear and area contraction process continued over the subsequent weeks and maximum contraction was noted at the last follow-up visit 24 weeks after the treatment.

Linear contraction observed at 6 months follow-up were much more significant than reported with any other technology, and varied from 12.7% up to 47% depending on the patient and treatment variables. It is important to note that soft tissue area contraction can be estimated as the square of the linear contraction and represents much higher numbers.

The measured linear contraction was then correlated using three parameters:

- Aspirated volume that was varied in the range of 0.5L to 3.4L with average volume of 2.0L.

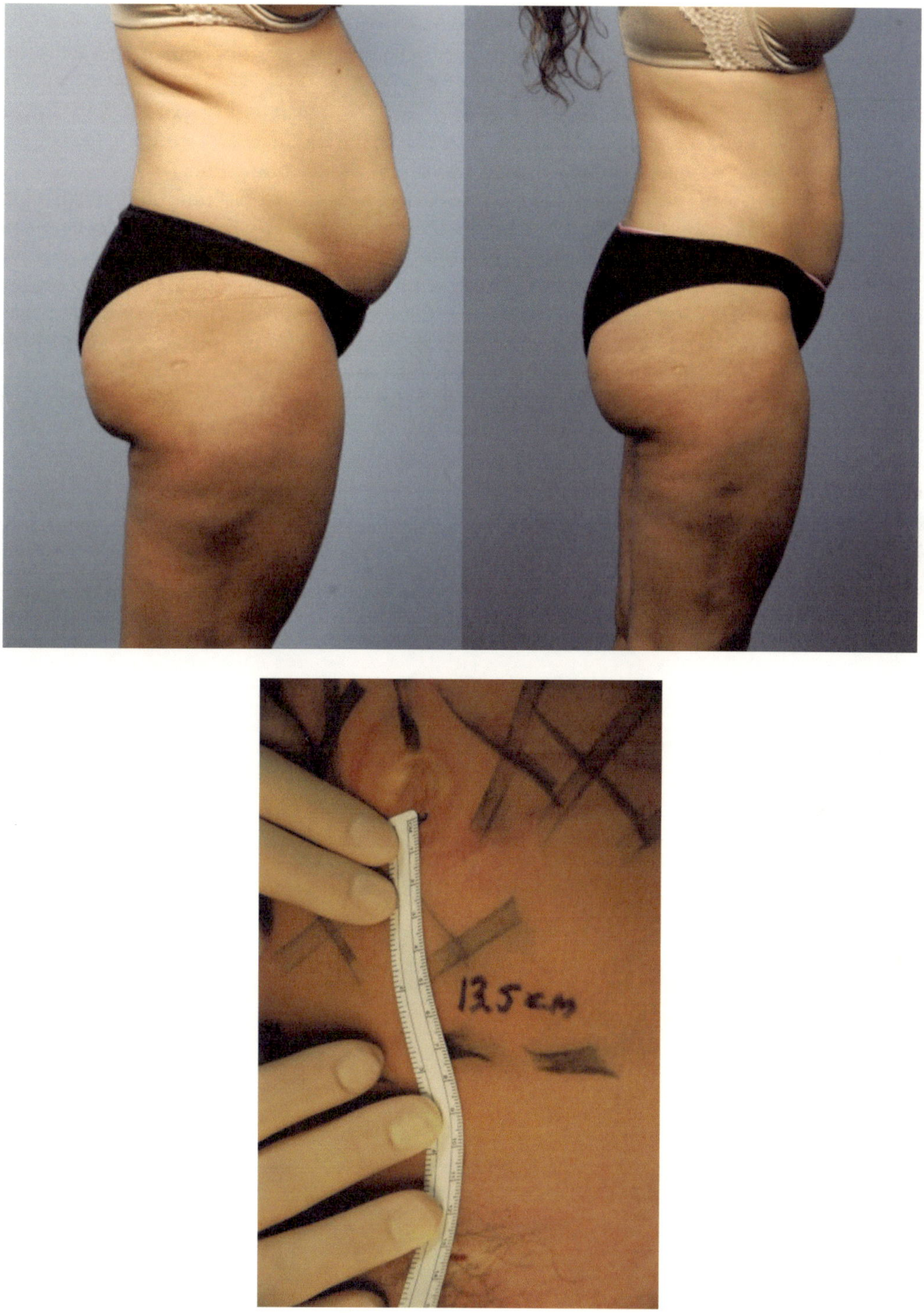

Fig. 10. Before and After RFAL and intra-operative two point linear contraction registration points from pubic RFAL incision point to the lower point of the umbilicus.

- BMI of the patients that varied from 20.8 to 31.7 with an average index of 25.7.
- Deposited RF energy that was varied from 60kJ to 96kJ per abdominal area with an average number of 72kJ.

For statistical analysis of the correlation between the measured variables and linear contraction, the coefficients were calculated. The closer the coefficient to the 1, the higher the linear correlation is between the measured variable and tissue contraction.

Analysis shows no or very weak correlation between aspirated volume and linear skin contraction. The Pearson coefficient is about 0.22. Figure 11 shows the correlation between these values, with a random distribution.

The Pearson coefficient for correlation between contraction and patient BMI is much higher and equals 0.64. It is easy to naturally come to the conclusion that a patient with a larger volume of adipose tissue would have more tissue available to undergo contraction thus providing a much stronger connection between these parameters [Figure 12].

The highest correlation (0.86) was obtained between deposed RF energy and skin contraction. Figure 13 shows the measured results that almost has a linear function between these two parameters. The more energy deposited, the more linear contraction that was observed.

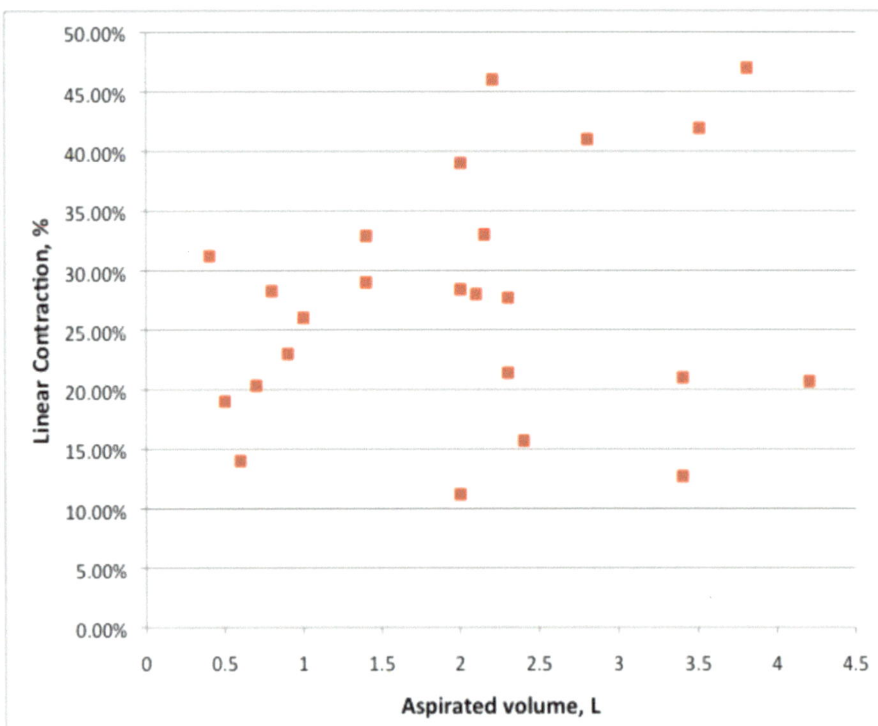

Fig. 11. Correlation between aspirated volume and linear contraction.

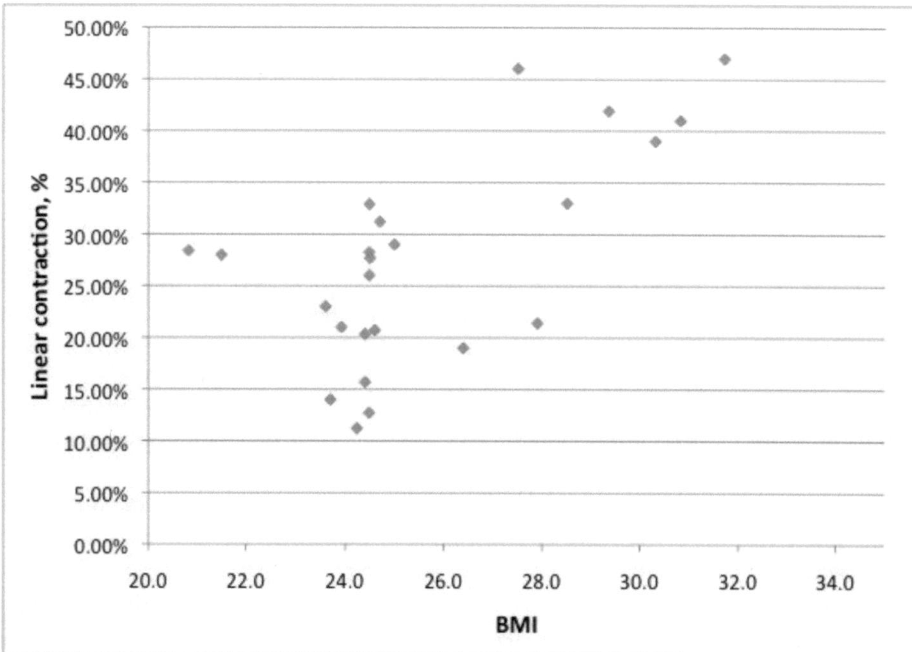

Fig. 12. Correlation between BMI and linear contraction.

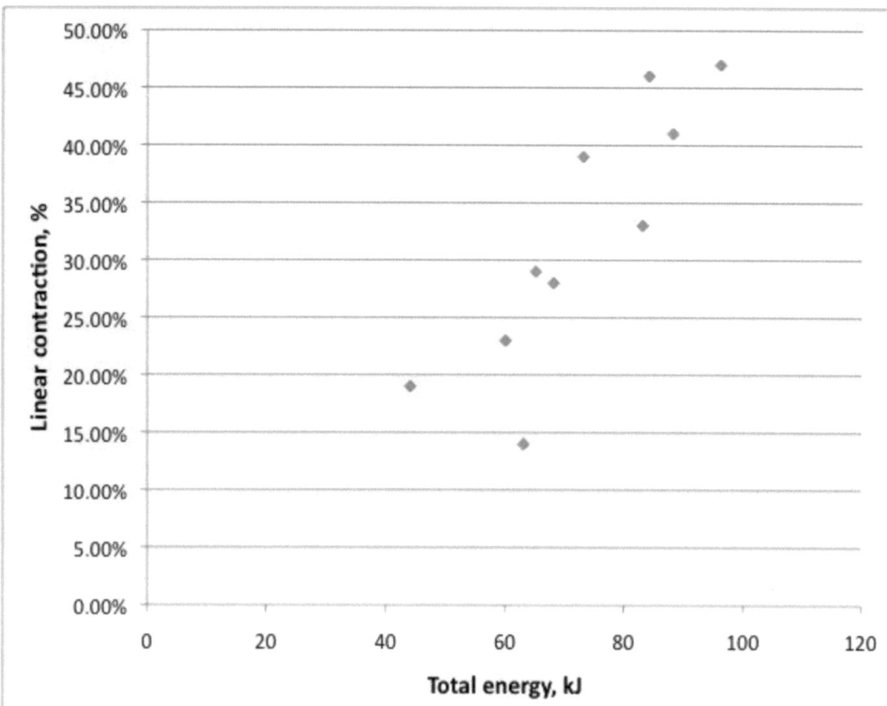

Fig. 13. Correlation between total energy and linear contraction.

In spite of improved contraction obtained at higher energies, the amount of energy during the treatment should be measured and controlled to avoid negative side effects such as seromas and skin burns while still achieving optimal linear and area contraction.

Features of an ideal liposuction procedure would include reduced ecchymosis, pain, and edema from pre-aspiration coagulation of adipose and vascular tissue, followed by less forceful and traumatic extraction forces, as well as a significant soft tissue contraction when host tissue elasticity is compromised. Thermal based lipoplasty appears to hold this potential.

In the present study based on volumetric heating we reached an average local linear contraction of 31%. This is statistically significantly higher than that reported with other energy emitting liposuction technologies. Overall area contraction was much higher than the linear contraction. These in-vivo results confirm the proposed mechanism of RF based tissue tightening and recruitment of the vertical and oblique fibrous adipose matrix.

About 30% of patients noted minor weight loss, however, it is premature to correlate it with treatment procedure. Further studies are recommended to explore this relationship.

The study reported one seroma, which was treated with closed serial aspiration. Seroma is not a rare side effect for energy-assisted liposuction, especially for high volume treatment and may necessitate a lower threshold for closed drainage systems in selected patients.

The RFAL is a versatile procedure and provides advantages for a myriad of treatment concerns. Similar to UAL, RFAL has the ability to work through more fibrotic tissue common in the male chest [Figure 14] or characteristic of secondary liposuction cases. In addition, its ability to offer the highest contraction rate of all energy treatments allows RFAL to be considered for large volume patients [Figure 15] or patients with compromised skin laxity. The varied number of hand piece configurations also permits RFAL to be used for fat aspiration in combination with tightening, such as the body and breasts [Figure 16], or pure skin tightening procedures, where fat removal is a secondary concern, as desired in areas as arms, neck and face treatments [Figure 17].

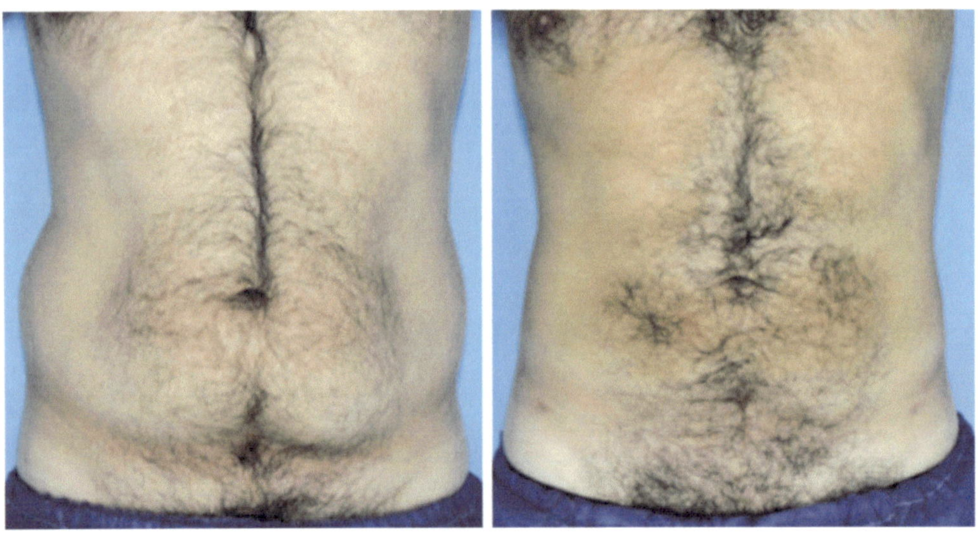

Fig. 14. Before and 3 months post treatment of a male patient with 13.6% reduction in waist circumference.

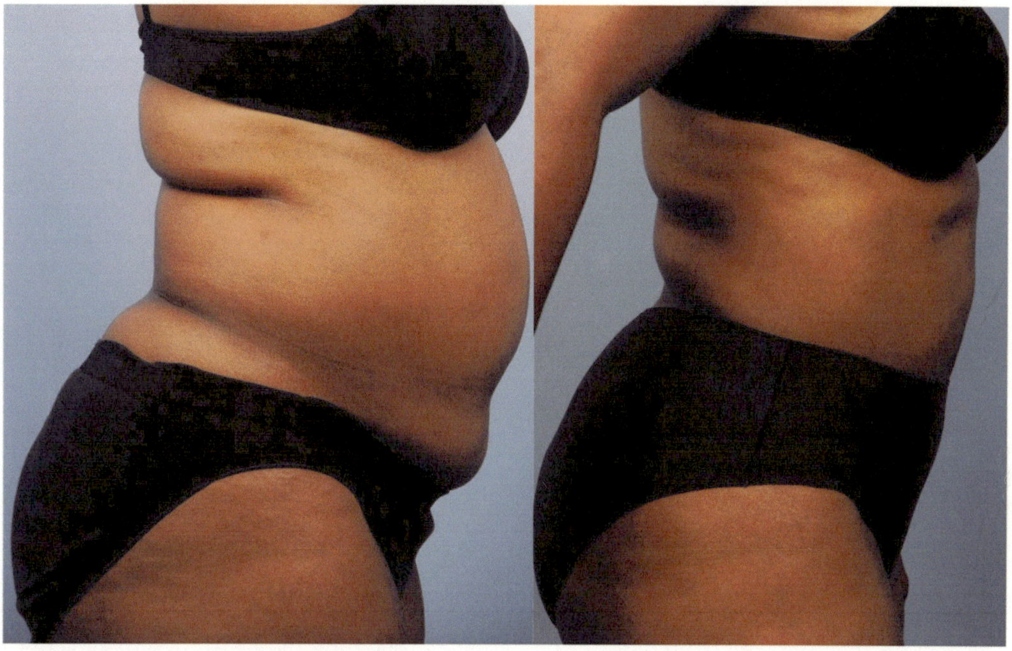

Fig. 15. Before and 6 months post treatment of a large volume female patient.

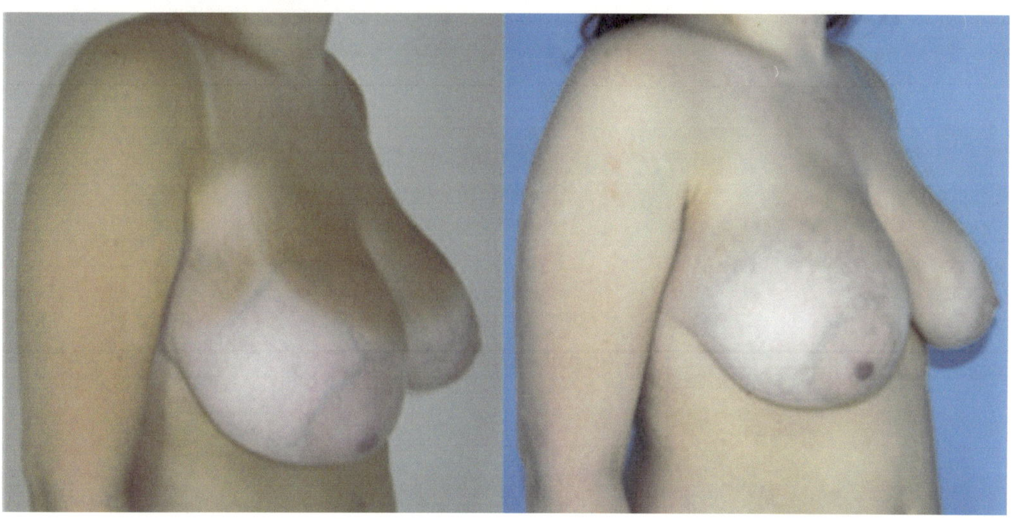

Fig. 16. Before and 4 months post treatment with 2500 cc removed to provide a breast lift.

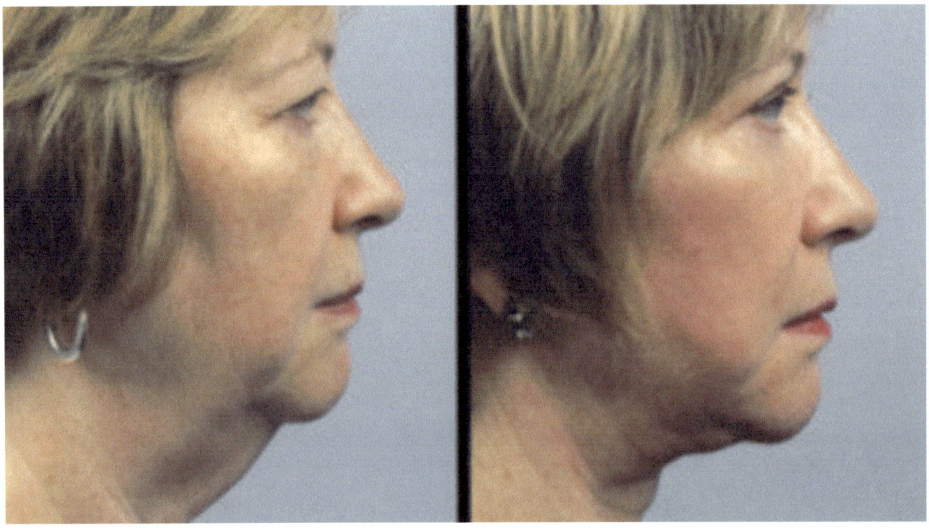

Fig. 17. Before and 3 months post treatment of the neck and face providing tightening and contour.

2.5 Histologic and MRI studies

Pre and post-operative photography, weight and circumferential reduction data were obtained on all patients.

The skin histologies taken from biopsies immediately following the RFAL treatment show a canal created by the cannula, which thermally destructed adipocytes around the canal [Figure 18].

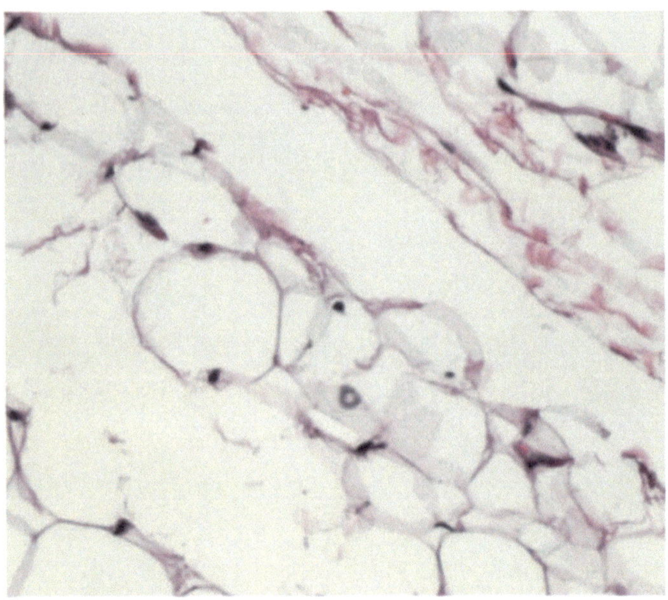

Fig. 18. After RFAL, channels in the fat tissue are observed and surrounded by disrupted fat cells.

Skin biopsies taken from an RFAL study patient at 12 months, show normal dermal architecture, with healthy collagen and elastin fibers in the deep reticular dermis with no evidence of scar tissue or abnormal collagen fibers [Figures 19, 20].
A magnetic resonance imaging study of five patients before and three months after RFAL [18] showed a reduction in the thickness of adipose tissue in treated area and an increase of collageneus tissue in subcutaneous fat [Figure 21]. Signals of remaining edema could be observed 90 days after treatment, signaling the continued persistence of the reparatory process.

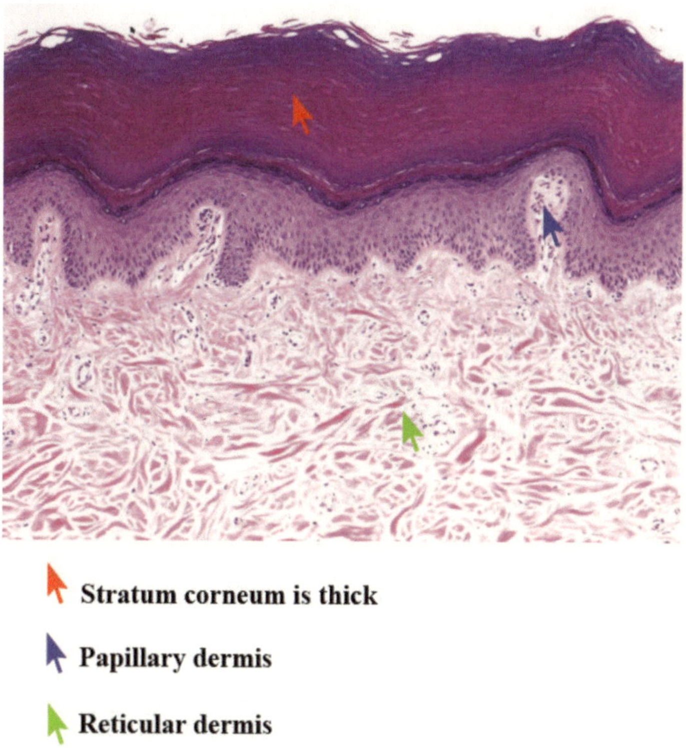

Fig. 19. Normal skin histology 12 months following optimal RFAL thermal endpoint.

3. Patient comfort and safety

Data and feedback compiled from a few hundred RFAL patients illustrate that the treatment is safe for small and large areas [3, 4, 16-19]. Most patients were able to return to a regular routine a few days following the treatment. In addition, for single or small zone procedures, the treatment can be performed under local anesthesia thereby reducing the risks related to general anesthesia. Most patients were drawn to RFAL as there was a reduction of downtime caused by bruising or pain.
The main safety precautions are:

- Limit deposited RF energy per zone of 150cm^2 by 6-8kJ for thin skin less than 2.5cm thickness and by 12kJ per thick fat layer.
- Observe skin reaction during treatment, the appearance of erythema indicates a strong effect for tumescent infiltrated tissue and should be considered an end point.

- In many cases skin temperature up to 36-38°C is enough to get good results, especially for thick skin layers.
- Avoid the return of the cannula to the same point. This can cause focal over-heating and can be prevented by moving the hand piece in a zig-zag pattern.
- Move the cannula slowly to control its position and maintain its thermal effect.

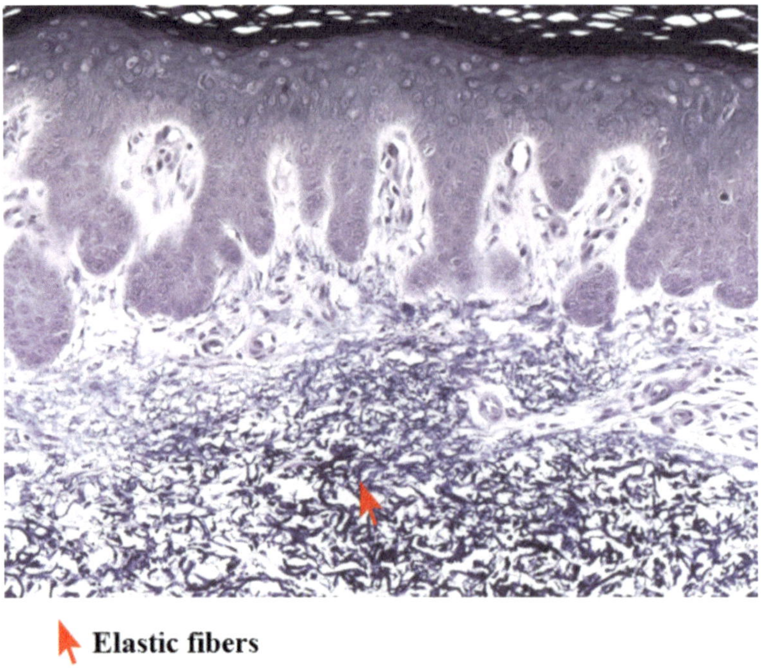

Fig. 20. The same RFAL patient as in Figure 12 with 43% contraction and normal elastic fiber content.

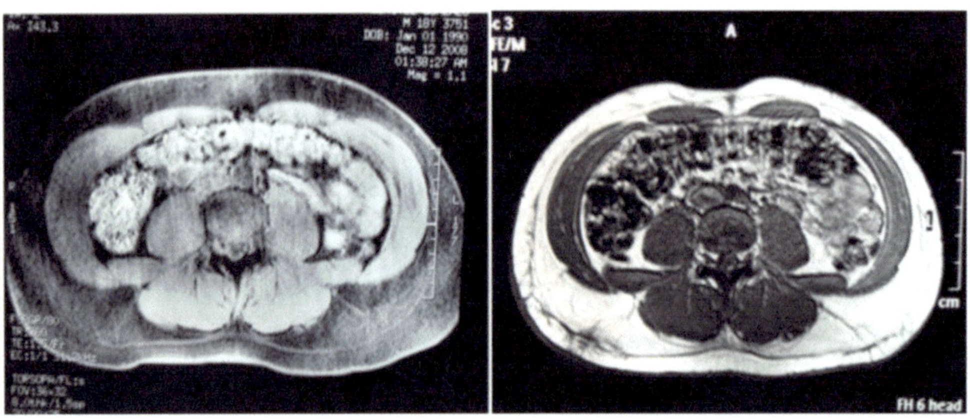

Fig. 21. Magnetic resonance imaging of the abdomen before (left) and 3 months after (right) RFAL, showing significant reduction of the abdominal fat thickness and mild edema. Note the indentation of the mid-abdominal line at 3-month follow-up, which was absent prior to the procedure.

4. Acceptance by physicians

Acceptance by physicians can be quite high as there are only a few changes to the standard liposuction technique, these include reducing the speed of cannula movement and ensuring the cannula does not return to the same return point.

A comparison of RFAL aspiration speed with a standard Mercedes liposuction cannula, each with the same diameter, conducted on a split body treatment demonstrated a 17% higher aspiration speed with RFAL compared to a regular cannula. Measurements of aspirated tissue volume after 20 minutes of treatment showed 490ml fat extracted with RFAL, compared with 420ml with the regular cannula. The increased speed of RFAL over standard liposuction is likely the result of the lower viscosity and increased flow following Poiseuille's law [3]. However, in a true treatment setting physicians using RFAL may see an increase in the treatment time by about 10-20% depending on number of treatment areas. Overall, the majority of energy based liposuction techniques require an increase in treatment time and thermal assisted procedures require more attention from physician to control in parallel thermal and contouring processes.

The skin tightening benefits demonstrated through the treatment results, is an advantage that standard liposuction and other thermal treatments are unable to reproduce. Often these results can only be provided with more extensive excisional surgeries. The ability of RFAL to provide the patient an alternative to abdominoplasty or brachioplasty provides the surgeon a highly sought after competitive advantage.

5. Conclusion

The main advantage of RFAL is consistent and substantial 3-dimensional tissue contraction resulting from the heating of subcutaneous tissue without significant increase in the length of the procedure. The tightening of the tissue with RFAL broadens the physicians ability to treat a more diverse population who may require stronger contraction in addition to fat reduction. It is the experience of the authors that RFAL provides a safe procedure with obvious tightening benefits for the aesthetic medical market.

There is potential of the RFAL technology in following specific cases where skin contraction is critical:

- Treatment of overweight patients
- Treatment of patients after weight loss
- Treatment of areas with saggy skin and low fat content such as the upper arms, neck and face
- High potential in the treatment of cellulite

While RFAL technology does not solve all the above mentioned problems, it greatly expands the horizon of liposuction technology to a broader patient demographic.

6. References

[1] Scuderi N, Tenna S, Spalvieri C, De Gado F. Power-assisted lipoplasty versus traditional suction-assisted lipoplasty: Comparative evaluation and analysis of output power-assisted lipoplasty versus traditional suction-assisted lipoplasty: Comparative evaluation and analysis of output. Aesth Plast Surg. 2005;29:49–52.

[2] DiBernardo B. ASAPS, The Best of Hot Topics – Lipo-Transfer and SmartLipo, May 6 2008.

[3] Mulholland RS. An in-depth examination of radiofrequency-assisted liposuction (RFAL). J Cosmet Surg Med. 2009, September;4(3):14-19.
[4] Paul M, Mulholland RS. A new approach for adipose tissue treatment and body contouring using radiofrequency-assisted liposuction. Aesth Plast Surg. 2009;33(5):687–694.
[5] Asbell P, Maloney RK, Davidorf J, Hersh P, McDonald M, Manche E. Conductive Keratoplasty for the correction of hyperopia, Tr. Am. Ophth. Soc. 2001; 99:79-87.
[6] Obrzut SL, Hecht P, Hayashi K, Fanton GS, Thabit G III, Markel MD. Effect of radiofrequency on the length and temperature properties of the glenohumeral joint capsule. Journal Arthroscopy Rel Surg. 1998, May-Jun;14(4):395-400.
[7] Lu Y, Edwards R III, Cole BJ, Markel MD. Thermal chondroplasty with radiofrequency energy, an in vitro comparison of bipolar and monopolar radiofrequency devices. American Journal of Sports Medicine. 2001, Jan-Feb;29(1):42-9.
[8] Lu Y, Edwards R III, Kalscheur VL, Nino S, Cole BJ, Markel MD. Effect of bipolar radiofrequency energy on human articular cartilage: Comparison of confocal laser microscopy and light microscopy. Journal Arthroscopy Rel Surg. 2001, Feb;17(2):117-23.
[9] Theodore H. Teruya, MD, Jeffrey L. Ballard, MD, New approaches for the treatment of varicose veins, Surg Clin N Am. 2004;84:1397–1417.
[10] Mayoral, Flor A. Skin tightening with a combined unipolar and bipolar radiofrequency device.(CASE REPORTS), Cosmet Laser Ther. 2005;7:11-15.
[11] Fatemi A, Weiss MA, Weiss RA. Short-term histologic effects of nonablative resurfacing: results with a dynamically cooled millisecond-domain 1320 nm Nd:YAG laser. Dermatol Surg. 2002, Feb;28(2):172-6.
[12] Mayoral FA. Skin tightening with a combined unipolar and bipolar radiofrequency device, J. of Dugs in Derm. 2007, Feb;6(2):212-215.
[13] Doshi SN, Alster TS. Combination radiofrequency and diode laser for treatment of facial rhytides and skin laxity. Effect of controlled volumetric tissue heating with radiofrequency on cellulite and the subcutaneous tissue of the buttocks and thighs. Journal Drugs Dermatol. 2006;5:714-722.
[14] Zelickson B, Kist D, Bernstein E, et al. Histological and ultrastructural evaluation of the effects of a radiofrequency-based nonablative dermal remodeling device: a pilot study. Arch Dermatol. 2004; 140:204-209.
[15] Hsu T, Kaminer M. The use of nonablative radiofrequency technology to tighten the lower face and neck. Semin Cutan Med Surg. 2003;22:115-123.
[16] Paul M, Blugerman, G., Kreindel, M., Mulholland RS. Three-Dimensional Radiofrequency Tissue Tightening: A Proposed Mechanism and Applications for Body Contouring. Aesth Plast Surg. 2010, Sept. [Epub ahead of print]
[17] Sandhofer M, Schauer P, Blugerman G, Schavelzon D, Paul MD. Sicherheits- und Machbarkeitsstudie einer neuen radiofrequenzassistierten Fettabsaugungstechnik. Journal Fur Aethetische Chirurgie. 2010.
[18] Blugerman G, Schavelzon D, Paul MD. A safety and feasibility study of a novel radiofrequency assisted liposuction technology. Plast Reconstr Surg. 2010;125(3):998-1006.
[19] Paul M, Mulholland RS. A New Approach for Adipose Tissue Treatment and Body Contouring Using Radiofrequency-Assisted Liposuction. Aesth Plast Surg. 2009;33: 5 687-694.

9

Ultrasound Assisted Liposculpture - UAL: A Simplified Safe Body Sculpturing and Aesthetic Beautification Technique

Nikolay P. Serdev
Medical Centre "Aesthetic surgery, Aesthetic medicine"
Head, International University Program in Cosmetic Surgery,
New Bulgarian University, Sofia
Bulgaria

1. Introduction

The use of ultrasound for cosmetic surgery has been introduced since the late 1980's, and the technique and equipment have been improved during the years.
Authors experience on 1300 patients since 1994 has proven that the ultrasound assisted liposculpture - UAL is a simplified safe procedure. UAL delivers ultrasonic energy directly to deep fat deposits through very tiny incisions in the skin. This technique enhances the current procedure in liposuction by adding ultrasonic waves to break down the magnified and giant fat cells in the deep fat deposits, preserving normal size microscopic fat cells in the superficial subdermal fat layer, which enables smooth results with UAL. This technique shortens the total multi-area operation time to about one hour or less and avoids possible mechanical damage to surrounding tissues.
We use the ultrasound assisted liposculpture with tumescent infiltration and UAL thin probes to precise location of deep fat deposits. UAL should not be used as a dry method. Blood vessels, muscle cells, and other small bodily structures remain unharmed by the selected ultrasound wave. Once the ultrasound liquefies the targeted fat area, we use a very gentle suction internally to remove the fat. UAL is particularly useful for areas affected by scar tissue, large areas, or areas with dense fields of fat, but for us UAL is the best method for very fine body reshaping in skinny patients seeking for beautification. It is also popular in the treatment of gynecomastia. The UAL requires more specialized equipment.
In the recent years the Vibration Amplification of Sound Energy at Resonance System[14] (VASER) became another method of liposuction using ultrasound and we use it with same atraumatic and aesthetic success in our practice in the last 3 years.
Important aspects of patient selection, markings, surgical technique, and postoperative care are outlined.

2. History

In 1921, Charles Dujarier, in France, attempted to remove subcutaneous fat using a uterine curette on a dancer's calves and knees. A tragic result occurred due to injury of the femoral artery leading to amputation of one of the dancer's legs. In 1964, Schrudde extracted fat from the lower leg through a small incision with a curette. Hematomas and seromas resulted from this technique. Pitanguy favored an to remove excess thigh adiposities. Significant noticeable incisions diminished the popularity of en bloc removal of both fat and skin. Arpad and Giorgio Fischer published first their results from aspiration of fat in 1976. Working in Rome, they developed a blunt hollow cannula equipped with suction. Some of their early cannulas also contained a cutting blade within them. They also developed the technique of crisscross tunnel formation from multiple incision sites [1,2]. Fewer complications such as hematomas and seromas were seen than with sharp curettage. In 1977, Pierre Fournier, working in Paris, showed an early interest in the Fischers' liposculpture technique. Later Fournier subsequently became a world leader in liposuction and fat transplantation, eventually recognizing the benefits of tumescent anesthesia and contributing greatly to teaching syringe liposuction to surgeons throughout the world [9-15]. Illouz [9-10] felt the solution was a "dissecting hydrotomy" which would facilitate the removal of fat and reduce trauma with less bleeding. Illouz was responsible for creating worldwide publicity for the new procedure. Julius Newman, an otolaryngologist and cosmetic surgeon, and his associate Richard Dolsky, a plastic surgeon, taught the first American course on liposuction in Philadelphia in 1982. The first live surgery workshop was held in Hollywood, California, in June 1983 under the direction of the American Society of Cosmetic Surgeons and the American Society of Liposuction Surgery. Newman first used the term "Lipo Suction" and established the American Society of Liposuction Surgery [53]. Initially, large cannulas were employed for liposuction, some up to 1 cm in diameter. In 1987, Jeffery Klein developed the tumescent technique, allowing nearly bloodless liposuction using only local anesthesia [3]. This innovation involved infiltration of a dilute solution of lidocaine with epinephrine to allow more extensive liposuction totally by local anesthesia, significantly reducing bleeding [16]. To date, there have been few complications and no fatalities when the tumescent anesthesia technique is employed as a local anesthetic approach without excess intravenous fluids or general anesthesia [29]. After having been used for many years in other medical specialties, selective ultrasound waves have been introduced to simplify and facilitate the liposuction, reducing the blood loss by first liquefying fat. In 1987, Scuderi et al. offered the use of ultrasound as an emulsifying modality for adipose tissue. Then Zochhi in 1988 first presented the ultrasonic liposculpturing, built on the Scuderri's concepts [7, 8], as a totally new technique, based on the surgical use of the ultrasound energy that allows for the selective destruction of excess adipose tissue, or rather of it's fluid fraction [18, 19, 23]. It was introduced to be combined with infiltration [3, 6, 8, 16]. UAL is effective because of its effect not only on fatty tissue but also on loosening the cell-to-cell structures, allowing easy removal of adipose cells [4]. Later external ultrasound (Hydrolipoclasis Ultrasound) was introduced for smaller fat amounts without or with liposuction [23, 25, 51, 52]. The firstly undue fear [20, 23, 39] of heat was later used in subsequent techniques like laser assisted liposuction [21]. So, in the recent years, lasers introduced the thermal lipolysis as a comparison to traditional techniques.

3. UAL

UAL is a type of liposuction that is primarily used for fat removal in hard-to-treat areas such as the chin, neck, cheeks, knees, calves, and ankles. It is best indicated in tumescent liposculpture for patients who require more precise body contouring.

Few studies conducted to compare classical liposuction with UAL[40, 46.]. The studies were done comparing ipsilateral traditional lipoplasty with contralateral ultrasound assisted lipoplasty on one or more body area. The ultrasound liquefies fat thus the aspirate is less bloody and contained more fat than tradition liposuction aspirate. Skin tightening and weight loss cannot be compared to traditional liposuction that is more traumatic. Classic liposuction does not achieve metabolic benefits of weight loss.[47] "UAL is not a replacement for suction-assisted lipoplasty - SAL; it is an extension of this technique."[40] The advantages of UAL are selective destruction of fat cells, the possibility of skin tightening of treated areas, and a reduction of physical strain on the surgeon[8, 28]. UAL uses high-frequency sound waves to liquefy fat beneath the skin surface before removing it with a gentle suction. Tumescent liposuction and traditional liposuction cannot liquefy fat cells, and this makes the fat more difficult to remove. There is less surgeon fatigue, allowing the surgeon to focus on true sculpting in body contouring and less tissue trauma.[28] UAL is also successful in breast surgery [48, 49] and as a very superficial ultrasound-assisted lipoplasty for the treatment of axillary osmidrosis.[50] UAL allows the trabecular system and elastic skin to retract, but the degree of skin tightening following UAL depends on the age and quality of skin.
Ultrasound waves in the infiltrated tissue cause fat tissue destruction via:

1. **Selective destruction of single adipose tissue fluid** - UAL uses chemo-physical effect of strong sound-waves in a fluid, formulated by Alfred Loomis, 1927 [8] ,
2. **Micromechanical effect** – Ultrasound displaces intracellular molecules, breakups up chromosome, and conglomeration of molecules caused by the breakup of intermolecular bridges, leading to cessation of DNA duplication, modification of the proteins spatial structure, formation of free radicals, denaturation of the cellular membrane components and electrochemical modifications of the cellular surface[18, 19, 21];
3. **Cavitation phenomenon** - strong cellular fragmentation and lipolytic effect;
4. **Thermal effect** if the techniques is properly used , this will be minimized and won't create collateral damages[21, 24, 25];
5. **Preservation of vascular and nervous structures** [21, 24];
6. **Reduction of blood loss.** [18, 26-28]

3.1 Alternatives

Many alternatives to UAL exist. These include diet and exercising, other liposuction techniques, excision techniques, removal of lipomas, breast reduction etc. External Ultrasonic Hydrolipoclasis[21, 24] and external UAL have been used for smaller amounts of fat, but external UAL has not provided the promised ideal of fat dissolution without surgery (suction).[51, 52]

4. Patients selection

Since 1994, we performed Ultrasound Assisted Liposculpture(UAL) on 1300 patients targeting a total of 5200 body areas with very good aesthetic results, short downtime, and a very low level of blood loss and bruising.
The author selected patients with localized excess adipose tissue in specific areas, even if the patient is at or below his or her ideal weight. Overweight patients may also benefit, but generalized obesity was excluded by author as is not in the scope of beautification [14, 41, 42].
The best results were achieved on healthy patients with good skin elasticity and localized deposits of excessive fat.[14] If patients have more fat than can be removed safely in one

operative setting, a second session or more was planned. Ultrasonic liposuction appears to be most useful in treating larger or more fibrous areas thus reducing blood loss and post operative pain.

4.1 Indications

We used UAL for the following indications: aesthetic beautification, removal of unwanted fat deposits and aesthetic body contouring, facial and double chin contouring, gynecomastia and breast reduction, correction of irregularities, calves elongation by reduction and change of the position of the inner knee fat, elongation of the thighs by reduction and reshaping fat surround the buttocks, removal of fat in very fine areas like ankles, calves, face, and total body contouring.

We did not use UAL for the treatment of general obesity (isolated areas can be treated in multiple sessions). UAL cannot be substitute of a balanced exercise and diet. However, it may help patients to remove areas not affected by diet and fitness or exercises. We also did not use UAL for the treatment of dimpled, uneven superficial fat surfaces of cellulite. UAL can be also used in bodybuilders to create the abdominal "six packs" which is increasing in demand, but patients have to be informed not to stop hard exercise as this will cause accumulation of visceral fat leading to abdominal "turtle shell" appearance.

5. Method

The author's UAL technique was performed on an outpatient basis under local tumescent anesthesia and i.v. monitored sedation. Dry technique was not used. In order of achieving the desired cosmetic aesthetic results, the author recommends to avoid using UAL superficially. The author's technique maintains the surface untouched "taboo area", to avoid surface irregularities.

5.1 Anesthesia

Our experience is very good when using local anesthesia - Klein's tumescent technique [3, 4, 6] combined with additional IV monitored anesthesia: mild sedation, iv analgesia with opioids and NSAIDs.

The recommended maximum safe dose of lidocaine (when used with epinephrine) is 35 mg/kg based on Klein's study [6]. However, lidocaine doses up to 64 mg/kg have been safely used by some authors.[16, 25-28]

Epinephrine is a critical component of the wetting solution. It has a vasoconstrictive effect that minimizes blood loss and delays the absorption of lidocaine. The total epinephrine dosage used in wetting solutions range from 1:200,000 to 1:1,000,000 [5].

Local anesthesia with sedation is a reasonable option especially in the ambulatory surgery and in procedures of shorter duration. The advantage of local tumescent anesthesia is shorter recovery period, decreased postoperative hypoxemia and lower rates of postoperative nausea and vomiting [29].

Infiltration has to be properly and uniformly distributed in the fat deposit in order to obtain smooth results after the suction!

5.2 Short time ultrasonic application

After infiltration of the areas to be treated, we introduce a selected ultrasonic probe into the specific body area and use the properly selected power no more than 4-6 minutes per ca. 200

cc adipose tissue.[28] The probe should be moved slowly uniformly all over the fat deposit. Once the feel of fat softening (liquefication) is achieved we stop. We never use hollow ultrasonic probes for ultrasound action and suction at the same time!

5.3 Anatomic approach

Ultrasound treatment should be applied onto the deep adipose tissue, below the superficial subdermal fascia. We never apply the ultrasound superficially as proposed for superficial classic liposuction![30-32] Ultrasound waves are effective for unstable increased in size and giant cells alone (in the deep localized fat deposits) and do not affect the normal microscopic cells in the superficial subdermal layer. Proper selection of both ultrasound power and probes is important and manufacturers guidelines should be followed. With the VASER® we never exceed 70% power. Application of inappropriate power of ultrasound and or the use of improper probes could be too damaging to tissue!

5.4 Low aspiration

After achieving the liquefication of fat, we use low-pressure suction of the liquid fat, which is easily done, in a manner of a violin play. Histological evaluations revealed that these parameters were associated with minimal effect on connective tissues and blood vessels.[33] Longer application times are associated with disruption of collagen and elastin structures. The lower suction of fluid could be compared to suction applied by drinking fresh juice with a straw, i.e. there is only a minimal trauma to the tissue, resulting in nearly no blood loss. It is advisable to end liposuction once the aspirate changes in color from yellow to pinkish red! It is important to create smooth transition between the area treated and the surrounding areas! At this moment we have to make sure that all deep fat is equally removed and the superficial fat layer is similar in thickness to the surrounding untreated areas.
The average blood loss is no more than 100 - 250 ml during the whole procedure even if multi-areas are addressed in one session. We have never had a case requiring blood transfusion.

5.5 Number of treated areas per session

The number of treated areas per session is limited on the first place by the maximum lidocaine dose allowed based on the patient's weight in kilos. The lidocaine dose ranges from 45 to 60 mg/kg without any serious lidocaine toxicity. We use the dosage below 35 mg/kg as "exceedingly safe" [6] and count the number of possible areas we can infiltrate with this amount of tumescent solution. Independently of the low blood loss, the patient's health and status evaluation at the time of operation will dictate the number of areas treated and maximum lidocaine dose used.

5.6 Pre operative consultation and evaluation

Initial consultation is scheduled to clinically assess the health status of the patient. This includes history, physical exam, and a psychological evaluation. Any health problem should be referred to a specialist and treated adequately. No patients will be operated on unless he or she obtains a medical clearance from a specialist. Pre-existing conditions should be checked and brought under control before UAL. This includes: history of heart problems, high blood pressure, diabetes, allergic reactions to medications, pulmonary problems, smoking, alcohol, drug use or abuse. If needed (in cases of presumable allergic reactions, history of uncontrolled diabetics etc.), we request the corresponding consultants to be present during surgery, and to manage the patient's medical condition peri-operatively. An anesthesiologist is always present in the operating theatre during surgery. In all our clinical cases we used IV monitored sedation and analgesia in addition to the local tumescent anesthesia.

Preoperative blood and urine testing should include basic blood chemistry evaluations (CBC, prothrombin time/activated partial thromboplastin time, bleeding time and general chemistry) to screen for any renal, hematologic, or hepatic disease before the procedure. ECG is needed in elderly and if indicated in younger patients. The results should be interpreted together with the anesthetist and if necessary with consultants. Health status should be checked again before surgery. Patients are asked one more time about using contraindicated medications and drugs. Before the procedure, no anticoagulants, anti-platelet , hormonal and NSAIDs medications should be taken for two weeks before and after surgery. Fasting is required for four hours before the operation to prevent from regurgitation and aspiration, which can provoke postoperative bronchopneumonia. Smoking should be avoided, as nicotine interferes with circulation and can result in hypoxemia and loss of tissue.[16, 20, 38]

In general, a good candidate for UAL (as well as other liposuction techniques) is a person with an average or slightly above average weight, in good health, with a localized area of fat that does not respond well to diet and exercise. Slim models are best candidates in our hands, because the UAL does not affect the normal size fat cells in the superficial subdermal fat layer. After surgery the even subdermal fat layer will tag along the usually aesthetic form of the muscular and skeletal frame. Patients with superficial fat layer affected by lipodystrophy are not good candidates for UAL.

Before surgery, patient's problematic areas and desired result will be discussed one more time. Patients must understand fully the pre-operative preparations, the procedure, the post-operative care and predicted aesthetic results, enhancing appearance and self-esteem. Patients who are not motivated and psychologically unstable are declined. After full understanding the risks and possible complications, the informed consent form and permission forms for photography should be fulfilled and signed.

Similar to traditional liposuction, the skin is marked in standing position to indicate the areas from which the fat will be removed. We mark only outer borders of the fat deposits as well as depression borders, keeping in mind that in horizontal position, the deposits will move in cephalic direction and downwards with minimum 2-5 cm. Too much marking is false, because fat deposits change their position from standing into horizontal position. Marking of highest bulges is also false in our experience. They will change much, due to gravity vectors. Photography in different positions and light angles are necessary, to visualize and document the status and irregularities, preoperatively.

In the operating theatre, a disinfection solution, such as Betadine, is applied to the relevant areas. The first step in the ultrasonic liposuction procedure is the uniform infiltration of tumescent fluid into the area being treated. The tumescent local anesthesia technique allows the patient to move intraoperatively into the exact position, needed for our work to treat and remove fat without difficulty. Lidocaine toxicity must be properly considered.

Patients should be monitored during the procedure. The patient should have an IV fluid line; the fluid balance must be kept intact. There are also monitoring devices in use to keep track of the blood pressure, heart rate, and blood oxygen level.

The surgeon should have a full understanding of the features of the ultrasound device used, its proper application of selective ultrasonic destruction of fat, as well the correct power and probes selection.

After the uniform tumescent infiltration in the selected level and area is done, the proper ultrasound power and ultrasonic probe are chosen and then the probe is inserted through small 11 blade incisions, each about 2-3 mm. The introduction of infiltration cannulas, ultrasonic probes, and aspiration cannulas through the skin and the superficial fat layer are done in a perpendicular direction through the superficial fat layer and then the direction is changed, in order to prevent the superficial layer from damage and aspiration. We have proven that the temperature on the probe lateral walls using the prescribed energy stays below 37 degrees Cs. We have never experienced any change in the skin temperature, higher than 37 degrees Celsius. The temperature at the ultrasonic probe lateral wall has been found below 37 degrees Cs in our first hundred clinical cases and all next regular tests. These findings allowed us to safely use the ultrasonic probes without skin protectors. It allowed us to widen the frontiers of ultrasound assisted liposculpture and we were able to use the UAL in very tiny areas like ankles, calfs, face etc. without leaving visible scars. Our clinical experience has proven the probe temperature safety at the skin level in all our clinical cases.

After introducing of the probe to the respective deep fat deposit, the probe is maneuvered in a crisscross pattern all around the deposit, while sound waves generate negative pressure, causing nearly the whole amount of fat cells in the deposit to implode, collapse, and liquefy. The huge difference with traditional and some other liposuction methods is that the wave is active some centimeters from the probe tip in front and lateral and destroys the fat three dimensionally, while the suction cannula is creating tunnels with unaffected fat between tunnels. Comparisons between equal aspirates in traditional liposuction and UAL are fake, because the UAL destroys more fat than aspirated and has a prolonged effect of fat desorption. In all our patients we have observed lose of volume not only in the area of procedure but also from all around the body during the first six months following the procedure (See Fugures). The slimming effect after UAL became one of the positive side effects in our practice along with skin tightening! Patients for UAL should not be asked to slim before the procedure because diet reduces body response to stress and has negative effects like skin drooping and decreases by number the indications for liposuction and increases indications for excision surgery.

5.7 Areas of the body treated by UAL

Ultrasound can help break up tough fibrotic fat in different areas of the body, like face, ankles, calves etc. that are difficult to remove with traditional liposuction. Fat in the leg are ideal for UAL because of the elongation effects and beautification achieved by this technique. Ultrasonic liposculpture is recommended in areas that require precision. Tumescent UAL is among the safest and most effective techniques in chin, cheeks and jowls, ankles. The areas that we treated with UAL include the following:

a. Face and neck: Cheeks and submental (double chin)
b. The abdomen is one of the most common areas requested by both men and women. It is divided with the fascia into lower and upper parts with different anatomical fat structure. In the lower part, we have to leave a very thin superficial layer of fat. The peri-umbilical fat has a "croissant" shape. Anatomically this is a separate superficial fat structure, divided from the rest of abdominal fat by a fascia and should be treated

separately. Upper abdomen requires skilled contouring to preserve normal concavities and six packs in body builders.

c. Tumescent UAL of upper arms gives the best cosmetic result of skin tightening.
d. UAL in female breasts as well as in localized "bra-fat" provides aesthetic improvement with usually a moderate breast lift, due to reduced tissue weight and good skin retraction.
e. Treatment of pseudogynecomastia due to fat accumulation is one of the most frequent indications in males together with abdominal, flank and pubic fat, as well as double chin.
f. The area where smooth results are extremely difficult to obtain is the anterior thigh, where maximal volume reduction easily produces irregularities.
g. UAL of the outer and inner thighs, and inner knee UAL provides the most significant aesthetic improvement of the leg silhouette, with a visible elongation and straightening of lower extremities and body proportions (Fig. 1, 2, 3, 4).
h. Buttocks UAL can achieve results with a pleasing lifting, roundness and reduction. It gives elongation of the legs and better proportion to body (Fig. 4.).
i. We obtained a dramatic aesthetic improvement in the ankles and crus. The localized fat in these areas is genetically predetermined, and is resistant to diet and exercise.
j. Crus localized fats are mostly reduced from laterally and often need fat transfer to the inner part.
k. Areas that have been previously treated with liposuction and where is need of further contouring, respond very well to UAL

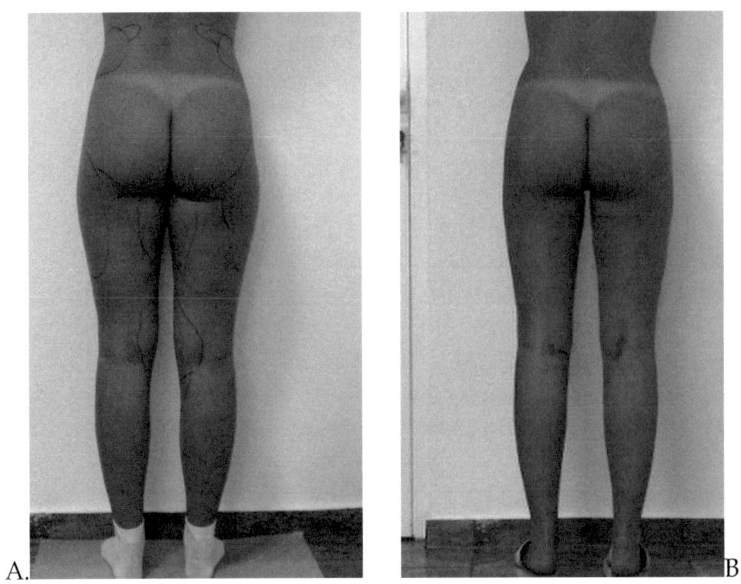

Fig. 1. A. Before, B. Result on day one after UAL of flanks, lower buttocks, outer and inner thighs, inner knees. Good effect of crus and leg elongation. Great loss of fat amount and minimal bruising.

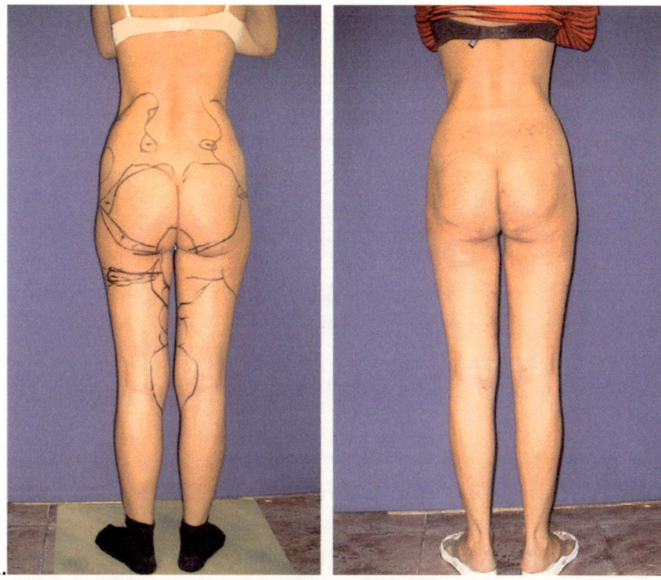

A. B.

Fig. 2. A. Before, B. Day one after UAL of flanks, lower buttocks, outer thighs, inner thighs and inner knees and buttock lift by Serdev suture technique. Surgical markings from the previous day are still visible. Note the relative elongation of the crus and legs. Buttocks look smaller, rounded and at a higher position due to body proportions changes.

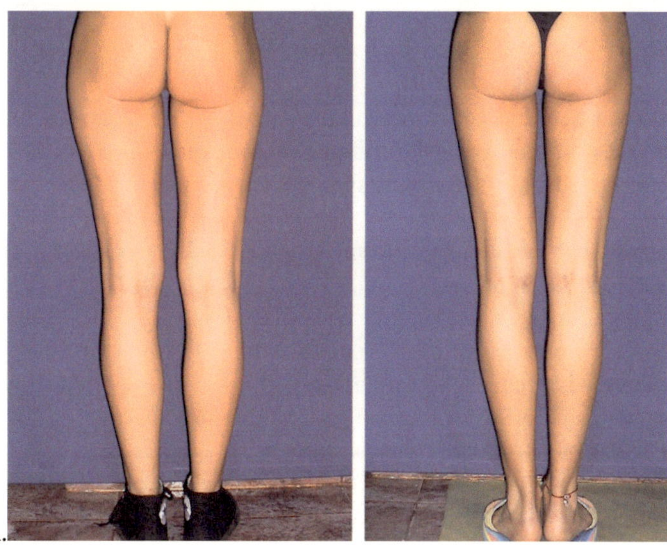

A. B.

Fig. 3. A. Before, B. After UAL of lower buttocks, outer thighs, inner thighs and inner knees. Result of straitening and legs elongation of a skinny model. Important volume reduction where needed, higher knee position for crus elongation along with smooth results and no surface irregularities.

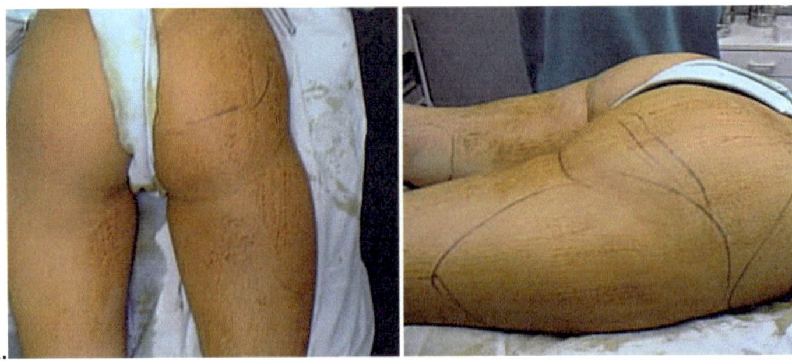
A. B.

Fig. 4. A. and B. Left buttock reduced using UAL. Right buttock still not treated. Effect of buttock's lift on the left side in different patients using UAL. Visible lift of 3-5 cm of the infragluteal sulcus.

5.8 No sutures

Since the incisions are small, we leave the incisions open, to drain the tumescent fluid. Drainage of the fluid allows the incisions to heal more quickly. Some surgeons suture them partially, leaving space for the fluid to drain out [34, 35, 36]. While the fluid is draining, dressings need to be changed daily. Patients take a daily shower in the clinic for about 7 days, and incisions are disinfected. It is important to open and drain the wounds for few days post-op as they are very tiny and could be occluded.

5.9 Outpatients procedure

As patients do not receive general anesthesia, after a time for stabilization, usually they are ambulatrory and can go home the same day, although they need someone else to drive them and stay with them in the first 24 hours.

5.10 Recovery

Depending on the extent of the UAL procedure, patients are generally able to return to work after two to three days. In the first 48 hours, pain is controlled by over the counter meds or by prescription medications, usually. Bruising dissipates in few days to weeks. Swelling subsides with time. Normal activities can be resumed after 2-3 days. The result is visible even on the first day post-op (Fig. 1, 2, 8) but will be much evident after six months when skin tightening and resolution of edema are attained (Fig. 5, 6, 8). Skin tightening, which is a positive side effect of UAL goes on for up to 6 months after surgery (Fig. 5, 6, 7). Weight loss in the first 6 months to normal is another very favorite side effect after UAL (Fig. 5, 6). The destructed and suctioned fat cells are permanently lost, however patients have to maintain a proper balance between calories intake and exercise regimen. Any positive intake balance causes the fat cells all around the body to enlarge.

5.11 Postoperative care

We administer antibiotics for 7-10 days. Patients apply elastic compression garments to areas that we have treated to prevent seromas, minimize bruising and decrease soreness in these areas. Patients are informed about postoperative leakage of tumescent fluid from incision sites for up to several days. Patients should be reassured that such leakage is common.

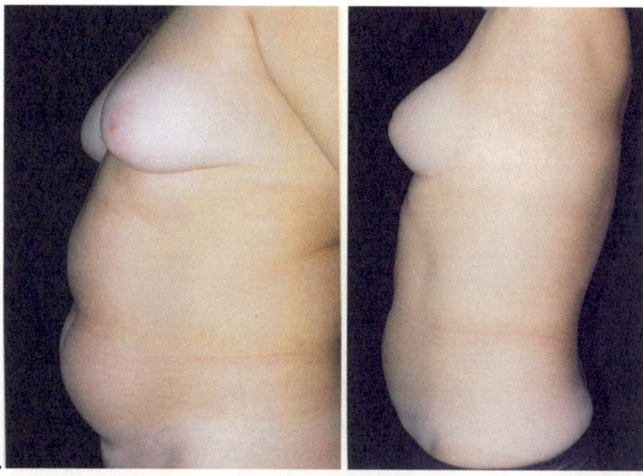

A. B.

Fig. 5. A. Before. A 90 kg female patient, B. Result 6 months after UAL of abdomen and flanks and removal of 2 liters of aspirate. The patient has lost 40 kg. Very good skin retraction.

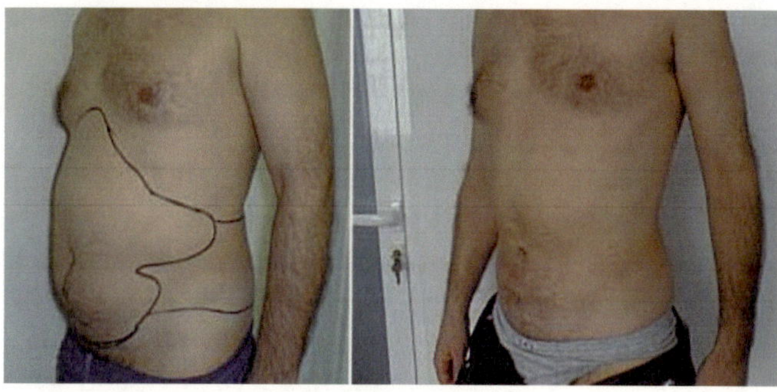

B.

Fig. 6. A. Before, B. Result after 4 months after abdomen and flanks UAL. Loss of fat all around the body - visible loss of volume in the upper arm.

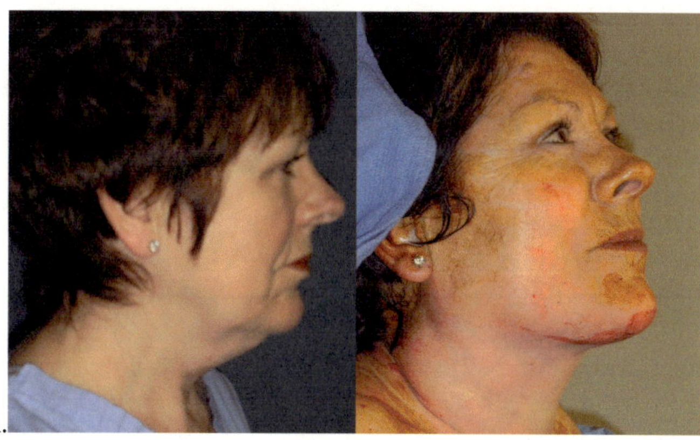

A. B.

Fig. 7. A. Before, B. At the end of the surgery, the skin still not cleaned from blood and brown colored Braunol. Immediate result after UAL of the lower face and neck - double chin. Immediate result of tightening of the skin.

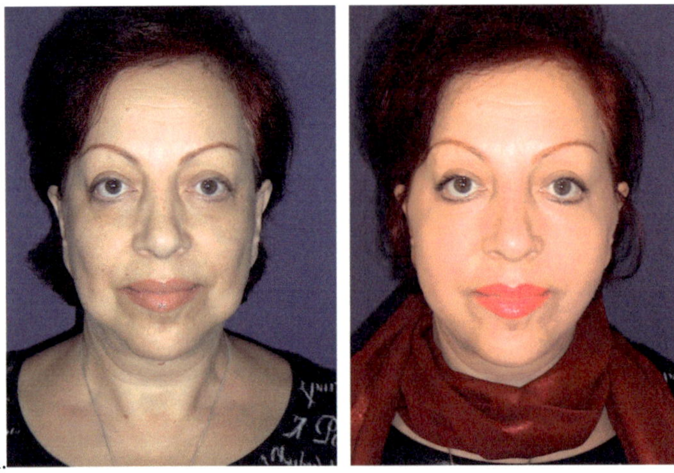

A. B.

Fig. 8. A. Before, B. Result after cheek UAL. Change from square face into oval. The beauty triangle is achieved.

Optimally, patients should wear these 24 h/d for approximately 4 to 6 weeks (depending on summer or winter times and on flabbiness of the skin and tissue). In our geographic area compression will be advised for about a month in summer time, and for a month and a half in wintertime. It will reduce swelling and results will be visible more quickly.

Patients are advised to walk as soon as possible after surgery! Exercising the treated areas should be avoided for about a month after the surgery. Patients are free to fulfill their daily duties, and work after 2-3 days. By exercising regularly and eating a healthy diet, patients will help maintain their new shape.

The treated areas appear to be swollen, but volumes are visibly reduced even on the first day post op (Fig. 1, 2, 7). Swelling augments in the first 7-10 days, and start receding in few weeks when the patients start noticing reduction of dress sizes.

6. Results and complications

Following risks in ultrasonic liposuction have not been observed in our cases:

1. No overheating and elevated temperature of targeted fatty tissue was observed. Temperature measured on the surface of the ultrasonic probe and on the surface of the skin was below 37 degrees Cs.
2. No skin necrosis or burns were observed in all cases.
3. No injury to peripheral nerves was found with UAL. Our patients' base appear to have no incidence of prolonged numbness consistent with injury to sensory nerves.
4. Any liposuction method can cause seroma. Seromas can persist for weeks or months if not treated. In our experience the strict daily patient follow up in the first 7 to 10 days after UAL and daily opening of the skin perforations has allowed us to minimize cases of seromas. Only in 3 cases (2 males and 1 female) we discovered one side seroma in the flanks that needed drainage for 2 days covered by antibiotic. The seromas were treated with suction through the operation incision using an infiltration cannula and healed in 4 days. The seromas were found deep in this area. Only once we were forced to use drainage for 2 days.

5. Due to our no sutures and good drainage technique, our patients experienced no hematomas, minimal ecchymoses and bruising.
6. Only one unilateral infection of the right inner knee wound was observed after the third day post op and was treated with widening of the wound from 2 mm into 5-6 mm, with the tip of a "mosquito" instrument for a daily drainage and daily change of bandages. The infection resolved in few days.

7. Discussion

In our experience, Ultrasound-assisted liposculpture (UAL) presents important advantages when compared to traditional liposuction we used before 1994. UAL, allowed us to deliver good aesthetic sculpting and contouring results with preservation of connective, vascular and lymphatic structures, low blood loss and minimal bruising, significant skin retraction capability and weight loss to normal in the first six months (Fig.5, 6, 7, 8), and shortened downtime. All surgeries were done as outpatient.

Highly satisfactory aesthetic results and tiny inconspicuous scars have led us to utilize UAL even in cases of highly pretentious patients like models (Fig. 3). The change of the inner knee fat form and position, visible relative leg elongation and beautification became one of the most requested procedures of UAL in our practice.

The excellent results supported new indications and future developments of "high definition" techniques.

In our experience the UAL has given the possibility to perfect our technique and results.

8. Conclusion

This study confirms other author's conclusions that UAL is an effective and safe ambulatory treatment technique in experienced hands when attention is given to proper regulations for application of ultrasound energy [20, 40].

The advantages of UAL are decreased bruising, reduced blood loss, overall faster healing, short downtime, and reduction in post-operative discomfort.

We have often used UAL as a "fine-tuning" to treat liposuction irregularities in secondary cases, since it allows for more precision. Using the ultrasound selection of fat cells, we can affect only the irregular fat collections and the superficial subdermal fat layer will be preserved.

UAL increases the safety and minimizes risks because of the reduced trauma and minimized amount of blood removed through UAL. Ultrasonic assisted liposuction is intended to create improved body contouring and harmony. It is safer technique for removing larger amounts of fat compared to other techniques or standard liposuction. Ultrasound action after surgery causes some weight loss all over the body with skin tightening that get noticed in the first 6 months, with remarkable tightening at the end of 18 months. One of the most important advantages of our method is the smooth result.

We believe that UAL is a safe, effective, and easily acceptable procedure for body contouring[18,, 20, 26-28].

9. References

[1] Fischer, A, Fischer GM, First surgical treatment for modeling body's cellulite with three 5mm. incisions. Bulletin of the International Academy of Cosmetic Surgery, September, 1976

[2] Fisher A, Fisher GM: Revised technique for cellulitis fat reduction in riding breeches deformity. Bull lnt Acad Cosmet Surg 1977; 2:
[3] Klein JA. The tumescent technique for liposuction surgery. J Am Acad Cosmetic Surg 4:263-267,1987.
[4] Klein JA. Anesthesia for liposuction in dermatologic surgery. J Derm Surg Oncol 14:11 24- 1132,1988.
[5] Stewart JH, Cole GW, Klein JA. Neutralized lidocaine with epinephrine for local anesthesia. J Dermatol Surg Oncol 15:1081-1083,1989.
[6] Klein JA. Tumescent technique for regional anesthesia permits lidocaine doses of 35 mg/kg for liposuction. J Derm Surg Oncol 16:248-263,1990.
[7] Scuderi N, De Vita R, D'Andrea F. Nouve prospettive nella liposuzione: La lipoemulsificazione. G Chir. 1987;2:1-10.
[8] Zocchi M: New perspective in lipoplasty: The ultrasonic assisted lipectomy (U.A.L.). Presented at the Congress of the French Society of Aesthetic Surgery, Paris, May 1988.
[9] Illouz YG: Body contouring by lipolysis. A 5-year experience with over 3,000 cases. Plast Beconstr Surg 1983; 72:591.
[10] Illouz YG: Surgical remodeling of the silhouette by aspiration lipolysis or se- lective lipectomy. Aesthetic Plast Surg 1985; 9:7.
[11] Fournier P: Liposculpture - Ma Technique. Paris, Arnette, 1989.
[12] Kesselring U, Meyer R: A suction curette for removal of excessive local deposits of subcutaneous fat. Plast Beconstr Surg 1978; 62:305.
[13] Agris J: Suction Assisted Lipectomy: A Clinical Atlas. Houston, Eclectic Pub- lishing, 1983.
[14] Avelar J, Illouz YG: Lipoaspiracao, ed 1. Sao Paulo, Editoria Hipocrates, 1986.
[15] Grazer FM: Suction-assisted lipectomy, suction lipectomy, lipolysis, and li- pexeresis. Plast Beconstr Surg 1983; 72:620.
[16] Kucera IJ, Lambert TJ, Klein JA, et al. Liposuction: contemporary issues for the anesthesiologist. J Clin Anesth. 2006;18(5).
[17] Pinto et al. Liposuction and VASER. Ibid, 108-110
[18] Baker ML, Dalrymple GV: Biological effects of diagnostic ultrasound. Badi- ology 1978; 126:479.
[19] Bartoletti, C.A., Ceccarelli, M., About the Use of Ultrasound at 3 MHz in the Treatment of Localized Adiposity, The Aesthetic Medicine, 1990, No. 1
[20] Baxter, RA. Histologic Effects of Ultrasound-assisted Lipoplasty Aesthetic Surgery Journal March 1999 , 19: 2: 109-114, doi:10.1053/aq.1999.v19.97391
[21] Bartoletti, C.A., Ceccarelli, M., Pignatelli, V., Hydrolipoclasis Ultrasound in the Treatment of Localized Fat Excess: a Modification of the Protocol and Further Evaluation, The Aesthetic Medicine, 1995, No. 2
[22] Apfelberg DB, Rosenthal S, Hunstad JP at al. Progress report on multicenter study of laser-assisted liposuction, , Aesthetic Plastic Surgery, Volume 18, Number 3, 1994 ,Springer New York
[23] Bartoletti, C.A., Ceccarelli, M., Localized Adiposity and Ultrasonic Hydrolipoclasis, The Aesthetic Medicine, 1992, No. 2

[24] Ceccarelli, M., Chimenti, S., Colantonio, A., Santarelli Marino, AR., Magnetic Resonance Imaging in Monitoring the Treatment of Lipomas with Ultrasonic Hydrolipoclasis, The Aesthetic Medicine, 1994, No. 2
[25] Ceccarelli M. The Hydrolipoclasis Ultrasound, The Aesthetic Medicine, 1997, No. 2
[26] Zocchi M: La liposculpture aux ultra-sons. Actes du Congres d'hiver de la Societe Vran g aise de Chirurgie Esthetique, Paris, Nov 1990
[27] Zocchi M: Liposcultura Ultrasonica. Torino, Italy, Edizioni Scienti6che Cor- tina, 1992.
[28] Zocchi M: Ultrasonic liposculpturing. Aesthetic Plast Surg 1992; 16: 287 - 298.Mark Laurence Jewell. Lipoplasty. In: M. Eisenmann-Klein, Constance Neuhann-Lorenz, eds. Innovations in Plastic and Aesthetic Surgery. Springer, Berlin Germany; 2006:439-444
[29] Haeck, P.C.; Swanson, J.A.; Iverson, R.E; Schechter, L.S.; Singer, R.; Bob Basu, C.; Damitz, L.A.; Glasberg, S.B.; Glassman, L.S.; McGuire, M.F. & the ASPS Patient Safety Committee (2009). Evidence-Based Patient Safety Advisory: Patient Selection and Procedures in Ambulatory Surgery. Plastic and Reconstructive Surgery, Vol. 124, No. 4S, (October 2009), pp. (6S-27S).
[30] Gasparotti M: Superficial liposuction for flaccid skin patients. Presented at the International Symposium on Recent Advances in Plastic Surgery, Sao Paulo, Brazil, March 28 - 30, 1990, p 443.
[31] Gasperoni C, Salgarello M, Emiliozzi P, et al: Subdermal liposuction. Aesthetic Plast Surg 1990; 14:137 - 142.
[32] Gasparotti M: Superficial liposuction: A new application of the technique for aged and flaccid skin. Aesthetic Plast Surg 1992; 16:141 - 153
[33] Baxter RA, Histologic Effects of Ultrasound-assisted Lipoplasty Aesthetic Surgery Journal March 1999 , 19: 2: 109-114, doi:10.1053/aq.1999.v19.97391
[34] Regnault P: Basic principles and indications of liposuction, in Regnault P, Daniel RK (eds): Aesthetic P l astic Surgery. Boston, Little, Brown, 1984, pp 679 - 692.
[35] Teimourian B: Suction Lipectomy and Body Sculpturing. St Louis, Mosby, 1987.
[36] Heymans O, Castus P, Grandjean FX, Van Zele D. Liposuction: review of the techniques, innovations and applications. Acta Chir Belg. Nov-Dec 2006;106(6):647-53.
[37] Schruddle J: Lipexeresis (liposuction) for body contouring. Clin Plast Surg 1984; 11:445.
[38] Pitman GH, Teimourian B: Suction lipeetomy: Complications and results by survey. Plast Reconstr Surg 1985; 76:65 - 72.
[39] Bruno, G, Amadei F, Abbiati G., Aesthetic Plastic Surgery, 1998, Volume 22, Number 6, Pages 401-403
[40] Gingrass MK, Kenkel JM. Comparing ultrasound-assisted lipoplasty with suction-assisted lipoplasty. Institute for Aesthetic and Reconstructive Surgery, Nashville, Tennessee, USA
[41] Serdev, N. Leg beautification and elongation using ultrasonic liposculpture, Int J Cosm Surg. 2009, Volume 9, Number 1, Pages: 1-84
[42] Serdev, N. Body beautification, straight and elongated legs using UAL, Int J Cosm Surg. 2010, Volume 10, Number 3, 1
[43] Ross, R.M. & Johnson, G.W. Fat Embolism After Liposuction. Chest, Vol. 93, June, 1988, 1294-1295

[44] Grazer, F.M. & de Jong, R.H. Fatal outcomes from liposuction: Census survey of cosmetic surgeons. Plastic and Reconstructive Surgery 105:436

[45] Illouz YG. 2006. Complications of liposuction. Clin Plast Surg. Jan;33(1):129-63

[46] Fodor, PB. Watson, J. Personal Experience with Ultrasound-Assisted Lipoplasty: A Pilot Study Comparing Ultrasound-Assisted Lipoplasty with Traditional Lipoplasty, Plastic & Reconstructive Surgery: April 1998 - Volume 101 - Issue 4 - pp 1103-1116

[47] Gottlieb, S. (2004). "Liposuction does not achieve metabolic benefits of weight loss". BMJ 328 (7454): 1457.

[48] Rohrich RJ, Ha RY, Kenkel JM, Adams WP Jr. Classification and management of gynecomastia: defining the role of ultrasound-assisted liposuction. Plast Reconstr Surg. Feb 2003;111(2):909-23; discussion 924-5.

[49] Góes JC, Landecker A. Ultrasound-assisted lipoplasty (UAL) in breast surgery. Aesthetic Plast Surg. 2002 Jan-Feb;26(1):1-9.

[50] Park S. Very superficial ultrasound-assisted lipoplasty for the treatment of axillary osmidrosis. Aesthetic Plast Surg. 2000 Jul-Aug;24(4):275-9.

[51] Lawrence N, Coleman WP 3rd. Ultrasonic-assisted liposuction. Internal and external. Dermatol Clin. Oct 1999;17(4):761-71.

[52] Lawrence N, Cox SE. The efficacy of external ultrasound-assisted liposuction: a randomized controlled trial. Dermatol Surg. Apr 2000;26(4):329-32.

[53] Flynn TC, Coleman WP III, Field LM et al. History of liposuction, Dermatol Surg. 2000; 26:515-520

Part 2

Lipotransfer and Stem Cell Enriched Fat Transfear

10

Advanced Lipotransfer Techniques

Guillermo Blugerman et al.*
Argentina

1. Introduction

1.1 Liposhifting: Treatment of post-liposuction irregularities

One of the most frequent complications after liposuction is the presence of residual fat accompanied by surface irregularities such as ridges, waves and depressions.
According to some statistics, about 15 to 20% of liposuction require some type of secondary correction to fill irregularities or should have a second session of liposuction to improve the result. Gerald Pittmann (1) states that a 15% required minor adjustments or lipofillings in office, and 9% required a second liposuction with or without lipofilling.
Until 2001, post-liposuction irregularities were attempted to be corrected by auto-graft of fat cells aspirated from other body areas, with varying results over time (2). Lipofilling as unique technique has not proven to be the correct solution for such irregularities. There is evidence that the transfer of large volumes of fat in an unfavorable area, as it occurs after liposuction does not survive. In our opinion this is not the best option to fill post-liposuction irregularities (3,4). In 2001, after many years of disappointment with fat fillings in post-liposuction irregularities, Dr. Ziya Saylan (5) decided to internally mobilize the surrounding fat tissue to the affected area without any vacuum, suction, contact with air or injection. He named this new technique liposhifting. With internal lipomobilization or liposhifting, the fat tissue is cut into micro grafts that are mobilized under the skin without any suction and without removing the fat from the body during the procedure. Avoiding contact with air lowers the risk of apoptosis promoted by dehydration of fat tissue. After the internal lipomobilization a special type of bandage and fixation is needed for the first 48 hours. The results obtained have been very satisfactory.

1.2 Our approach

Our experience is that the lipofilling of small liposuction irregularities can be useful, but never offers a long-term outcome for large irregularities or undulations. After a few months, a great quantity of the injected fat disappears and sometimes patients complain of new

* Roger Amar[1], Diego Schavelzon[2], Marco A. Pelosi II[3], Marco A. Pelosi III[3], Javier A. Soto[4], Anastasia Chomyszyn[2], Maurizio Podda[5], Andrea V. Markowsky[4], Jorge A. D'Angelo[4] and Rodrigo Moreno[4]
[1]*Amar Clinic, Marbella, Malaga*
[2,4]*Centros B&S "Excelencia en Cirugía Plástica", Buenos Aires, Argentina*
[3]*Pelosi Medical Center, Bayonne, NewYersey*
[5]*Department of Dermatology of Darmstadt Hospital,German,*
[4]*Universidad Nacional del Nordeste, Corrientes, Argentina*

undulations at the donor site. In liposhifting, as published by Saylan, avoiding suction (which causes tissue damage), by not removing the tissue from the body (no pressure, no contact with air) and no re-injection (applied external force on the fat to be grafted), ensures the production of adipose tissue micro-grafts of excellent quality and vitality.
Based on this work, in 2001 we began to apply the technique originally described by Saylan, with good results but, looking for a more predictable result, in 2002 we therefore designed a set of specific instruments for this useful technique [6,7,8,9]. (Fig. 1)

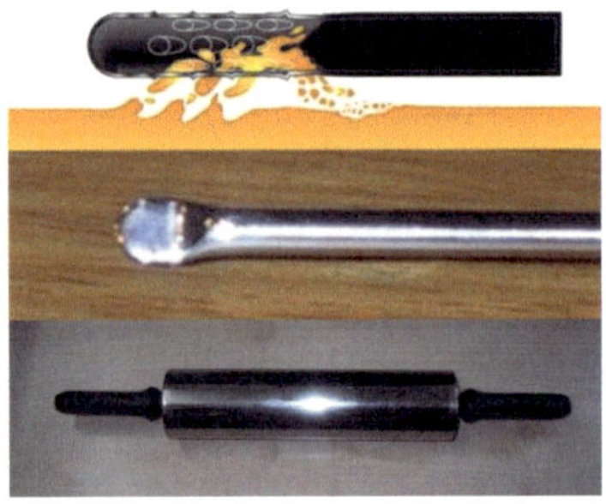

Fig. 1. Liposhifting instruments set.

This set of instruments has three basic elements.

- A spatula dissector with atraumatic flat and round tip to make pre-tunelization of the receptor area with minimal bleeding given that hematoma formation diminishes the possibility of "engraftment of fat."
- A tubular knife cannula named Micro Graft Fat Cutter, (MGFC) with multiple cutting edge holes of 1.5 mm in diameter, distributed in the first 2 centimeters from the tip and two holes of 3 mm in diameter located proximately to allow the output without damaging the fat tissue micrografts. This instrument looks similar to a liposuction cannula, its main difference is that it has no connection to the vacuum pump, and operates as a "cheese grater" in the fatty tissue, cutting and releasing microscopic portions of adipose tissue in the donor areas, which remain floating in the tumescent solution.
- The third element is a roller that is used over the skin surface in order to mobilize these grafts in the spatula creating tunnels in the recipient area.

1.3 Patient selection

Patients that can be favored with this technique are those with a localized deficit of adipose tissue, with available donor areas around them.
This group includes:

- Sequelae of liposuction.
- Fat atrophy from application of steroids.
- Circular fat atrophy.
- Depressed scars or scars adhered to deep planes.
- Sequels of abscesses or hematomas drainage.
- Traumatic fat atrophy.
- Irregularities after lipofilling.

1.4 Technique

This procedure must meet the following stages:

- Pictures with frontal and tangential light. (Fig. 2)
- Marking the skin with the patient standing.
- Tumescent Anesthesia.
- Creation of receptor tunnels in the depressed zones (receptors).
- Preparation of adipose tissue micrografts with MGFC in the donor area.
- Mobilizing micrografts.
- Tunneling
- Stabilization of mobilized tissue. (Microporing and Reston foam for fixing)

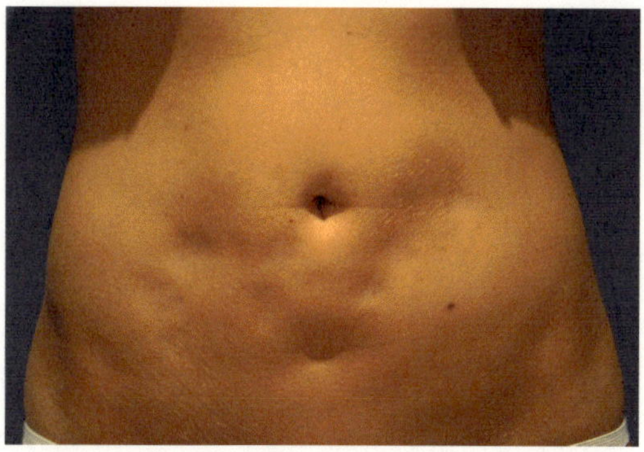

Fig. 2. Taking photographs with a tangential light is an important key to document the patients defect. See patient post-op in Fig. 5.

1.4.1 Marking the skin

The marking of the skin is very important because the tumescent anesthesia hides the fat irregularities. The markings have to be done while the patient is standing, which allows the surgeon to locate appropriate sites for liposhifting. Edges, elevations and undulations should be marked with different colors. Do not forget that when the patient lies on the operating table fatty deposits surrounding depression can change their position. The place where the fat is required should be marked (receiving area) with one color and the surrounding area where the tissue is obtained (donor area) with a different one. Photographic documentation of marking is very important for future comparison (Fig.3)

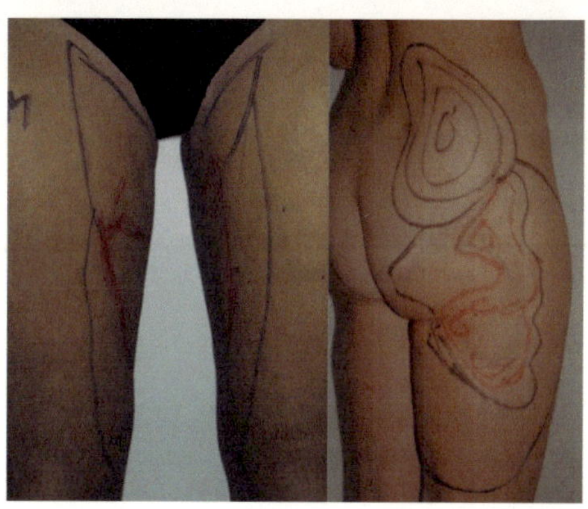

Fig. 3. A previous marking and photograph is important for an optimal result.

1.4.2 Anesthesia

We perform this type of procedures under tumescent anesthesia [(10)] given that the presence of fluid facilitates the internal mobilization of the micrografts, and this also allows us to vary the position of the patient during the procedure for the proper location of the fat to be mobilized.

1.4.3 Tumescent technique

The tumescent solution is used to lubricate the adipose tissue, to provide anesthesia, to stabilize tissues and also to re-expand the collapsed areas by excessive resection of adipose tissue in previous liposuction.
After infiltration of tumescent solution, time is required to diffuse into the tissues, lending the necessary vasoconstriction to reduce the risk of hematoma and allowing the instrument to glide smoothly cutting accurately the micrografts.

1.4.4 Tunneling or tunnel creation in the target tissues

The spatula is inserted through a two mm incision in the skin held from the edges of the marking, at least 3 cm to prevent graft loss during mobilization maneuvers. Multiple tunnels must be made throughout the thickness of subcutaneous tissue (SCT). These tunnels will be used as beds for fat grafting receptors.
It is important to use the spatula's flat tip perpendicular to the skin surface to diminish trauma of the vascular plexus that runs along the walls of the SCT from the muscles to the skin. (Fig.4)

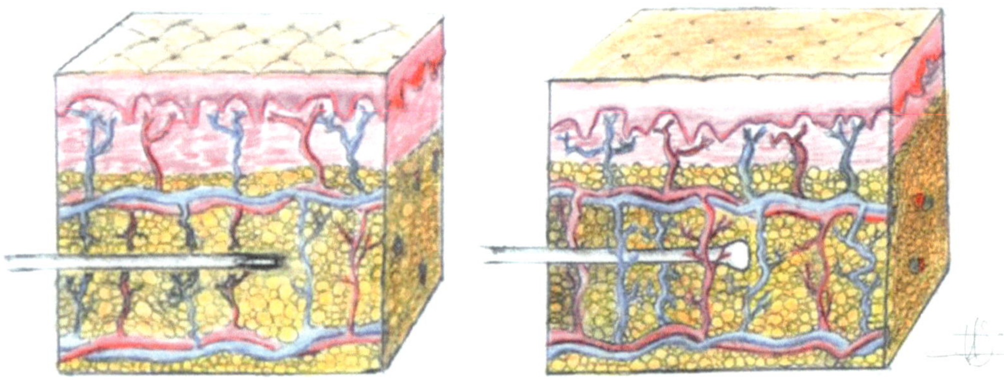

Fig. 4. Incorrect way of using the spatula cannula when doing the tunnels, will lead to damage the blood vessels.

The correct way of using the spatulated cannula is perpendicularly regarding the skin, thus preserving the vascular plexus.

1.4.5 Preparation micrografts

Tumescent anesthesia stabilizes the fatty tissue of the donor area allowing the fat to acquire consistency enough so it can be cut with the edge of the holes of the cannula. For this purpose, we introduce the MGFC through the same incision, to be mobilized under the skin in a criss-cross technique to produce grafts from the donor areas.

1.4.6 Quality of the micrografts

To assess the quality of micrografts and their ability to survive, Dr Maurizio Podda (11) in 2003 conducted a study in the Department of Dermatology at the Goethe University of Frankfurt. The study consisted of the separation of fat cells obtained from different types of cannulas and a portion cut with a scalpel with collagenase. They measured total lipids and DNA. Lipolysis was stimulated in these cells with Isoproterenol and Fosfokin, and the production of glycerol was spectrophotometrically measured.
These evaluations established that grafts taken with a scalpel, with Liposhifting cannula and vibrating cannula tip were the ones which showed greater survival rate.
The results have shown that micrografts obtained with cannula Liposhifting have the same quality and percentage of survival than those obtained with a scalpel and were better than those obtained with vacuum suction (fig.4).

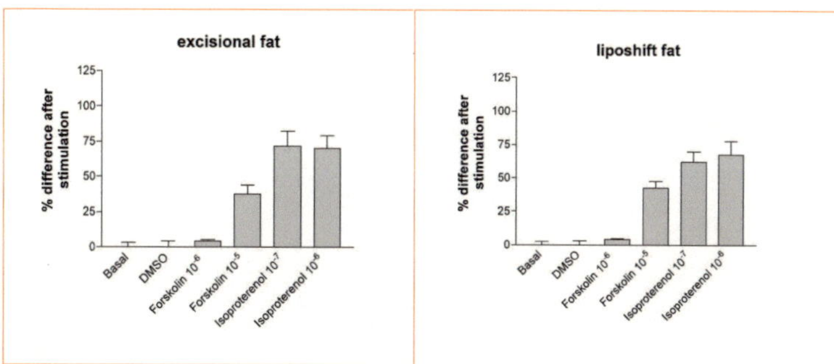

Fig. 4. Dr Maurizio Podda´s study showing similar survival rate from the grafts taken with the scalpel and the MGFC.

1.4.7 Mobilization

The mobilization of fat under the skin is effected by rolling maneuvers and massages on the skin directed from the donor to the recipient areas.
A 6-9mm thick cannula may be useful for this purpose. The cannula is held in the surgeon's hands like a rolling pin, and the fatty tissue under the skin will move to the imperfection that is to be filled. The place to fill must be watched very carefully and when the pit is full it reaches the same level of the surrounding skin, overcorrection of 20-30% is is thought to represent the amount of tumescent solution which will be absorbed in a few hours. During these maneuvers the entrance hole should be closed with a suture to prevent loss of micrografts.

1.4.8 Fixation

After fat mobilization into the depressed area, a Micropore® tape fastening and Reston® are placed to keep the fat in its new site. Pressure is applied to the donor parts and no compression is left in the receiving areas. The film and the setting can be removed after 72 hours.

1.5 Results

We have applied this technique in 140 patients over a period of seven years. Some cases with large defects should be treated more than once. This should be explained to the patient before surgery. An interval of 4 to 6 months is recommended between treatments. The final results are not ready before 3-6 months. The rate of patient satisfaction was nearly 90%. The same results were obtained by other authors [12] (Fig.5, 6 and 7).

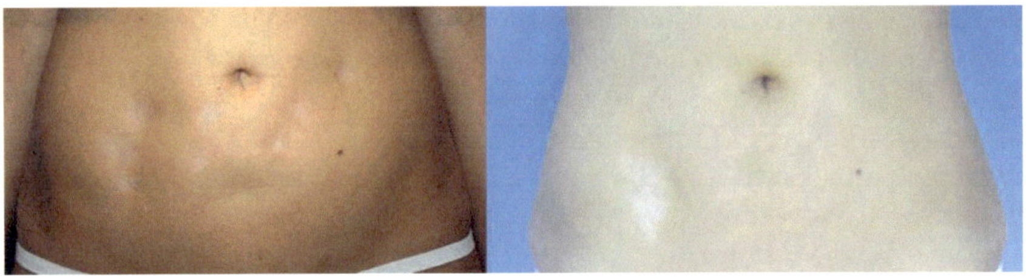

Fig. 5. Pre-operative and post-operative results of liposhifting after 10 months, in a patient with fat and dermal atrophy after intralesional steroid injection.

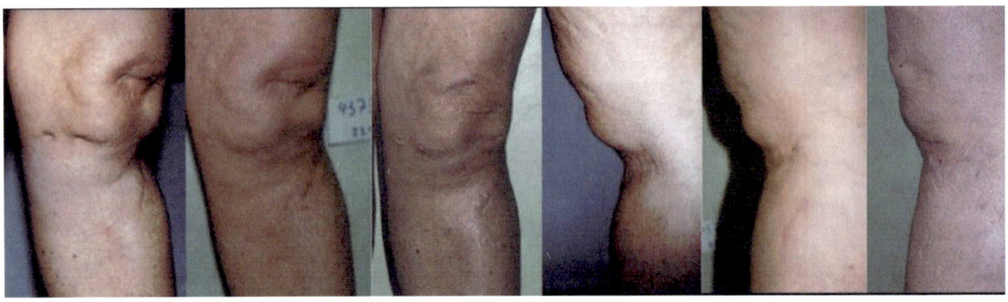

Fig. 6. Pre-operative and post-operative results in traumatic scaring in knee.

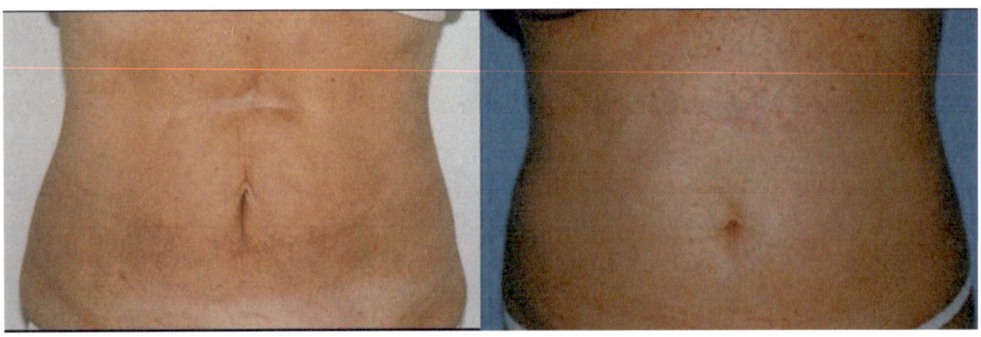

Fig. 7. Before and after liposhifting of a post-liposuction defect.

1.6 Complications

The most common complication was hematoma at the recipient site when we used sharp prongs for tunneling, the incidence decreased markedly with the use of a spatula perpendicularly to the skin.

We had no cases of infection. Hypoesthesia was more often seen than in liposuction, but it disappears after a few months.

Hemosiderin pigmentation (pigmentation of the superficial dermis by the iron in the blood) was seen in two cases that had bruises and remained between 6 and 9 months. In these cases we used a gel with heparinoids that enhances resolution.

1.7 Conclusions

We believe Liposhifting is a very good technique to eliminate extensive and deep subcutaneous tissue irregularities caused by liposuction or due to trauma and previous surgery. As a single procedure it reduces the volume of surrounding tissue and fill the central defect, so that ultimately a smaller volume of tissue is moved and so the success rate rises considerably.

It is useful both in the limbs and in the abdominal region. It is practical and safe. The risk of contamination of the fat transplant, having no contact with air, is impossible. The fixation of the treated region is very important to stabilize the mobilized fat and to raise its survival.

2. Enriched adipose micrografts with autologous plasma (EAM)

2.1 Summary

Liposuction fat transfer used to fill facial and body areas is now one of the most fascinating treatments of plastic, reconstructive, and cosmetic surgery.

Still today it is common to have reports of failures with the traditional technique of harvesting by liposuction, which is why we have refined the technique in each step in order to obtain Micrografts of adipose tissue that are of better quality to ensure a good survival of these once grafted into the recipient area.

Micrografting implantation in combination with Total Plasma (TP) or Platelet Rich Plasma (PRP) has allowed in our hands to achieve more predictable and permanent results opening a wide range of therapeutic possibilities, ranging from cosmetic to reconstructive procedures.

Plasma from the patient is an autologous non-toxic, non allergenic preparation, easily obtained by centrifugation of blood. Once the platelets are activated and mixed with the collected micrografts, you obtain a gel that is a natural support for the transplanted tissue, favoring the formation of extracellular matrix, collagen fibers and angiogenesis in an accelerated way. It promotes neovascularization and decreases the reabsorption of the grafted adipose tissue.

In our opinion, Enriched Adipose Micrografting (EAM) is now the ideal material for the restoration of aesthetic or postraumatic subcutaneous tissue defects of the face and body.

2.2 Introduction

The use of autologous fat as a filler has been around for over 100 years. In 1983 [13,14], fat grafts were made to achieve tissue remodeling and improve asymmetries with good results. In 1910 Erix Lexer [15] used autologous fat to improve depression made from zygomatic fractures with acceptable results and stable for years, and later, Peer [16] reaffirmed the use and survival of these grafts. The biggest problem remained the need for extirpation of adipose tissue through acceptable skin incisions.

The introduction of liposuction in the 80's opened new possibilities of obtaining fat and subsequent grafting, without scarring sequelae in the donor area. Our first results were presented at the Brazilian Congress Belho Horizonte in 1986 [17]. Since then we continue to improve our technique, looking for the best protocol to cover all aspects of this procedure, despite being easily reproducible, it has a high rate of failure if the basic principles of tissue transplantation are not respected [18].

This chapter summarizes our current technique of EAM, based on the results of the last 5 consecutive years of its application.

2.3 Healing and growth factors

Healing is a process that takes time and compliance with a series of steps that begin with the activation of multiple growth factors. The increased availability of these factors during this process shortens time and improves results, reducing inflammatory reaction and scarring sequelae.

The availability of growth factors (GF) at the tissue level may be increased using autologous platelet concentrate obtained from the patient's own blood.

Growth Factors (GF) are polypeptides of amino acids that form a globular protein and belong to the group of cytokines. They are produced in greater quantities by macrophages and platelets [19, 20].

These cytokines have the ability to join cell membrane receptors that activate or inhibit cellular functions by target cells on which they act.

The most studied growth factors are:

- The epithelial growth factor. It was the first to be discovered. It induces proliferation of epidermal cells in-vitro. It is a peptide of 52 amino acids produced by keratinocytes, platelets, the kidney, the gastrointestinal tract and the brain. It stimulates the synthesis of DNA and RNA from keratinocytes and fibroblasts, and helps in wound repair.
- The Growth Factor of Fibroblasts is a peptide derived from fibroblasts. It increases the division of the keratinocytes, promotes epithelialization of the tissues and provides tensile strength to collagen matrix.
- The Growth Factor, Platelet-derived is the one with the highest participation in wound repair. Its effect is vasoconstriction and stimulation of mitosis and chemotaxis of polymorphonuclear cells, monocytes, keratinocytes, fibroblasts and endothelial cells. The arrival of platelets to the site of injury causes a rapid activity of this factor and therefore an early wound repair.
- The use of growth factors was initiated in the field of maxillofacial surgery and dentistry as a biological material to stimulate bone remodeling, and then its use was expanded to other areas of medical science.

2.3 EAM Indications

2.3.1 Facial corrections

- Poorly defined jaw line.
- Naso-labial fold, looking sad or tired.
- Lip augmentation to correct thin lips achieving greater volume and more youthful appearance-[21, 22, 23].
- Asymmetries or lack of volume on cheeks and malar or chin area.
- Facial lipo-dystrophy in patients with HIV treatment or Romberg Syndrome [24].

2.3.2 Body corrections

- Surface defects by subsidence, posttraumatic sequelae or scarring.
- Imperfections or asymmetries from previous surgical procedures.
- Hand defects, reaching its rejuvenation [25].
- Buttock contour deformities [26, 27, 28].
- Any type of asymmetric atrophy or hypotrophy of soft tissue.
- Correction or lengthening of the penile region [29].
- Post-Mammary Implant deformities, with or without removal of implant placed.

- Breast deformities such us: Tuberose breast, micromastia, Poland Syndrome, breast tissue damage by radiation therapy.
- Post-surgical chest deformities.
- Defects caused by conservative or reconstructive breast treatment using implants and/or flaps (latissimus or rectus abdominis).
- Cosmetic-gynecological procedures.

2.4 Surgical technique

2.4.1 Documentation and marking [30]

The recognition of the problem areas must be made initially (donor and recipient) by the surgeon, in consultation with the patient, documenting them with pictures. Patient selection and the realistic expectations of possible outcomes are important points to arrive at a good percentage of satisfied patients. Photographs, as well as the marking of the patient, are made standing so that the posture does not change the default. In some surface defects, a tangential light on the skin is useful for a better documentation and marking of the defects. It is important to use natural colored long-term markers to avoid erasure during the procedure. The main issue to consider when choosing the donor site is to approach a site with adequate tissue volume, which is specific to each patient, and also taking into account the surgeon's preference. There is no heavy evidence on the choice of the donor site in the efficacy of fat grafting, but some studies suggest that there are areas with a higher number of stem cells than others.

2.4.2 Obtaining inactive plasma

Before starting the procedure, obtain a blood sample from the patient, and then process it, to obtain the TP, or PRP, given that, after the surgical procedure has started, there is going to be a lower platelet count in the patient´s blood.

Following our protocol we proceed to extract the blood with a 20 ml sterile syringe in cases where the treatment was carried out in the facial region and a 40 ml of blood when the treatment was performed in a body area. (Fig. 8)

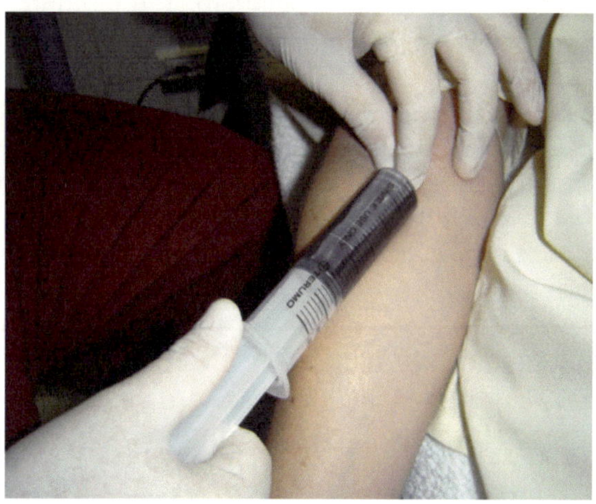

Fig. 8. Obtaining the patient's blood before the surgery is important to maintain a good platelet count.

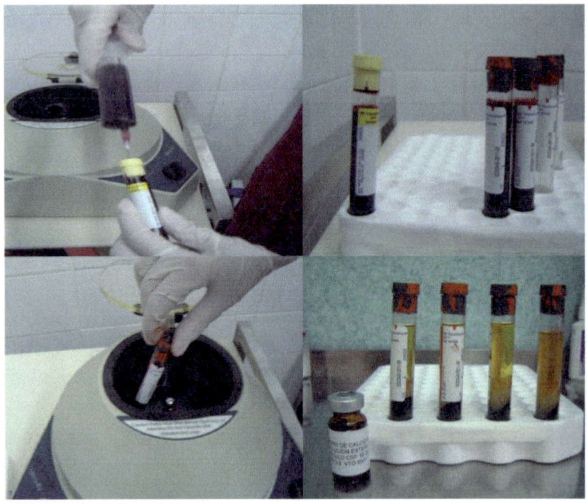

Fig. 9. Blood components separation process.

The blood is collected in tubes of 8.5 ml. each, containing calcium citrate (BD Vacutainer ® ACD Solution A) to prevent activation of the coagulation process. Then the anticoagulated blood is passed to other special tubes that contain a separation gel (BD Vacutainer ® SST) that allows mechanical separation of red cells and plasma during centrifugation. The separation process is performed at 3000rpm for 10 minutes using our equipment, so this step will be adaptable to the functionality of each centrifuge. (Fig.9.)

2.4.3 Anesthesia of the donor area

The use of epinephrine or lidocaine in the donor site, has been acused to affect the viability of the graft, but there is not much research about it. Following the previous markings anesthetic infiltration of the donor site is performed using tumescent anesthesia with a solution composed of 0.06% lidocaine with epinephrine 1:1000000 and 12.5 meq of sodium bicarbonate for each liter of saline (0.9%Na Solution). The infiltration is performed using Klein cannulas connected to the B&S peristaltic pump [31].

2.4.4 Anesthesia of the receiving area

Likewise, through microcannulas or selected needles according to the graft area, we proceed with local anesthesia of the receiving area previously marked. Same concentrations of tumescent anesthesia are used without infiltrating large quantities of liquid, so it does not modify the area to be corrected, achieving only anesthetic effect. In the face we prefer the nerve blocks as described by Amar [32].

2.4.5 Preparing micrografts of adipose tissue [33, 34, 35, 36, 37, 38, 39]

The main points to consider when taking the tissue are the degree of tissue invasiveness (patient safety) and tissue viability (efficiency). With this in mind, mechanical damage is minimized in this step.

In our protocol, the procedure requires the use of specific instruments, which we called MGFC (Micro Graft Fat Cutter) or BGC (Blugerman Graft Cutter). (Fig.10)

In the study by Dr. Maurizio Podda, University of Frankfurt [40] it was found that the micrografts obtained with our instrumental had the same characteristics and survival rate than grafts cut with a scalpel, surpassing those obtained with liposuction cannulas. This instrument could be defined as a tubular multiscalpel that works without suction or vacuum, cutting edge micrografts by presenting the holes, which act similarly to those of a grater, aided by external compression of the fingers pushing the adipose tissue into the holes to facilitate the splitting of the tissue.

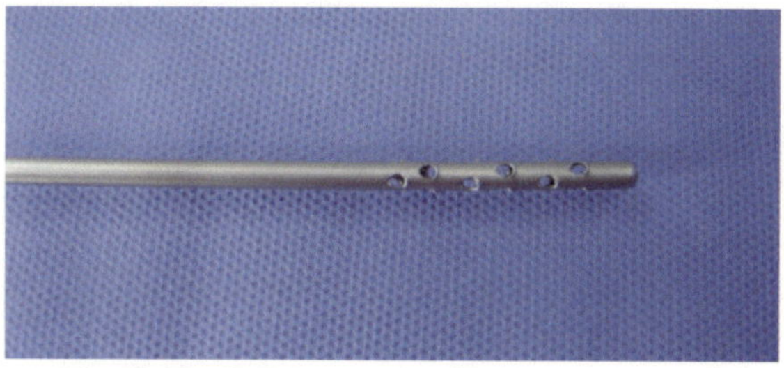

Fig. 10. Blugerman Graft Cutter (BGC).

Micrografts produced by the actions of MGFC remain suspended in the tumescent solution in the donor area, ready for collection.

2.4.6 Collection of manufactured micrografts

To collect the micrografts we prefer to use a 3 to 4 mm large hole atraumatic blunt cannula. This step is performed by sucking the material with 10 ml syringes at low vacuum pressure, when the volume required is small, or with a B&S peristaltic pump when volume is larger.
In our hands, using the B&S peristaltic pump to recover micrografts in the donor site allows us to work in a closed circuit, minimizing the risk of contamination, preventing the entry of large volumes of contaminated air and avoiding the "Cyclone" effect inside the bottle.
Reduced air contact also avoids fat dehydration with a consequent decreased rate of apoptosis, thus ensuring a better vitality of micrografts.

2.4.7 Settling or centrifugation of the material [41, 42, 43, 44, 45, 46, 47, 48]

When we work in the facial region, the material obtained is centrifuged at 3000 rpm for 3 minutes to separate the micrografts from the tumescent fluid and the oil resulting from the rupture of adipocytes.
When using volumes exceeding 100 cc. we prefer to decant the material, without any filtering or transfer.
The special features that our system has, allow the tissue to be sucked in through a hole in the bottom of the collector and immediately there is an automatic washing of grafts in the previously sucked fluid, making the process of separation by gravity faster and more efficient than using a top hole bottle. This avoids the need of any material washing before implanting and minimizes the risk of contamination.
Finally, by reversing the direction of rotation of the peristaltic B&S pump, tumescent fluid is removed leaving only the concentration of micrografts ready to use.

2.4.8 Plasma activation

The platelet concentrate (600,000 to 1,500,000 x mm) obtained from blood centrifugation has a first supernatant that corresponds to the platelet-poor plasma (PPP), and the second corresponding the Platelet Rich Plasma (PRP), which is the portion closest to the Red Blood Cels (RBCs). (Fig.11)

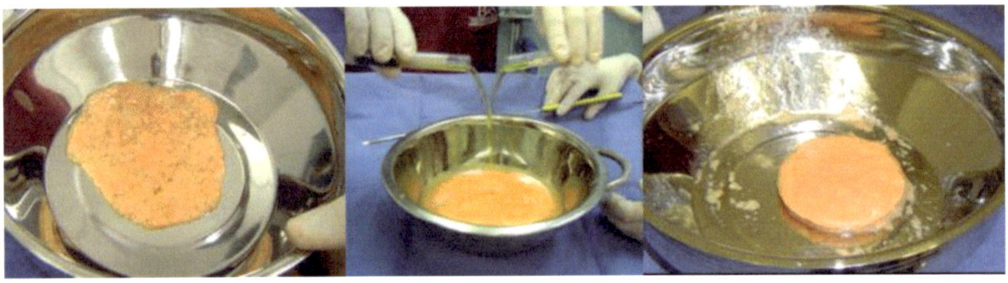

Fig. 11. Enriching the adipose tissue micrografts with plasma. EAM gelification.

When using facial EAM, in which precision in milliliters is important, we use only the PRP to prevent dilution of micrografts.
When working in the body area, we use TP, as we add the PRP properties to the PPP, which is the residual plasma and contains clotting factors, mainly fibrinogen, thrombin and calcium molecules that stabilize the blood clot and contribute to a rapid and effective healing of the soft tissues.
In our experience the use of total plasma (PPP + PRP) in the process has submitted satisfactory and comparable with the use of PRP only, while this allows simplifying the procedure and reduces material handling with the risk of contamination.
Technically you activate the PRP or PT by adding 10% CaCl (0.05 cm3 of CaCl per 3 ml), thereby activating the coagulation cascade.

2.4.9 Preparation of the recipient's site [49]

Antisepsis of the recipient area and placement of surgical wraps are performed. If the local anesthesia of the recipient region has not been previously performed, this is the moment to do it, before the infiltration of the micrografts. Depending on the region to be treated micro-incisions are carried out taking into account the location of the defect and the aesthetic result on the skin.

2.4.10 Injection technique of EAM [50, 51]

To optimize the viability of enriched adipose micrografts the mechanical damage of the implanted tissue has to be minimized.
In the face we follow the basic principles of the FAMI technique.
In the body, we prefer subcutaneous implantation of the grafts instead of the muscular implantation, thus lowering the risk of fat embolism.
Prior to the implantation of micro grafts, the technique of pre-tunneling of the subcutaneous tissue (SCT) is done with the spatulated cannula (Fig. 12). By using the spatulated cannula it creates paths or tunnels on several levels where the micrografts will be deposited for better distribution.
This pre-tunneling should be done with the bevel of the spatulated cannula perpendicularly in respect to the surface of the skin in an attempt to preserve the sub-dermal plexus, which is highly needed to ensure rapid revascularization and consistent implementation of micrografts.

The preservation of the vascular elements also reduces the risk of hematoma, which if present leads to necrosis due to the loss of oxygenation and nutrition of micrografts in their early stages.

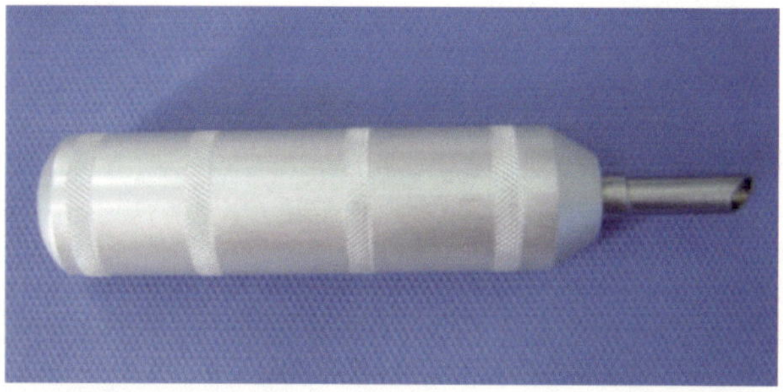

Fig. 12. Luer-loock cutter.

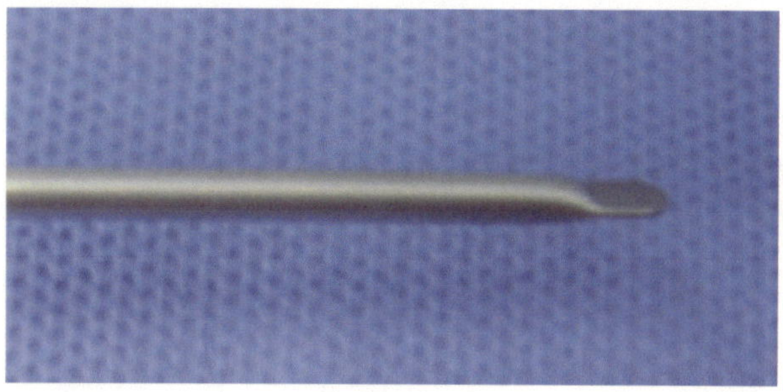

Fig. 13. Spatulated cannula.

From the mixing of micrografts and PRP or TP a gel is obtained (EAM) that is placed in 1 ml syringes when implemented in the facial region and in 5, 10 or 20 ml when used in the body. The syringes should have a Luer-Lock receptor. Using a special tool, the central portion of the beak is removed to increase the diameter of the hole through which the micrografts must pass. (Fig. 13)

Material injection in the facial area is performed using a set of micro-cannulas designed by Dr. Roger Amar, specific to each area and depth of the tissue following the FAMI technique parameters (fig 18).

When working in the body area we prefer the 1.5 to 3mm Tulip spatulated cannula (Fig. 14).

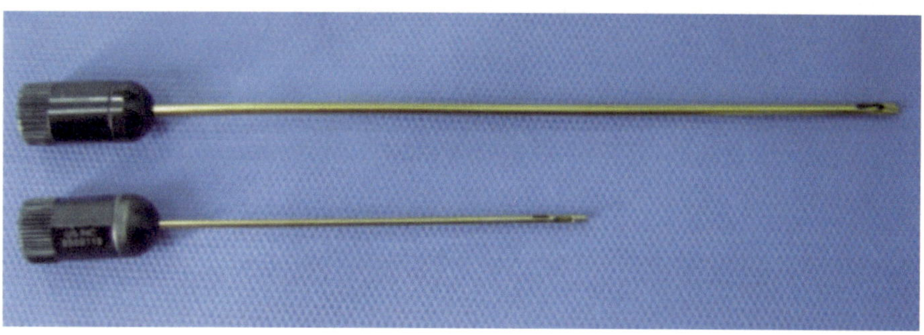

Fig. 14. Long and short tulip spatulated cannulas.

2.4.11 Retunelization

After the implementation of the micrografts, the spatula is reintroduced and new re-tunneling maneuvers are done using the same instrument that will continue to work perpendicularly to the skin. This maneuver will redistribute the grafted tissue more evenly and will reduce the compression exerted from the surrounding tissues to the micrografts.

2.4.12 Post-operation bandage

At the end of the procedure a bandage of the micro-incisions with sterile Micropore® tape is done in the recipient's area, exposing the treated area and leaving it free of compression. In special cases Reston® may be applied to keep the implanted areas free from external pressure. The donor site incisions are left opened to promote drainage of the tumescent solution, sterile dressings are placed and compressive bandaging is applied.

2.5 Risks and complications associated with fat grafts

- There were no reported cases of complications related to anesthesia and the use of fat grafting. These complications are rare considering that most cases are performed under local anesthesia with or without sedation, which minimizes the risk of surgery.
- Some cases were reported of patients with prolonged inflammation, Staphylococcus infection and septic shock, most treated with antibiotic therapy (52, 53).
- Regarding blood loss there were reported cases of seroma or hematoma associated with this procedure, but none were severe or unresolved (52, 53).
- Poor results or expectations that do not cover expected are rare (52, 53, 54,, 55). In general the results of this procedure are reported as excellent or good. Most cases reported as unsatisfactory, are due to the volume loss of the grafted tissue due to necrosis or reabsorption.
- Cases of graft hypertrophy or overgrowth have been documented on rare occasions.
- Other complications include the formation of calcified and non calcified masses.
- As for its relationship with breast cancer, although there is no strong evidence of interference, fat grafting is not recommended in patients potentially biased (56, 57, 58).
- Two cases of breast cancer were reported after the completion of fat grafts; however, this procedure did not interfere with the detection and treatment.
- Imaging studies (ultrasound, mammography and MRI) can identify fatty tissue grafts as micro-calcifications or the presence of suspicious lesions, determining the need for a biopsy to clarify the diagnosis if required.
- Based on the limited number of cases reported, we can establish that fat graft does not interfere with breast cancer, but further studies still needed to confirm.
- Other risks that should be taken into account are the level of invasiveness during the procedure, the experience of the surgeon and unforeseen complications during the procedure.
- The potentially severe or fatal cases are rare, considering the invasiveness of the procedure and the frequency with which it is performed.
- Patients should know the risks and potential complications, and sign an appropriate informed consent of the procedure (52, 53, 54, 55).

2.6 Results

We have used this EAM protocol over the past 5 years. (Fig. 15, 16 and 17)

During this period we have performed a total of 945 EAM procedures. 234 corresponded to facial applications and 711 to body applications. The patient satisfaction was high in all procedures. Our complication rate was less than 10 %.

It is important to inform patients about the possibility of re-implantation of new micrografts in the treated area, based on the concept of a progressive increase in volume, so that the patient is prepared for this eventuality.

In our case the need for further sessions of EAM depended on the degree of the defect and the results achieved, with a maximum of 3 sessions in the most complex cases which corresponded to 15% of the treated cases.

It is clear that in most cases the second procedure corresponded to minor corrections or minimum volume of tissue irregularities.

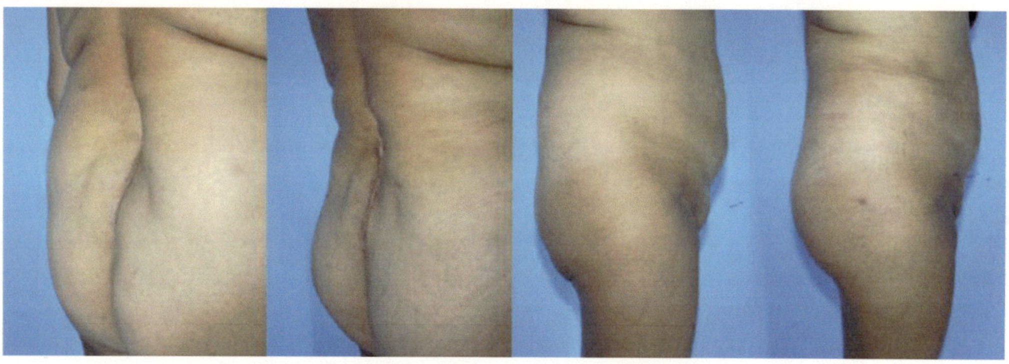

Fig. 15. Before and after RFAL in upper and lower back combined with 250cc of subcutaneous EAM in each buttocks.

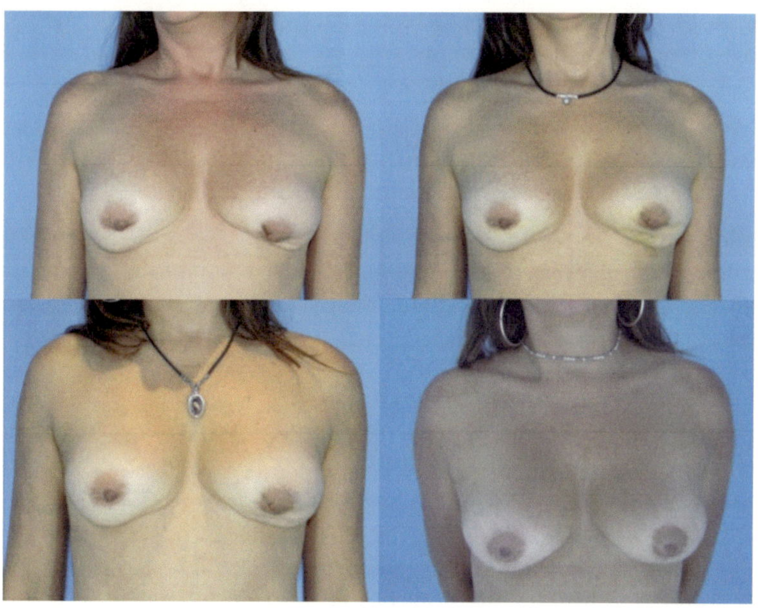

Fig. 16. Patient with multiple mammary implant replacement due to implant rejection, which later on is treated with EAM for breast augmentation and correction of the sequelae.

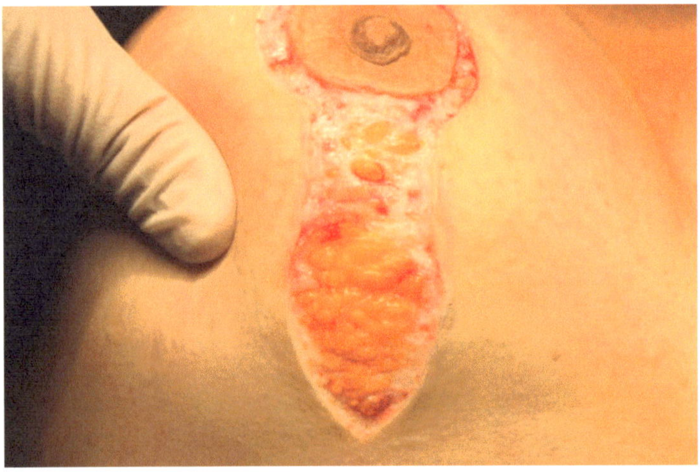

Fig. 17. Same patient, 6 months later from the last EAM, when doing a vertical mastopexy we found the good quality of the previously grafted adipose tissue.

2.7 Conclusions

The combination of adipose tissue micrografts with concentrate PRP or PT allows us to accelerate the restoration of facial and body tissues, with a low risk of complications when using autologous material.

We noticed that the resulting gel is easier to enter through the cannula, creating less friction and requiring less pressure for the passage of the micrografts through the syringe to the prefabricated tunnel. Prefabrication of these tunnels reduces the resistance of the tissues to the entrance of the micrografts, facilitating transplantation and uniform distribution.

In our experience the use of EAM has increased fat graft survival in all body areas, further improving the quality of skin in patients with radiation dermatitis or skin atrophy and achieving greater satisfaction for our patients.

3. The FAMI procedure (fat auto-grafting muscle Injection): an anatomically based pan-facial rejuvenation with adipose stem cells

3.1 Introduction

The use of autologous fat for facial augmentation has been advocated for over a century (59, 60). Interest in facial fat grafting intensified twenty years ago with French authors using rough decanted lipo-aspirates to correct facial deformities due to age, trauma or surgery(61,62).

Subsequent innovators introduced modifications such as centrifugation, to purify the samples and blunt- tipped cannulas to make the injection less traumatic (63, 64, 65, 66, 67).

Fat injections relied more on artistry and technique than on a precise anatomical algorithm and often gave unpredictable outcomes, necessitating repeated engrafting sessions to achieve good results. A recent survey showed that current techniques still do not consider specific anatomic targets, but refer only to general areas related to surface topography (68).

FAMI (Fat Auto-grafting Muscle Injection) has been in development by the author for 14 years (69) and addresses atrophic aging changes using the patients underlying anatomy as the template (70, 71). The central thesis of this technique is that the placement of autologous lipo-aspirates and their adult mesenchymal stem cells, into the appropriate microenvironment will have the restorative effects that are sought: sub-periosteal for bone, intramuscularly for muscle reshaping, and into the fat pads to restore contours. Graft survival, predictability, and symmetry are greatly enhanced by targeting the rich vascular bed of the muscles of facial expression. Augmenting regressed boney surfaces with subperiosteal injections as well as the deep and subcutaneous fat pads leads to a more natural restoration of youthful contours and volumes.

3.2 Methods

3.2.1 Instrumentation

In 1998 10 reusable 18 gauge cannula were designed to approach the facial musculature from their origin to their insertions or conversely, following the skull curvatures to make the injection less traumatic. Their 7 main curvatures duplicate the contours of the skull with 3 different lengths, 2 different blunt tips - round and spatula-like. More recently, to insure sterility, disposable cannulas are used which are lighter and more precise. The tumescent local anesthesia is performed with a 17gauge disposable infiltration cannula leaving the reusable ones as a backup (Fig. 18). Each blunt-tipped cannula is made for a muscle or group of muscle or bone surface (Table 1).

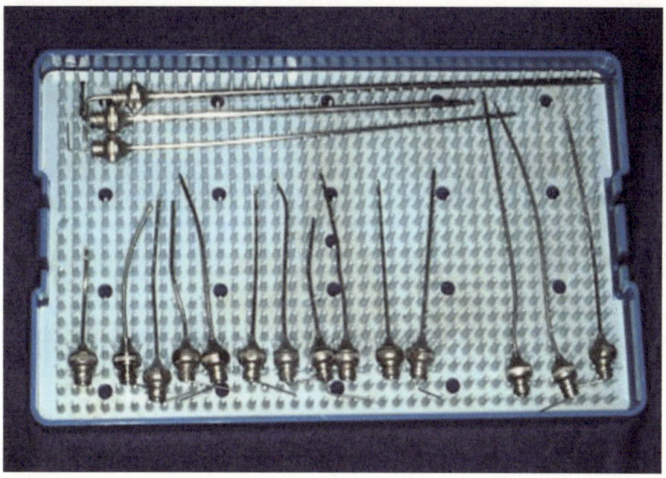

Fig. 18. The set of reusable cannulas is made of 14 injecting cannulas, plus 1 for injecting the tumescent anesthesia.

3.2.2 Procedure

Many articles have been published on fat injection; therefore we will only describe the points that make FAMI so specific.

Centrifugation: To prevent any leakage and air mixture during the spinning process an aluminum cap seals the 10 cc syringes. After removal the syringe from the centrifuge we can observe, on top, a layer of less density, yellow in color, mainly composed of the oil from destroyed fat cells; this layer can be up to 5cc after applying 13,000 G. In the bottom, the pink layer is mainly constituted of blood, Lidocaine, and saline with debris. The middle layer is composed by an accumulation of tissues: free fat cells, fat cells within a stromal vascular network containing mesenchymal stem cells, and a lower white crescent of pure collagen.

17 Cannulae	Target
Cannula # I:	for the Levators Labii superioris
Cannula # II:	for the Orbicularis oculii
Cannula # III:	for the Risorius muscle
Cannula # IIIA:	for the Pillars of the Cheek
Cannula # IV:	for the Zygomaticus minor cheek part and SOOF
Cannula # IVA:	for the Zygomaticus minor lip part and cupid's bow
Cannula # V:	for the Frontalis, Buccinator, Depressor Anguli Oris
Cannula # VA:	for the Platysma and neck bands
Cannula # VI:	for the Corrugators and Procerus
Cannula # VIA:	for the Temporal extension of the Bichat fat pad
Cannula #VII:	for the Depressor Labii inferioris, Mentalis, and LAO
Cannula #VIII:	malleable cannula for testing
Cannula # IX:	dissecting solid tube for scar undermining
Cannula # X:	for the Zygomaticus major and Platysma origin
Cannulae P1,P2,P3:	for Subperiosteal injections

Table 1. Cannulas list developed for a full face FAMI on the basis of one cannula for one specific muscle.

Different spinning speeds are used according to the facial tissue to be augmented: bone, muscle or fat pad (Table 2).

Spinning speed / 1or 2 minutes in G Force*	Tissue to repair
10,000 to 13,000 G	Subperiosteal
5,000 to 6,000 G	Muscles
1,000 G	Fat pads

Table 2. This table shows the different G force applied on lipo-aspirates to obtain purified tissues for restoration of bone, muscle and fat pads.

Lipo-aspirates centrifuged at higher G force (13,000) tend to be more liquid and are injectable sub-periostealy. Lower G force (1000) processing is done when larger volume corrections with lobulated fat aggregations are desired, such as in the fat pads.

3.2.3 Anesthesia

Complete trigeminal sensory nerve block is administered using Naropin 0.5% (Ropivacaine 5mg/100ml - Astra-Zeneca) along with cervical sensory branches if neck bands are to be addressed. Lorazepam 0.5mg PO or similar sedative, and Clonidine 0.1 - 0.2mg are useful adjuncts preoperatively.

3.2.4 The graft placement

The processed lipo-aspirates are transferred into 1cc and 3 cc Luer-lock syringes for injection with the appropriate cannula. Acquired technical skill and a detailed knowledge of the anatomy are necessary to successfully place the grafts (Table 3).

Correct intramuscular placement is associated with no resistance when the plunger is depressed, injecting with each withdrawal, for the 1-3 passes used for each muscle. The systematization of the injections, from periosteum to skin, plane after plane, is one characteristic of the FAMI procedure.

Approach site	Subperiosteal	Muscle	Fat pad
1.Frontal		*Frontalis Corrugator Procerus*	
2.Temporal	*Temporal crest*		*Superficial temporal*
3.Orbital	*Orbital rim*	*Orbicularis oculii Zygomaticus minor*	*Brow / Charpy's/ ROOF SOOF*
4.Zygoma	*Zygoma, Zygoma orbital process, Zygomatic arch*		
5.Nasal	*Nasal frame, nasal spine*	*Levator Labii superior, Lev Labii sup alaque nasi*	
6. Oral commissure	*Alveolus superior and inferior*	*Levator Anguli Oris Zygomaticus major Orbicularis Oris Buccinator Platysma*	*Bichat / buccal FP* *Buccinator FP*
7.Mandibular	*Mandibular body*	*Platysma (neck bands) Depressor Anguli Oris Depressor Labii inferioris, Digastric*	
8.Mental	*Chin*	*Mentalis*	*Submental FP*

Table 3. This table shows the detailed anatomy of the face to successfully place the grafts.

3.3 Complications

In our 726 cases the FAMI procedure has been remarkably free of complications. No cytosteatonecrosis, pseudocyst formation, or infections have been noted in 14 years of practice. Nerve injury, sensory or motor, has never occurred.

3.4 Conclusion

The FAMI Technique achieves a true facial volume correction with natural and proper vectors to return a youthful appearance to the aging face appearance of the aging face. The time is coming where injecting the face disregarding the micro-anatomy of the underlying tissues will no longer be tolerated. By aiming principally on the 30 muscles of facial expression, the FAMI technique has proved to be gratifyingly effective to rejuvenate and/or restore facial contours without creating deformities. (Fig.19)

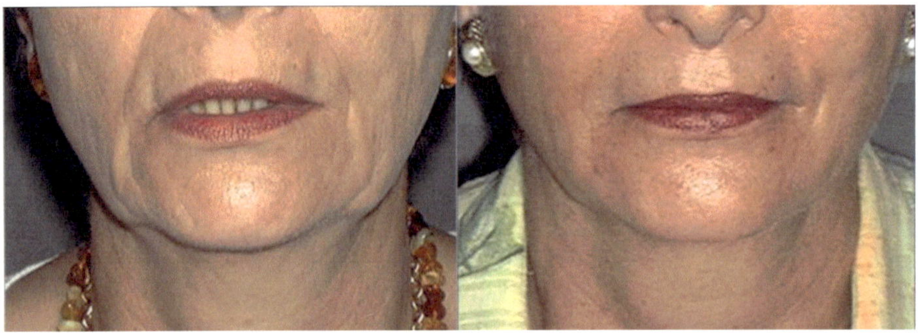

Fig. 19. Patient with 33cc of fat injection in depressor of labbi inferioris, platysma, and depressor anguli oris. Previous the injection and 6 months later.

4. Labia majora cosmetic volume enhancement with autologous fat transfer

4.1 Introduction

The surgical aesthetic management of the vulva is poorly understood and as a result it is often neglected by gynecologists and cosmetic surgeons. Factors explaining the reluctance to treat these women include the scarcity of medical literature detailing operative techniques for the cosmetic enhancement of the labia majora and mons pubis and the surgeon's concern of creating sexual dysfunction as a result of the surgery.

Women seeking cosmetic improvement of the labia majora and mons pubis can be divided into two distinctive groups. The first group includes those women who request the correction of large and ptotic labia majora and mons pubis related to unsightly fat deposits that may persists even after dramatic weight loss, as is frequently seen after bariatric surgery. The second group are those who seek cosmetic surgical help to improve labia majora volume loss, secondary to both age and weight loss that result in ptotic and deflated labia majora with looseness and wrinkling of the overlying skin. Patients belonging to the second group can be effectively treated using autologous fat transfer for the volume enhancement of the labia majora.

4.2 Anatomical considerations

The vulva is composed of the labia majora and the mons pubis. The labia majora consist of skin and appendages, including hair follicles, sebaceous glands, sweat gland, and two prominent swellings on both sides of the vulva - the result of sub-dermal fat deposits. The two labia come together in the midline creating the anterior commissure, and posteriorly at the perineum the two labia also come together creating the posterior commissure.

The majority of the tissue beneath the skin of the labia majora is fat (95 %) through which course numerous superficial vessels and nerves. The next layer is composed by a fibrocondensation of fat called the Colles's fascia. The thin bulbo-cavernosus muscle is found beneath the Colles's fascia. The bulbocavernosus muscles cover the very vascular vestibular bulbs. These vascular structures have a typical bluish hue - the result of the venous blood held within the sinuses. The Bartholin's glands are partially covered by the posterior ends of the vestibular bulbs. The vascular and neural supply of the vulva originates from both the internal and external pudendal arteries and nerves. The posterior femoral cutaneous, ilioinguinal and genital femoral nerves also supply areas of the vulva. [72]

4.3 Technique

4.3.1 Fat harvesting

Tumescent anesthesia (a combination of lidocaine, epinephrine, and sodium bicarbonate in a bag of saline solution) is infiltrated in the area were the fat will be removed. Typical donor sites are the medial aspect of the knee, the abdomen, and hips A sufficient amount of fat is harvested from a suitable site under sterile conditions by liposuction under low negative pressure using 3 mm suction cannulas or by syringe . When the syringe technique is used, a small diameter (2 mm) blunt cannula with a lateral distal opening is connected to a 10 cc or 20 cc Luer-Lok syringe for the fat harvesting.

4.3.2 Fat preparation

After sufficient fat is harvested, the fat is placed in 10 cc syringes after the syringe plungers have been removed. The syringes are then centrifugated at 3000 rpm for 3 minutes. At the end of the centrifugation, 3 levels are present: an upper level with oil from broken fat cells, a middle level with the fat tissue, and a lower level with blood and residual tumescent fluid. The upper and lower levels are discarded.

Autologous platelet-rich-plasma (PRP) is then prepared. The PRP is a platelet concentrate that contains numerous protein and growth factors that has demonstrated to accelerate and improve the healing process. It has been used extensively to accelerate soft and hard tissue healing. The PRP is prepared using a small volume of blood taken from a peripheral vein. We use a self-contained disposable kit (Selphyl. Cascade Medical Enterprises, LLC. Princeton, New Jersey) to process 18 cc of peripheral blood. Recent studies have shown excellent results when autologous fat is combined with PRP in aesthetic plastic surgery [73, 74, 75]. In order to increase the potential for autologous fat graft acceptance and retention we mix the harvested fat with the autologous PRP in a 4:1 ratio. The PRP mixed with the fat tissue is then aseptically injected in the labia majora.

4.3.3 Fat Injection

The labia majora areas to be treated with the autologous fat injections are drawn. The procedure is performed under local tumescent anesthesia. The solution includes lidocaine, epinephrine, and sodium bicarbonate diluted in one liter bag of saline solution. The solution creates complete local anesthesia and optimal hemostasis. Approximately 15-20 ml are carefully injected in the subcutaneous layer of each labia majora. Approximately 20 ml of the autologous fat mixed with the PRP are injected subcutaneously in a fan-like pattern through bilateral 1 mm labia majora incisions with a 15 cm long, 14 gauge, blunt cannula. Deep injections must be avoided as they may disrupt and traumatize the deep vascular structures of the vestibular bulbs. In some patients the injection of the fat may be difficult due to the presence of sheets of connective tissue in the subcutaneous layer (Figures 20 a-d).

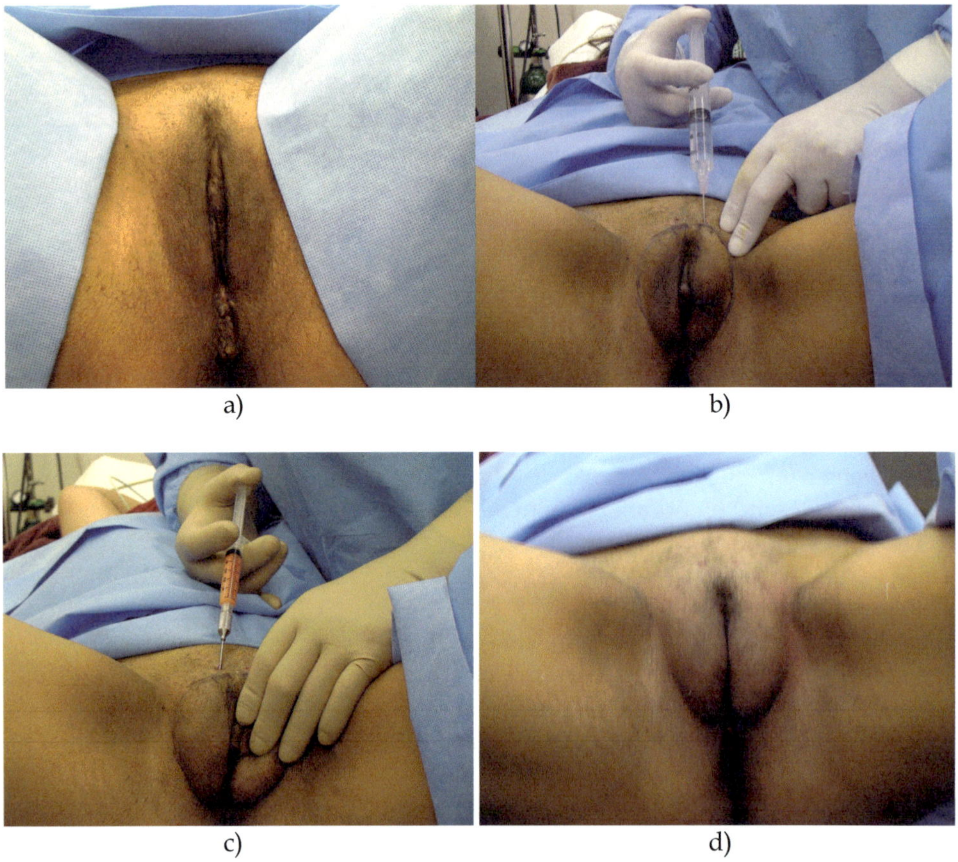

Fig. 20. a. Following significant weight loss a 49 year old requested cosmetic correction of the labia majora. Notice the deflated appearance of the labia majora and the associated looseness of the underlying skin, b. Local tumescent anesthesia is infiltrated bilaterally in the labia majora, c. Following the infiltration of tumescent solution, a autologous platelet enriched plasma fat is injected in each labia for volume enhancement, d. Notice the cosmetic improvement of the labia majora as a result of the fat transfer.

4.4 Labia majora convergence improvement using autologous fat transfer

In the young woman the two prominent subdermal fat swellings of the labia majora converge anteriorly creating the anterior labial commissure, and posteriorly creating the posterior labial commissure. With age or weight loss some women find that their labia majora diverge away from the clitoris or away from the perineal body and they find cosmetically unacceptable that their anterior and/or posterior commissures do not come together.

The convergence of the labia majora can be obtained using reduction surgery with a moderate excision of inner labia majora to pull the labia towards the midline to give a more aesthetically appealing contouring of the labia majora above and below the vaginal openings. The use of autologous fat transfer avoids the need to perform reduction surgery and can achieve a significant improvement of the labia convergence. The technique of fat transfer to correct this problem is similar to the procedure to create labia majora enhancement. It requires a careful pre-injection drawing of the anterior and posterior labia commissures in order to place the fat in the correct areas to recreate the commissures. (Figures 21a-d)

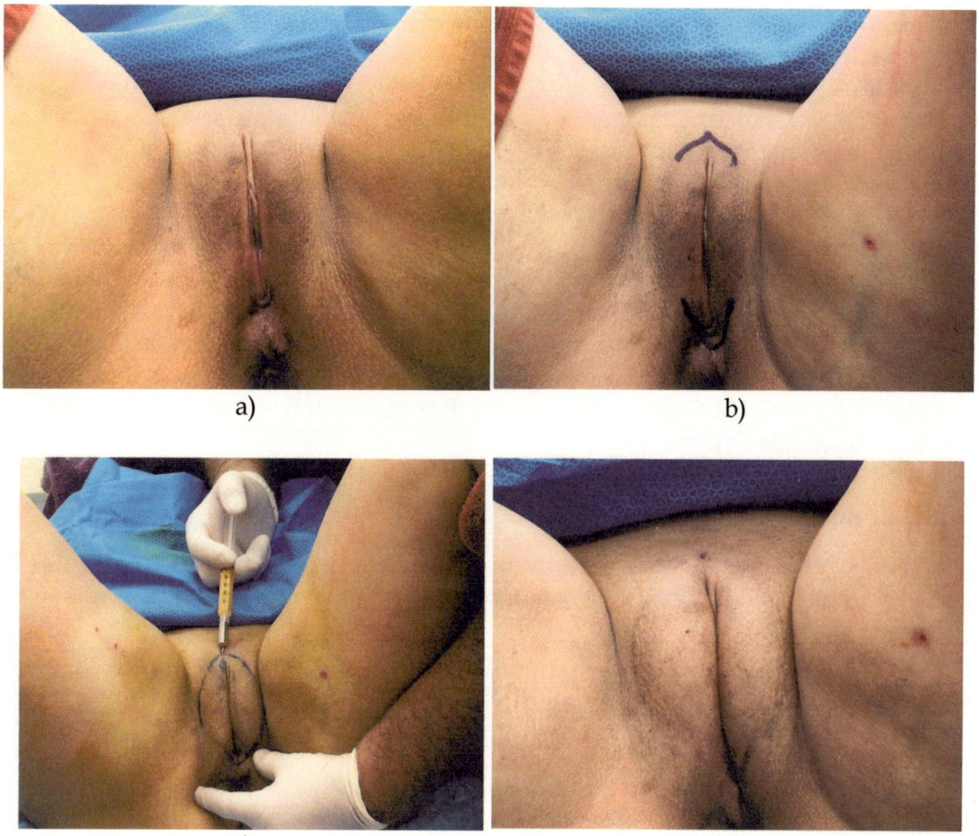

a) b)

c) d)

Fig. 21. a. Patient requested labia majora volume enhancement and that the right and left labial fat swellings meet in the midline, b. The anterior and posterior labial commissural angles are marked, c. Autologous platelet enriched plasma fat is injected bilaterally to achieve adequate volume and convergence. Approximately 25 ml were placed in each labia majora, d. Notice the cosmetically improved appearance of the labia majora following the injection of fat for volume replacement and the more aesthetically appealing contour of the labia in the midline.

4.5 Conclusions

Prophylactic antibiotics are routinely used. Patients are advised to refrain from intercourse for 6 weeks. Standard instructions for the care of the small labia incisions are given.

We have performed over 100 consecutive cosmetic volume enhancements of the labia majora using the technique described here. The minimal follow -up has been 12 months.

We have not encountered hematomas, infections, persistent pain, the development of irregularities or nodulations in the subcutaneous layer of the labia or anatomical distortions requiring correction. The retention of the transplanted fat has been excellent. Only 3 patients, approximately 6 months later have required a second fat injection to replace volume. In approximately one third of the cases undergoing labia majora volume enhancement with autologous fat transfer, additional cosmetic vaginal procedures were performed at the same time (vaginal rejuvenation/tightening, labia minora labiaplasty, and mons pubis liposuction or fat injection). The addition of the labia majora fat grafting did not compromise the performance or the recovery of the other vaginal cosmetic procedures. The satisfaction rate of the patients has been 100 % and all of them stated that they will recommend the surgery to others. (76)

In our experience labia majora cosmetic volume enhancement using autologous fat transfer has been an effective and safe cosmetic vaginal procedure with a very high patients' satisfaction rate.

An additional advantage of volume enhancement and correction of labia convergence using fat grafting in some patients is the ability of the procedure to conceal an associated labia minora enlargement or distortion, thus avoiding the need to perform a labia minora labiaplasty .In those situations, following the completion of the fat transfer to the labia majora the excessive labia minora protrusion or distortion will be effectively covered by the volume enhanced labia majora.

6. Final conclusions

The authors have presented different approaches in advanced lipotransfer techniques. The common pattern is to take advantage of adipose tissue as an autologous filler to obtain safe and consistent results.

7. References

[1] Pittman, Gerald, MD; Liposuction and Aesthetic Medicine, QMP Inc. St. Louis, Missouri, 1993

[2] Niechajev, I., and Sevcuk, O. Long-term results of fat transplantation: clinical and histologic studies. Plast Reconstr Surg 94:496-506,1994

[3] Boschert MT, Beckert BW, Puckett CL, Concannon MJ. Analysis of lipocyte viability after liposuction. Plast Reconstr Surg 109:761-5 766-7, 2002

[4] Shiffman MA, Mirrafati S. Fat transfer techniques: the effect of harvest and transfer methods on adipocyte viability and review of the literature. Dermatol Surg 27:819-26, 2001

[5] Saylan Z; Liposhifting instead of Lipofilling; Treatment of the Post-Liposuction Irregularities. Aesthetic Surgery Journal, March/April 2001, Volume 21 Number 2

[6] Blugerman G: Liposhifting. Vortrag auf dem Kongress der Deutschen Gesellschaft für Ästhetische Chirurgie, Heidelberg 2002

[7] Blugerman GS, Schavelzon DE, Liposhifting para el Tratamiento de las Irregularidades Post-liposuccion y Celulitis, Procedimentos Esteticos Minimamente Invasivos Capitulo 55: Santos Livraria Editora Sao Paulo Brazil 2005, 425-430

[8] Shiffman MA, Blugerman GS, Fat Shifting for The Treatment of Skin Indentrations, Liposuction Principles and Practice, Chapter 53 Springer- Verlang 2006: 353-356

[9] Blugerman G, et all. Movilización adiposa interna (Liposhifting) con espátula y cortador de microinjertos de grasa. Dermatologia CMQ Abr- Jun 2007; 5 (2):105-111.

[10] Klein J.A.: Tumescent technique chronicles. Local anesthesia, liposuction and beyond. Dermatol surg 1995; 21:449-457
[11] Blugerman G, M. Podda. Movilización adiposa interna (Liposhifting) con espátula y cortador de microinjertos de grasa. Dermatologia CMQ Abr- Jun 2007; 5 (2):105-111.
[12] Sommer B. Liposuktion und Eigenfett-Transplantation: Update 2004 Haut 3/2004 Band XV / 112-116
[13] Mojallal A, Foyatier J-L. Historical review of the use of adipose tissue transfer in plastic and ronstructive surgery [In French]. Ann Chir Plast Esthet 2004;49(5):419-25.
[14] Van de Graaf RC, Korteweg SFS. Gustav Adolf Neuber (1850-1932) and the first report on fat auto-grafting in humans in 1893. Hist Plast Surg 2010;1(1):7-11.
[15] Lexer E. Die Freien transplantationen, 1 Teil. Stuttgart: Verlag von Ferdinand Enke 1919:264-547.
[16] Peer, L. A. Transplantation of Fat. In Transplantation of Tissue. Baltimore: Williams & Wilkins, 1969. Pp. 165–244.
[17] Blugerman G. y col. Metodología actual para Lipoinjerto Autólogo. Actas del XXIII Congreso Brasileiro de Cirugía Plástica. Noviembre 1986. Belho Horizonte. Brasil.
[18] Kaufman MR, BradleyJP, DickinsonB, et al. Autologousfat transfer national consensus survey: Trends in techniques for harvest, preparation, and application, and perception of short- and long-term results. Plast Reconstr Surg. 2007; 119: 323.
[19] Serra-Renom,JM y Fontdevila,J: "Treatment of Facial Fat Atrophy Related to Treatment with Protease Inhibitors by Autologous Fat Injection in Patients with Human Immunodeficiency Virus.Infection" Plast. Reconstr. Surg. 2004,114:551.
[20] Eppley, B Woodell, J.Higgins, J.: "Platelet Quantification and Growth Factor Análisis from Platelet-Rich Plasma: Implications for Wound Healing". American Society of Plastic Súrgeons 2004; 114(6): 1502.
[21] Duskova M, Kristen M. Augmentation by autologous adipose tissue in cleft lip and nose: Final esthetic touches in clefts. Part I. J Craniofac Surg. 2004;15:478.
[22] Bertossi D, Zancanaro C, Trevisiol L, et al. Lipofilling of the lips. Arch Facial Plastic Surg. 2003;5:392.
[23] Fulton JE Jr, Rahimi AD, Helton P, et al. Lip rejuvenation. Dermatol Surg. 2000;26:470.
[24] Iñigo F y col.: Tratamiento estético de la enfermedad de Romberg. Cir Plast 2001;11(2):67-75
[25] Coleman SR. Hand rejuvenation with structural fat grafting. Plast Reconstr Surg. 2002;110:1731.
[26] Harrison D, Selvaggi G. Gluteal augmentation surgery: Indications and surgical management. J Plast Reconstr Aesthet Surg. 2007;60:922.
[27] Restrepo JCC, Ahmed JAM. Large-volume lipoinjection for gluteal augmentation. Aesthet Surg J. 2002;22:33.
[28] Roberts TL, Toledo LS, Badin AZ. Augmentation of the buttocks by micro fat grafting. Aesthet Surg J. 2001;21:311.
[29] Panfilov DE. Augmentative phalloplasty. Aesthet Plast Surg. 2006;30:183.
[30] Rohrich RJ, Sorokin ES, Brown SA. In search of improved fat transfer viability: A quantitative analysis of the role of centrifugation and harvest site. Plast Reconstr Surg. 2004; 113:391.

[31] D. Bergfeld, B. Sommer, G. Sattler. Technik der Infiltration. Tumeszenz-Localanästhesie: praktische Awendung. Springer. 1999, pg 50.
[32] Amar O, Bruant-Rodier C, Lehmann S, et al. [Fat tissue transplant: Restoration of the mammary volume after con- servative treatment of breast cancers, clinical and radiolog- ical considerations.] Ann Chir Plast Esthet. 2007;53:169.
[33] Coleman SR, Saboeiro AP. Fat grafting to the breast revis- ited: Safety and efficacy. Plast Reconstr Surg. 2007;119:775.
[34] Guyuron B, Majzoub RK. Facial augmentation with core fat graft: A preliminary report. Plast Reconstr Surg. 2007;120:295.
[35] Coleman SR. Structural fat grafting: More than a permanent filler. Plast Reconstr Surg. 06;118:108S.
[36] Burnouf M, Buffet M, Schwarzinger M, et al. Evaluation of Coleman lipostructure for treatment of facial lipoatrophy in patients with human immunodeficiency virus and param- eters associated with the efficiency of this technique. Arch Dermatol. 2005;141:1220.
[37] Gonzalez AM, Lobocki C, Kelly C, et al. An alternative method for harvest and processing fat grafts: An in vitro study of cell viability and survival. Plast Reconstr Surg. 2007; 120:285.
[38] Piasecki JH, Gutowski KA, Lahvis G, et al. An experimental model for improving fat graft viability and purity. Plast Reconstr Surg. 2007;119:1571.
[39] Ozsoy Z, Kul Z, Bilir A. The role of cannula diameter in improved adipocyte viability: A quantitative analysis. Aesthet Surg J. 2006;26:287.
[40] Blugerman G, M. Podda. Movilización adiposa interna (Liposhifting) con espátula y cortador de microinjertos de grasa. Dermatologia CMQ Abr- Jun 2007; 5 (2):105-111.
[41] Pu LL, Cui X, Fink B, et al. The viability of fatty tissues within adipose aspirates after conventional liposuction: A compre- hensive study. Ann Plast Surg. 2005;54:288.
[42] Karacalar A, Orak I, Kaplan S, et al. No-touch technique for autologous fat harvesting. Aesthet Plast Surg. 2004;28:158.
[43] Jackson IT, Simman R, Tholen R, et al. A successful long- term method of fat grafting: Recontouring of a large sub- cutaneous postradiation thigh defect with autologous fat transplantation. Aesthet Plast Surg. 2001;25:165.
[44] Shiffman MA, Mirrafati S. Fat transfer techniques: The ef- fect of harvest and transfer methods on adipocyte viability and review of the literature. Dermatol Surg. 2001;27:819.
[45] Fagrell D, Enestro ̈m S, Berggren A, Kniola B. Fat cylinder transplantation: An experimental comparative study of three different kinds of fat transplants. Plast Reconstr Surg. 1996;98:90.
[46] Rose JG Jr, Lucarelli MJ, Lemke B, et al. Histologic com- parison of autologous fat processing methods. Ophthal Plast Reconstr Surg. 2006;22:195.
[47] SmithP,AdamsWPJr,LipschitzA,etal.Autologoushuman fat grafting: Effect of harvesting and preparation techniques on adipocyte graft survival. Plast Reconstr Surg. 2006; 117:1836.
[48] Karacaoglu E, Kizilkaya E, Cermik H, et al. The role of recipient sites in fat-graft survival: Experimental study. Ann Plast Surg. 2005;55:63.

[49] Hu S, Zhang H, Feng Y, et al. Introduction of an easy technique for purification and injection of autogenous free fat parcels in correcting of facial contour deformities. Ann Plast Surg. 2007;58:602.
[50] Kuran I, Tumerdem B. A new simple method used to prepare fat for injection. Aesthet Plast Surg. 2005;29:18.
[51] Lacy EL, Bartness TJ. Effects of white adipose tissue grafts on total body fat and cellularity are dependent on graft type and location. Am J Physiol Regul Integr Comp Physiol. 2005; 289:R380–R388.
[52] Valdatta L, Thione A, Buoro M, et al. A case of lifethreatening sepsis after breast augmentation by fat injection. Aes- thet Plast Surg. 2001; 25:347.
[53] Guaraldi G, De Fazio D, Orlando G, et al. Facial lipohyper- trophy in HIV-infected subjects who underwent autologous fat tissue transplantation. Clin Infect Dis. 2005;40:e13–e15.
[54] Miller JJ, Popp JC. Fat hypertrophy after autologous fat transfer. Ophthal Plast Reconstr Surg. 2002;18:228.
[55] Coleman SR. Lower lid deformity secondary to autogenous fat transfer: A cautionary tale. Aesthet Plast Surg. 2008; 32:415.
[56] Yoshimura K, Sato K, Aoi N, et al. Cell-assisted lipotrans- fer for cosmetic breast augmentation: Supportive use of adipose-derived stem/stromal cells. Aesthet Plast Surg. 2008;32: 48.
[57] Hang-FuL,MarmolyaG, FeiglinDH.Liposuctionfat-fillant implant for breast augmentation and reconstruction. Aesthet Plast Surg. 1995;19: 427.
[58] Pierrefeu-Lagrange AC, Delay E, Guerin N, et al. [Radiological evaluation of breasts reconstructed with lipomodeling.] Ann Chir Plast Esthet. 2006; 51:18.
[59] Neuber. Fettransplantation. Bericht über die Verhandlungen der deutschen Gesellschaft für Chirurgie. Zentralbl Chir. 1893;22:66.
[60] Lexer E. Fett transplantation,. Dtsch Med.Wochenschr 1910;36:640.
[61] Illouz YG. The fat cell "graft": a new technique to fill depressions. Plast Reconstr Surg 1986;78(1):122-3.
[62] Fournier PF. Microlipoextraction et microlipoinjection,. Rev. Chir. Esthét. Lang. Fr 1985;10:p. 40.
[63] Carraway JH, Mellow CG. Syringe aspiration and fat concentration: a simple technique for autologous fat injection. Ann Plast Surg 1990;24(3):293-6; discussion; 297.
[64] Coleman WP, 3rd. Autologous fat transplantation. Plast Reconstr Surg 1991;88(4):736.
[65] Bircoll M, Novack BH. Autologous fat transplantation employing liposuction techniques. Ann Plast Surg 1987;18(4):327-9.
[66] Ellenbogen R. Free autogenous pearl fat grafts in the face--a preliminary report of a rediscovered technique. Ann Plast Surg 1986;16(3):179-94.
[67] Matsudo PK, Toledo LS. Experience of injected fat grafting. Aesthetic Plast Surg 1988;12(1):35-8.
[68] Coleman SR. Facial augmentation with structural fat grafting. Clin Plast Surg 2006;33(4):567-77.
[69] Amar RE. Adipocyte microinfiltration in the face or tissue restructuration with fat tissue graft. Ann Chir Plast Esthet 1999;44(6):593-608.
[70] Amar RE, Fox DM, Balin A (2010) Cannulation and injection of the muscles of facial expression: a cadaver study. Dermatol Surg 36:1–8

[71] Amar RE, Fox DM. The Facial Autologous Muscular Injection (FAMI) Procedure: An Anatomically Targeted Deep Multiplane Autologous Fat-Grafting Technique Using Principles of Facial Fat Injection. Aesth Plast Surg, Online First™, 5 February 2011.
[72] Baggish MS . Vulvar and Perineal Anatomy. In Baggish MS, Karram MM (editors): Atlas of Pelvic Anatomy and Gynecologic Surgery. Second edition. Elsevier. Philadelphia, PA. Chapter 62: 835-850
[73] Azzena B, Mazzoleni F, Abatangelo G, et al. Autologous Platelet-Rich Plasma as an Adipocyte In Vivo Delivery System: Case report. Aesth Plast Surg 2008; 32: 155-158
[74] Sclafani AP. Applications of Platelet-Rich Fibrin Matrix in Facial Plastic Surgery. Facial Plast Surg 2009; 25:270-276
[75] Cervelli V, Gentile P, Grimaldi M. Regenerative Surgery: Use of Fat Grafting Combined with Platelet-Rich Plasma for Chronic Lower-extremity Ulcers Aesth Plast Surg 2009;33:340-345
[76] Pelosi MA II, Pelosi MA III. Cosmetogynecology. In Jay N. (editor):State of the Art, Atlas of Endoscopic Surgery in Infertility and Gynecology. Second Edition. Jaypee Brothers Medical Publishers, London (UK) 2010; Chapter 39: 422-439

11

Processing of Lipoaspirate Samples for Optimal Mesenchymal Stem Cells Isolation

Leandra Baptista, Karina Silva, Carolina Pedrosa and Radovan Borojevic
Universidade Federal do Rio de Janeiro (UFRJ) –
Campus Xerém - Programa de Bioengenharia, Diretoria de Programas
Instituto Nacional de Metrologia Normalização e Qualidade Industrial (Inmetro)
Brazil

1. Introduction

Over the last 10 years, huge advances have been made worldwide in the adult stem cell field. Several donor sites can be used for harvesting mesenchymal stem cells (MSC), bone marrow and adipose tissue being the most frequent. The latter is easily harvested by liposuction and, in most patients, a large quantity of MSC can be obtained without harm to the donor (Casteilla et al., 2004). In 2001, Zuk and co-workers showed that a human lipoaspirate contains multipotent cells and may represent an alternative stem cell source to bone marrow-derived MSC. Adipose-derived MSC are capable of proliferation in monolayer culture and multilineage differentiation in response to inductive conditions, and thus have potential clinical application (Bailey et al., 2010; Fraser et al., 2008; Rigotti et al., 2009;).

However, research and clinical groups have distinct protocols to isolate and manipulate these cells, differing in the type and concentration of the enzyme used, time and conditions of incubation for adipose tissue digestion and methods of cell culture. These methodological differences result in diverse characteristics of the cells isolated and varied functional results. Therefore, the development of a standardized and reproducible method of isolating MSC as well as standard techniques for functional characterization is fundamental to validate cells for its use in therapeutic protocols.

A temptative for functional characterization of MSC was recently proposed by the International Society for Cellular Therapy (ISCT) (Dominici et al., 2006). According to this statement, MSC must: (i) be plastic-adherent in standard cultures; (ii) express a mesenchymal set of surface molecules; (iii) differentiate into osteoblasts, adipocytes and chondroblasts *in vitro*. The detection of these mesenchymal set of surface molecules as well as the differentiation assays can be performed on adipose-tissue MSC population after their isolation in laboratory and will be carefully described in this chapter.

2. Cell physiology of adipose tissue and mesenchymal stem cells

Only recently, the white adipose tissue has been identified as an endocrine organ besides acting in energy storage and, in humans, it can be found mainly in two sites: visceral and subcutaneous. By secreting bioactive molecules, called adipokines, this tissue plays an active role in the regulation of several functions in the organism (Gregoire, 2001; Trayhurn, 2005).

The white adipose tissue is composed by connective tissue, nerve endings and a rich vascular network (Figure 1). Cellular content includes specialized cells, the adipocytes, and a stromal vascular fraction composed by pre-adipocytes (which differentiate into adipocytes), fibroblastic cells, endothelial cells, macrophages (Casteilla et al., 2004) and lymphocytes (Caspar-Bauguil et al., 2005). A subset of cells that is associated with blood vessels, called MSC, exhibits developmental potential beyond angiogenesis. MSC are found throughout fetal and adult tissues. They are members of the pericyte cell family and may be defined as progenitor cells capable of giving rise to a number of differentiated mesenchymal cells and also contribute to tissue homeostasis (Baptista et al., 2007; da Silva Meirelles et al., 2008).

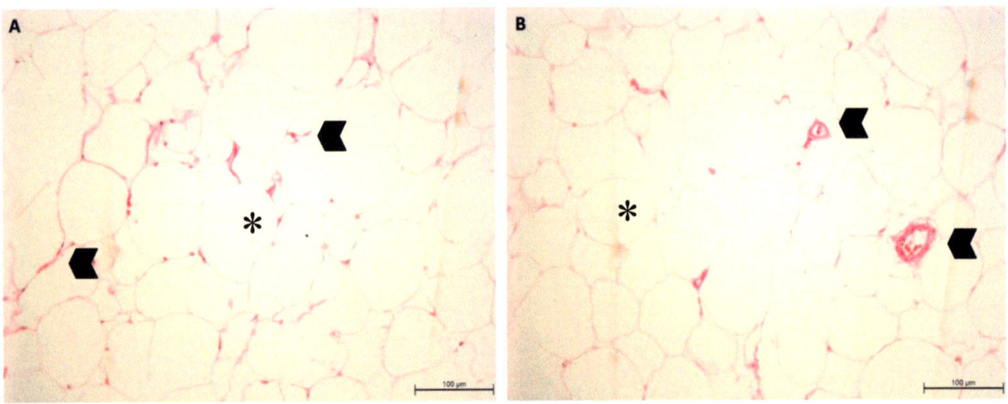

Fig. 1. Histological analysis of subcutaneous adipose tissue. Adipose tissue fragments were fixed in formaldehyde and processed for paraffin embed. Histological sections were stained by hematoxylin and eosin (H/E). Because histological process involves the use of xylol, the fat inside adipocytes are dissolved and the inclusions appear as its negative image, that is the area occupied by fat inside adipocytes (asterisks). Note the significant network of blood vessels (arrowheads) composed by small (A) and large ones, surrounded by multiple layers of cells (B), where the population of MSC dwells. Bar size=100 µm.

The term "mesenchymal stem cell" was introduced by Caplan (1991), after the studies of Friedenstein and co-workers, who isolated and characterized these cells from bone marrow (Friedenstein et al., 1968, 1974). MSC were distinguished from hematopoietic cells by plastic adherence and fibroblastic morphology. Besides that, when cultivated at a clonal density (few cells per cm^2) these cells adhere to the plastic and discrete colonies are established, initiated by a single proliferative cell, termed the Colony Forming Unit Fribroblast (CFU-F). These fibroblastic colonies, under adequate experimental conditions, give rise to differentiated cells of distinct types of connective tissue, like adipocytes, osteoblasts and condroblasts (Friedenstein et al., 1974). These cells have also the potential to differentiate into myoblasts (Wakitani, Saito & Caplan 1995; Ferrari et al., 1998, Zuk et al., 2001, Mizuno et al., 2002, Crisan et al., 2008), as well as into fibroblasts, and possibly, tendon (Caplan, 2007; Chamberlain et al., 2007).

Although bone marrow MSC-like cells can be isolated from different tissues, adipose tissue have been proposed to be an alternative to bone marrow, since fat tissue is abundant, easily harvested by liposuction and adipose tissue MSC, like bone marrow MSC, can differentiate towards mesenchymal lineages (Zuk et al., 2001).

Long-term cultured MSC maintain their differentiation capacity towards osteo-, chondro-, adipo- and myogenic lineages, also expressing MSC markers. Many reports have described stable phenotype after extensive expansion (Zuk, et al., 2001, Crisan et al., 2008, Khoo et al., 2008, Poloni et al, 2010). However, there is a growing body of literature demonstrating murine MSC transformation after long-term culture (Qin et al., 2009, Miura et al, 2010, Ahmadbeigi et al, 2011). To our knowledge, no *in vitro* spontaneous transformation of human MSC has been reported under usual conditions of culture. Although Rubio an co-workers (2005), have described this event, this group recently reported the contamination of MSC with tumor cells in his laboratory (Garcia et al, 2010).

Recent studies showed that MSC actively migrate to and proliferate in tumor progression. Moreover, MSC could undergo transformation into malignant cells and tumor formation *in vivo* (Muehlberg et al, 2009, Karnoub et al, 2007). Others suggest that MSC should not affect the status of dormant cancer cells (Zimmerlin et al, 2011). The possibility of tumor growth and metastasis induced by MSC has an effect on the safety of their use for clinical applications. Nevertheless, three research groups have now found contamination of the MSC with tumor cells used for other projects in their laboratories. In addition, over 1,000 patients were transplanted with MSC, and no tumor formation related to MSC has been reported (for a review, see Klopp et al, 2010)

There are no irrefutable studies about the role of MSC in stimulating or inhibiting tumor progression and metastasis. Discrepant results obtained by investigators are probably due to variations in MSC origin (humans or animals), MSC tissue source, individual donor variability, timing of MSC injection as many other factors. Studies considering the role of these factors are necessary to lead to new insights to resolve this important issue.

3. Adipose tissue harvesting and preparation for isolating mesenchymal stem cells

Surgeons have distinct techniques for harvesting adipose tissue and also to prepare them in the operating room. Liposuction can be performed using standard or vibro-assisted techniques. Vibro-assisted liposuction has already been reported to reduce the duration of surgery because of its large rate of aspiration (Viterbo & Ochoa, 2002). We were able to isolate MSC from lipoaspirates harvested by standard or vibro-assisted techniques, using a mechanic method (see topic 4). The total number of MSC obtained from vibro-assisted lipoaspirate samples was superior to that obtained from the standard one, but no differences in adhesion or proliferation in culture was observed (Baptista et al., 2009).

When taking into account the isolation of MSC with high cell quality, the use of a defined method of tissue harvesting and preparation in the operating room is crucial. Centrifugation of the adipose tissue harvested by liposuction has been used for nearly three decades. It is one of the preferred methods of fat processing for soft tissue augmentation.

We then investigated how the manipulation of lipoaspirate samples influences in the yield and quality of MSC subsequently isolated in the laboratory (Condé-Green et al., 2010). We have examined lipoaspirates prepared by centrifugation (1228*g* for 3 minutes) and decantation (30 minutes under the action of gravity). Centrifuged lipoaspirates had a lower yield of isolated MSC. Moreover, they were less capable to proliferate *in vitro*, probably due to the centrifugation forces suffered by cells in lipoaspirates. Also, centrifuged samples showed a fraction of cells in the bottom of the syringe, in the pellet, which was not identified in decanted samples. This fraction had a significant quantity of MSC.

In the majority of published reports, adipocyte viability analysis is qualitative, and only a few groups showed a more reliable analysis using quantitative methods.
Possible architectural alterations of adipose tissue caused by these methods was quantified based on the degeneration of adipocytes, staining tissue histological sections with Hematoxilin & Eosin (Condé-Green et al., 2010) or with antibodies against perilipin, an abundant protein in the adipocyte cytoplasmic membrane (Figure 2). Another histological quantification was performed by Rose and colleagues (Rose et al., 2006), showing that decanted samples had twice the quantity of intact adipocytes as compared to centrifuged and washed samples. Our study showed similar histological results. We observed that the adipose tissue resulted from centrifuged lipoaspirate samples contained most of adipocytes with disrupted membranes and general extracellular matrix disruption, whereas decantation maintained the adipocytes´ integrity (Figure 2; Condé-Green et al., 2010).

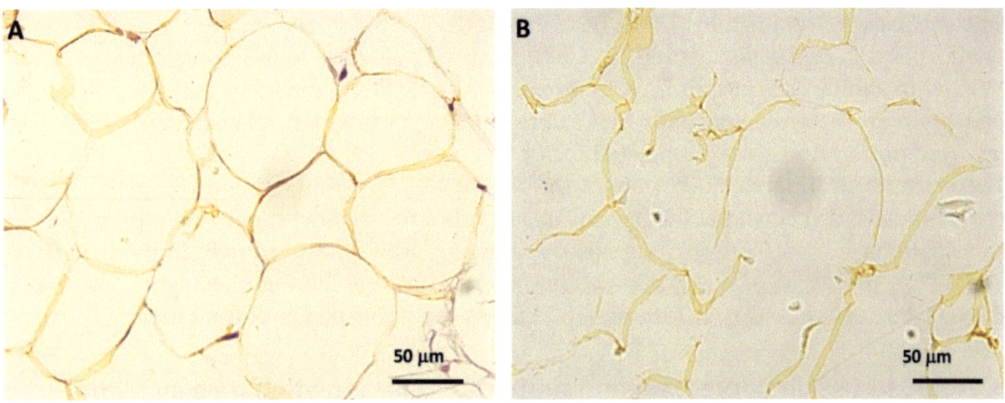

Fig. 2. Microscopic aspect of adipose tissue obtained from lipoaspirate samples. Adipocytes were specifically identified in histological sections of decanted (A) or centrifuged (B) lipoaspirates by staining with the commercially available policlonal antibody Perilipin to evaluate the impact of both methods on tissue architecture. Decanted lipoaspirate shows relatively intact, nucleated adipocytes with minor trauma and overall normal morphology (A). Centrifuged lipoaspirate clearly shows a reduced number of intact, nucleated adipocytes with more extensive trauma (B). Bar size 100 μm.

We cannot exclude the fact that reducing centrifugation forces will improve MSC recovery on centrifuged lipoaspirates samples, as already described (Kurita et al., 2008). The authors tentatively recommend 1200 g as an optimized centrifugal force, lower than used in our study, for obtaining good short- and long-term results in adipose transplantation. However, MSC content by surface marker expression was not evaluated on centrifuged adipose tissue samples of this study. Various speeds and time intervals for centrifugation have been recommended, but some reports demonstrated histologically a destruction of the most living fat (Chajchir et al., 1993; Rose et al., 2006).
These observations demonstrate that the centrifugation of adipose tissue harvested by liposuction have a negative effect on tissue architecture and morphology, losing its stem cell content, as MSC are lost in the pellet, as well as on the yield and quality of MSC subsequently isolated from the resulted tissue. On the other hand, decantation resulted in no harms to tissue structure and allows a substantial quantity of cells isolated, with a good proliferation rate and morphology.

The future of autologous fat transplantation seems to lie in stem cell research, specifically in adipose MSC. However, the use of adipose MSC raises numerous concerns, including the choice of harvesting and processing, cell isolation and culture. Scientific research is emerging to address these issues.

Membranes of adipocytes were disrupted when adipose tissue was submitted to forces generated during centrifugation, probably due the fact that adipocytes are very fragile cells with only a thin cytoplasmic envelope surrounding large fat droplets. On the other hand, MSC are smaller and more resilient, make them more practical to work than adipocytes (Suga et al., 2008).

4. Human adipose tissue mesenchymal stem cells: author´s protocol

4.1 Mesenchymal stem cell isolation

The commonly used method of isolating MSC from adipose tissue is enzymatic digestion (Gimble & Guilak, 2003; Jing et al., 2007; Bunnell et al., 2008), that consists of at least four main steps: digestion, washing, centrifugation and red blood cell lysis. Adipose tissue from lipoaspirate samples is incubated with collagenase for up to 1 hour. Then, the digests are washed, and centrifuged to separate the floating adipocytes from the pelleted stromal cells. The pelleted stromal cells are finally incubated with red blood cell lysis solution and centrifuged one more time. This enzymatic procedure generates tissue fragments that should be removed before cell plating through a 100–150 µm nylon mesh. Irrespective of the source of tissue, enzymatic digestion is time consuming and expensive, especially when applied to large volumes of tissue (Baptista et al., 2009); decreased cell viability due to lytic activity is also a problem with this method (Ishige et al., 2009).

We have described a novel method of isolating MSC from lipoaspirate samples, based on mechanical tissue dissociation. Despite the major differences between the enzymatic and mechanic methods, similar populations of MSC have been isolated. The population of cells derived from mechanic process was positive for mesenchymal surface markers such as CD90 and CD105. They were also positive for CD34, which is reported only in adipose tissue-derived mesenchymal cells (Planat-Benard et al., 2004). They also were able to accumulate lipid droplets, deposit extracellular calcium and cartilage extracellular matrix, under specific stimuli for each differentiation event (Baptista et al., 2009). Their proprieties support their use for diverse therapeutic applications. Techniques used on these assays will be detailed below (See topic 4.2).

MSC derived from mechanic process can be isolated easily from lipoaspirate samples and provide a significant quantity of cells with minor time and costs for the procedure. As commented above, the enzymatic procedure for adipose tissue consists of at least four main steps. Conversely, mechanical dissociation consists basically of two steps: dissociation of adipose tissue concomitantly with red blood cell lysis, followed by centrifugation. There are no visible tissue fragments, and it is not necessary to the filter cell suspension. The ease of mechanical digestion reduces considerably both time and cost, and does not interfere with cell viability (Figure 3). Furthermore, MSC culture derived from mechanic process gave higher yield of cells than digestion method after primary culture.

Besides taking advantages in time and cost when using mechanic process, their reproducibility makes it a preferred method for larger volumes of samples. We observed a large standard derivation among cell numbers isolated with the enzymatic digestion process, in opposition to mechanic process (Baptista et al., 2009). However, the most advantage of this innovative process is the possibility of cryopreservation of freshly isolated MSC cells. Interestingly, another study has investigated a method for cryopreserving human adipose-derived stem cells isolated by an enzymatic process. Fresh human cells were cryopreserved using Me_2SO as the cryoprotective agent at a density of 10^6 cells/mL (Liu et al., 2008), 10 times lower than the cell quantity cryopreserved in our study.

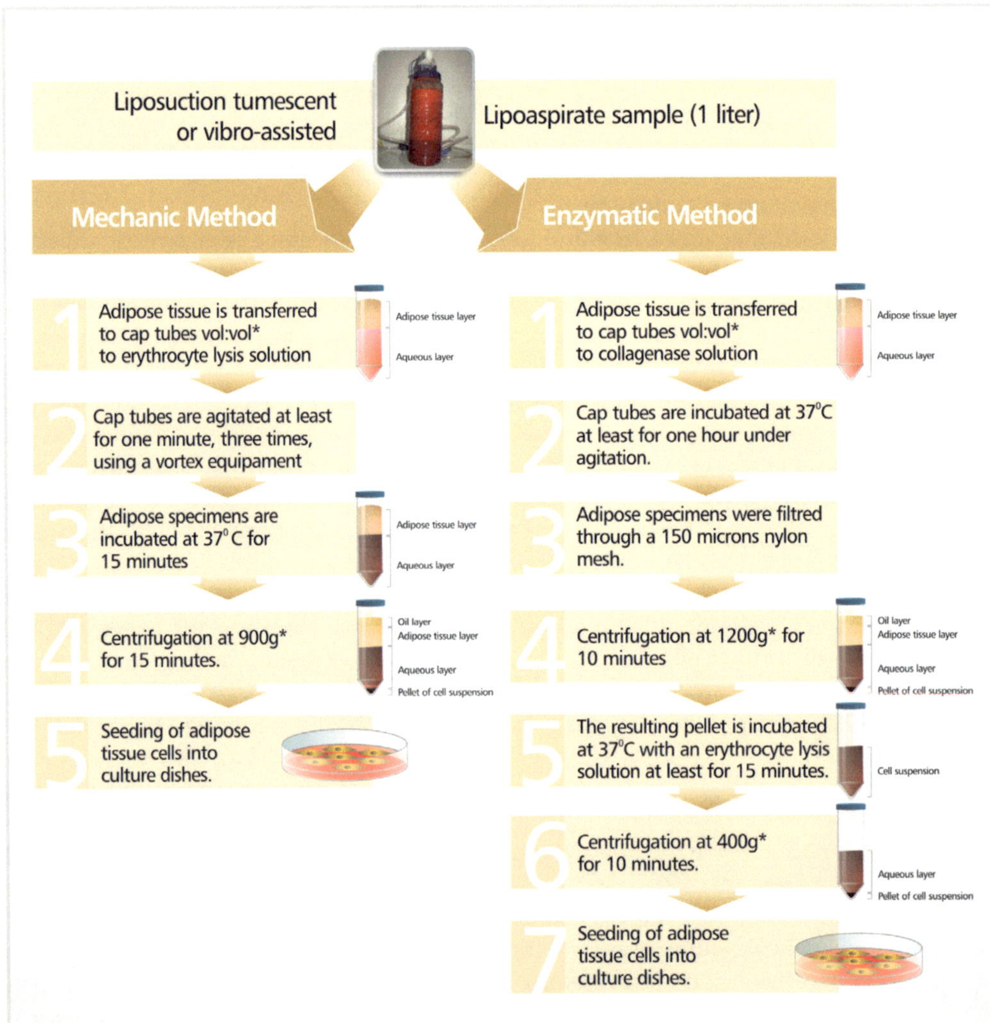

*vol:vol - volume to volume - the adipose tissue volume added should correspond to the same volume of solution.
*g = (gravities, the standard unit of centrifugation speed).

Fig. 3. Comparing mesenchymal stem cell isolation by mechanic and enzymatic methods.

Note that the enzymatic method consists of at least six main steps and the mechanic method basically of four. The centrifugation step (four in both methods) is used to separate cells from adipose tissue fragments, oil and debris. Resulting pellets - step four in mechanic and six in enzymatic - must be resuspended and seeded into culture dishes in suitable cell culture medium containing at least fetal bovine serum and antibiotics. Only the pellets obtained by mechanic method can be alternatively resuspended in fetal bovine serum supplemented with 10% dimethylsulfoxide (DMSO) for cryopreservation and storage at -196°C until thawing (see topic 4.2.1 Cell Culture).

Cryopreservation is interesting because it reduces labor costs and avoids possible loss of cell viability and senescence after long-term cultures (Serakinci et al., 2004; Rubio et al., 2005).

Another approach to isolate cells is based on primary explants culture (Klingbeil et al., 2009; Vunjak-Novakovic et al., 2006; Zhang et al., 2005). A simple small fragment of any tissue that adheres to the growth surface will usually give rise to an outgrowth of cells. Since the 1970s most studies of adipose tissue metabolism were carried out by explants methods (Smith, 1974). In the 1990s was documented the first evidence for preadipocyte proliferation during culture of adipose tissue explants (May, 1994), but there are few reports on the scientific literature regarding this method for isolation of adipose tissue stem cells.

Recently, Jing and co-workers (2010) described the explants culture as a time-saving and cost-effective method for isolation of adipose tissue MSC. They showed that adipose tissue fragments could adhere onto the growth surface of culture flasks after plating and MSC migrated from the explants reaching confluence after a while. Following *in vitro* expansion, this population of MSC was successfully induced into adipogenic, osteogenic, and chondrogenic lineages which demonstrated their multipotency. Despite the cost advantages of explants method, the techniques that are employed to adhere successfully adipose tissue fragments onto surface of flasks depend exclusively on the manual skills of the laboratory technician, which makes it a non reproducible method.

The Celution System is a medical device marked for processing adult adipose tissue stem cells for autologous re-implantation or reinfusion, and is currently being used in cosmetic & reconstructive surgery in Europe and Japan, but is not yet available in the United States because U.S. Food & Drug Administration rules. This system enables beside access to adipose stem cells by automating the extraction, washing, and concentration of a patient's own cells for immediate use.

The suctioned adipose tissue is introduced into the Celution cell-processing device and being enzymatically digested into a single cell suspension, which contains a combination of MSC, endothelial progenitor cells and other adipose tissue stromal cells. The cell suspension is washed and all lipid-laden adipocytes and matrix fragments are separated from it. The whole procedure is in a closed circuit and this reduces the chance of cell suspension contamination by fungus and bacteria (Duckers et al., 2006).

This automated closed circuit system would facilitate translational of bench research ideas and results to technologies for bedside use. However, this system has as a disadvantage the use of an enzymatic procedure to obtain a cell suspension. There is a concern over immunological reactions caused by enzyme-derived animal proteins (Spees et al., 2004).

4.2 Mesenchymal stem cell characterization for quality control

4.2.1 Cell culture

The ability to isolate, expand, criopreserve and differentiate MSC is an important step in the development of cell therapy approaches for therapeutical proposes of chronic-degenerative diseases, as well as for their application in plastic or reconstructive surgery. It was suspected that inconsistent data about therapeutical potentials of mesenchymal MSC is a result from different cell culture practices.

Based on our experience, we had set up a standardized protocol for the culture of human adipose tissue MSC and microbiological quality control procedures. Standards for the culture system included the use of alphaMEM (without nucleotides) containing 10% of fetal bovine serum selected for cell growth and 100U/mL penicillin and 100µg/mL streptomycin. After isolation, cultures of cells (10^5 cells/cm^2) were maintained at 37°C in a humid atmosphere containing 5% CO_2. A subset of plated cells could adhere to the culture dish, developing a spindle shape morphology (Figure 4A). Non-adherent cells were removed by washing 24 hours after plating. The medium was changed every 3-5 days for proliferation until cells reach pre-confluence, which means 90% of the culture area covered by cells (10 to 15 days after plating - Figure 4B). Adherent cells were detached with 0.78mm EDTA and 0.125% trypsin and cell suspension was centrifugated 400 *g* (gravities) for 7 min. For cell expansion, cells were re-plated into culture dishes (10^4 cells/cm^2). This procedure was considered to be 'one passage'. Typical morphology of proliferating cells can be visualized during cell expansion when the cultivation conditions are adequate (Figure 4B - arrows). Cells isolated by the mechanic method maintained the ability to proliferate and the fibroblastic morphology even after 10 passages. No stress actin bundles were visualized (Baptista et al., 2009).

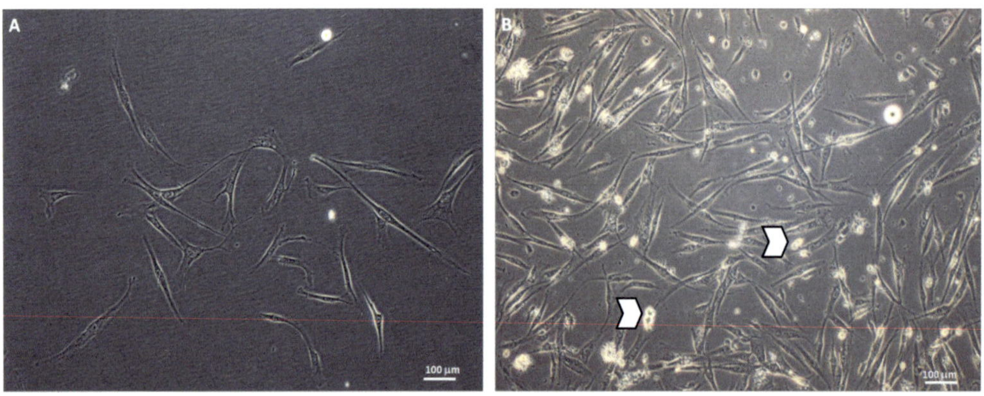

Fig. 4. Culture of human adipose tissue mesenchymal stem cells isolated by mechanic method. Immediately after isolation, cells were resuspended in alphaMEM (without nucleotides) containing 10% of fetal bovine serum and 100 U/mL penicillin and 100 µg/mL streptomycin and seeding at 10^5 cells/cm^2 into culture dishes. Cultures were maintained at 37°C in a humid atmosphere with 5% CO_2, and the medium was changed every 3-5 days until cells reach pre-confluence. (A) After 5 days of culture, the monolayer of cells showed typical fibroblast morphology, and after 15 days (B) proliferation events can be observed (arrowheads). Bar size 100 μm.

For cell cryopreservation, cell suspension was centrifugated 400 g for 7 min and pellet was ressuspended in cryopreservation medium consisting of 90% fetal bovine serum and 10%DMSO (dimethyl-sulfoxide). This cell suspension was distributed in cryotubes in the ratio of 10^6 to 2 x 10^6 cell/tube. Cell freezing was performed for 24 hours in -70°C freezer, the cryotubes were then transferred to the gas phase of liquid nitrogen (-196°C) for long term storage. Analyses carried out after thawing showed that cells maintain their typical fibroblastic morphology and high viability. The ability to differentiate into mesodermal (adipogenic, osteogenic and chondrogenic) lineages was also attested.

Cells used both for clinical or experimental purposes must be free of microbiological contamination. Standards to monitor this type of contamination includes the use of hemoculture like tests and molecular biology. Cultures are daily observed under an optical microscope as for the presence of structures similar to microorganisms. Before detaching cells with tripsin for cell expansion or cryopreservation, an aliquot of the culture medium is collected to perform hemoculture like tests, which can detect the presence of both bacteria and fungi. However, mycoplasm is a not visible bacteria and also not detectable by this test. Its identification in the culture medium can only be performed using RT-PCR (Reverse Transcriptase-Polimerase Chain Reaction - Figure 5). For details about the basis of PCR, see Alberts et al., 2002. Detection kits are comercially available to identify several species of mycoplasm. If tests show the presence of a microorganism, an antibiogram is done to indicate the best antibiotic or antifungal to be used for decontamination.

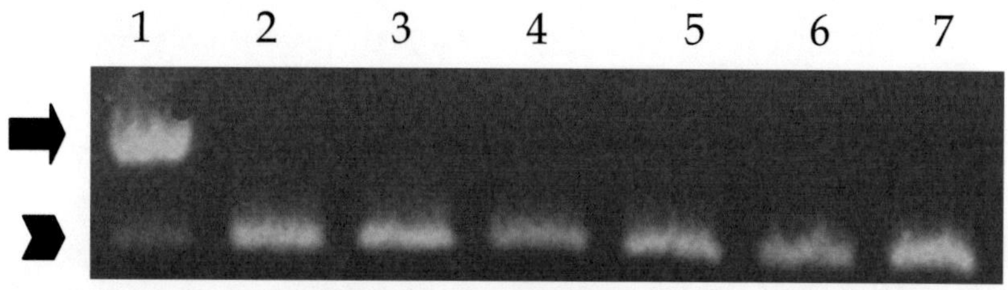

Fig. 5. RT-PCR to detect mycoplasm. RT-PCR was performed to monitor the presence of mycoplasm in the supernatant of mesenchymal stem cell cultures. We used a commercially available Detection Kit, which contains positive and negative samples used as reaction controls and reference. It is able to identify a range of mycoplasm species. Image was captured from a agarose gel with controls and experimental samples. Line 1: Positive control. First band is the detection of mycoplasm (arrow). Second band is the detection of a mRNA which serves as an internal control of the reaction (arrowhead), meaning that no intercurrences have occurred during sample preparation for analysis. Line 2: Negative control, absent of the mycoplasm band, but with internal control band presented (arrowhead). Lines 3 to 7, five different samples of the supernantant of cultured cells, free of mycoplasm. Note that the internal control band is present.

4.2.2 Flow cytometry

Standardized methods are necessary to assess the presence, viability and functional quality of MSC on the cell preparation obtained after the isolation procedure and after *in vitro* cell expansion. Fluorescence-activated flow cytometry is a very interesting tool to be used for this purpose. This is a technology based on the use of laser radiation, hydrodynamic fluid, optics, fluorochromes and computing resources. It is used to determine some structural and functional characteristics of biological particles, like cells. It is the most used technique to detect cellular antigens, called cluster of differentiation (CD) antigens, having a broad field of application in hematology, pharmacology, immunology, oncology, microbiology, genetics and stem cell research.

CD antigens are proteins expressed on cell membranes. They are commonly used as cell markers, allowing cells to be defined based on which molecules are present on their surface. However, CD antigens are not merely markers of cells. They usually act as receptors or ligands which initiate a signal cascade, being responsible for different cell behaviors. Besides cell signaling, some of CD antigens have different functions, like cell adhesion. A nomenclature is used to describe different monoclonal antibodies against specific antigens, using the term CD plus a number. For example, an antibody that detects a specific glycoprotein on the surface of T helper lymphocytes is named CD4.

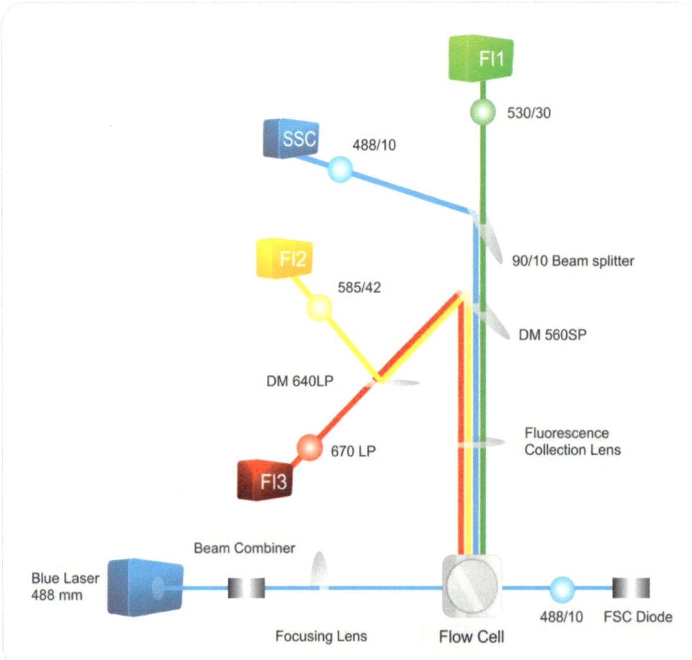

Fig. 6. Schematic representation of a flow cytometer. Flow cytometers aspire cells from a suspension and force them to pass by the flow cell, using a system of pressurization. A laser intercept cells individually. The modifications that occur in this light beam due to cell characteristics are detected and measured by sensors (detectors) disposed adequately. Dispersed light is collected by an optical system which allows to identify cells by their size and complexity (The FSC and SSC Detectors). Fluorescence emitted by fluorochromes are also collected. To select these luminous signals emitted by fluorochromes, optical filters are used to block certain incident light wavelengths and let pass only the desired one. Each fluorescence emission is identified by different detectors (FL1, FL2, FL3), which convert luminous signals in electrical pulses and amplify this signal.

Flow cytometer, the equipment used to this end, is prepared to aspire cells or particles in a previously prepared suspension and force them to go through a special chamber, centralized in a continuous flow of liquid (sheath fluid) and leaving this chamber one after another so that a single cell is intercepted by a laser. After laser interception, physical phenomena occurs, giving information about cells: First, part of the light is scattered according to structural and morphological cell characteristics. The Forward Scatter (FSC) is related to cell size and the Side Scatter (SSC) is related to cell granularity/complexity. Second, cells previously stained with fluorochomes coupled with antibodies are excited by the laser and a light emission occurs according to their fluorescent characteristics. Different fluorochromes absorbs the light and emit it in a higher and specific wavelength. Each fluorochrome has a spectral pattern of absorption and emission, allowing up to three light colors to be optically separated by selectively filters in common cytometers. Lenses are placed in series closed to the area of laser interception. They collect the light scattered and send it to photomultipliers that convert luminous signal in electrical pulses, which are proportional to the quantity of light dispersed or fluorescence captured by the photomultipliers (Figure 6).

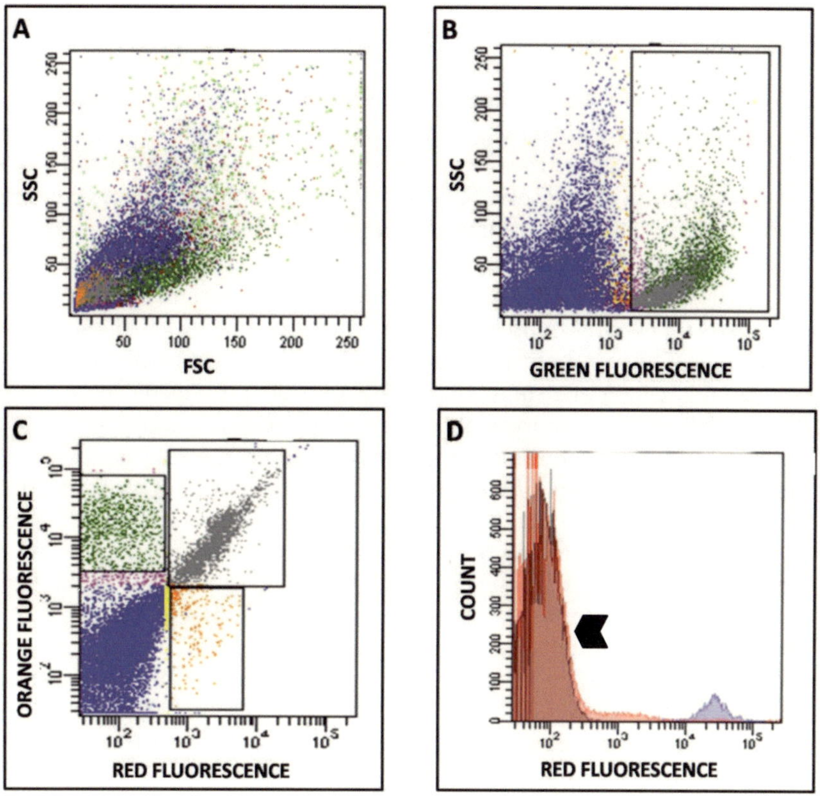

Fig. 7. Usual representation of data generated by the flow cytometer. Dot-plots (A - C) and Histogram (D) graphs are showed and represent the number of events or cells acquired. (A - C) Each dot is representative of one cell, (D) the number of cells is represented in y axis (counts). (A) Graph represents cell complexity in y axis (Side Scatter - SSC) and cell size in x axis (Forward Scatter - FSC). Parameters are presented in a linear scale. Cells with different degrees of complexity and size can be observed (A). Three-color immunofluorescence (green, red and orange) data were also collected from this sample and are presented in a log scale. (B) Side Scatter - SSC - is represented in y axis and green fluorescence channel in x axis. Only part of cells is positive for this green fluorescence parameter (box). (C) Graph represents two fluorescence channels (orange and red) simultaneously. We can identify at least four different cell populations. Cells exclusively positive for orange fluorescence parameter (box upper left), positive for both fluorescence parameters (box upper right), positive only for red fluorescence parameter (box lower right), and negative for both (cells outside boxes) (D) In this histogram it is possible to separate three populations of cells: Negative cells for red fluorescence parameter, which is overlaid with experimental negative control (arrowhead), positive cells with an intermediate staining (in red) and positive cells with a high staining (in blue).

To select and capture these luminous signals, optical filters are used to block specific incident light wavelengths and let pass only the desired wavelength. The electrical signs generated by the photomultipliers are amplified, converted to digital sign and sent to a computer. The data sampling, analysis and interpretation can then be performed using a specific software. Data generated by the flow cytometer can be represented in the form of mono- or biparametric histograms (Figure 7). By this way, it is possible to detect 10000 cells (called events) per second. Five parameters are considered basic and can be measured simultaneously: cell size, cell complexity, green fluorescence, red fluorescence and orange fluorescence.

To be detected by flow cytometry, cellular antigens must be labeled by immunofluorescence techniques. The antibodies against the antigens must be conjugated to fluorochromes. There are many fluorochromes, each of them with different ranges of excitation and emission light wavelengths. The most used are those that can be excited by the emission wavelength of the lasers available in flow cytometers. Some of them are Fluorescein, Phycoerithrin, Rodamin, Texas red, Cianins etc. There are fluorochromes with properties to attach directly to biological molecules, like the DNA stains: Propide Iodide (PI) and Ethidium Bromide (EB). PI is not able to cross a healthy cytoplasmic membrane. So, only dead cells stains with PI. EB can cross the cytoplasmic membrane, but only attach to DNA when cells are dead, because a transport system that expels the stain is off (Midgley, 1987). By using these or other DNA markers, it is possible to ascertain the viability of cells in a cell preparation.

It is possible to combine, in the same sample, two or more fluorescent stains if they emit light in different wavelengths and if the system is able to excite all of them and discriminate each emission. The most used multiple dying technique is green-red, by applying the fluorescein with maximum emission at 520nm, and phycoerithrin which emits at 576nm. Both can be excited by an Argon laser at 488nm, the most used laser in flow cytometers. Nowadays, studies are undertaken using 4 and 5 antibodies conjugated to different fluorochromes with different light wavelength emission. The most sophisticated cytometers can discriminate the information of up to 17 fluorescent markers, allowing the analysis of multiple possibilities of cell characteristics (Perfetto et al, 2004). This versatility is called multiparametric analysis. In cell biology, this property allows selective discrimination of subpopulations, based on the combination of many fluorochromes.

Cells isolated by the mechanic method contained two different major mononuclear cell subpopulations, CD45 positive and CD45 negative cells. Cells positive for CD45, a pan-hematopoietic marker, were also positive for CD16, CD14, CD31, surface markers of granulocytes, monocytes-macrophages and endothelial cells, respectively (Baptista et al., 2009). MSC do not have a hematopoietic origin, but a stromal one. So these cells are essentially CD45 negatives (Figure 8A). In this fraction, we could identify MSC, which are $CD146^+$ (Figure 8B).

After seeding the initial cell suspension, culture dishes were washed with saline solution, removing the CD45 positive peripheral blood contaminant cells, remaining only a fraction of adherent cells. MSC that must be plastic-adherent into culture dishes, are a part of this fraction. Not surprisingly, this adherent cells were negative for CD45 and positive for CD44, CD90, CD105 (Baptista et al., 2009) and CD73 (Figure 8D), surface markers described in MSC populations of different origins (Dominici et al., 2006). They were also positive for CD34, (Figure 8C), a glycoprotein reported to be present only in adipose tissue MSC (Planat-Bernard et al., 2004). After expansion *in vitro*, we and others detected a progressive increase of mesenchymal markers expression like CD73 and CD90, while the expression of CD34 decreases until being completely loss (McIntosh et al., 2006; Mitchell et al., 2006; Baptista et al., 2009; Bernardo et al., 2009).

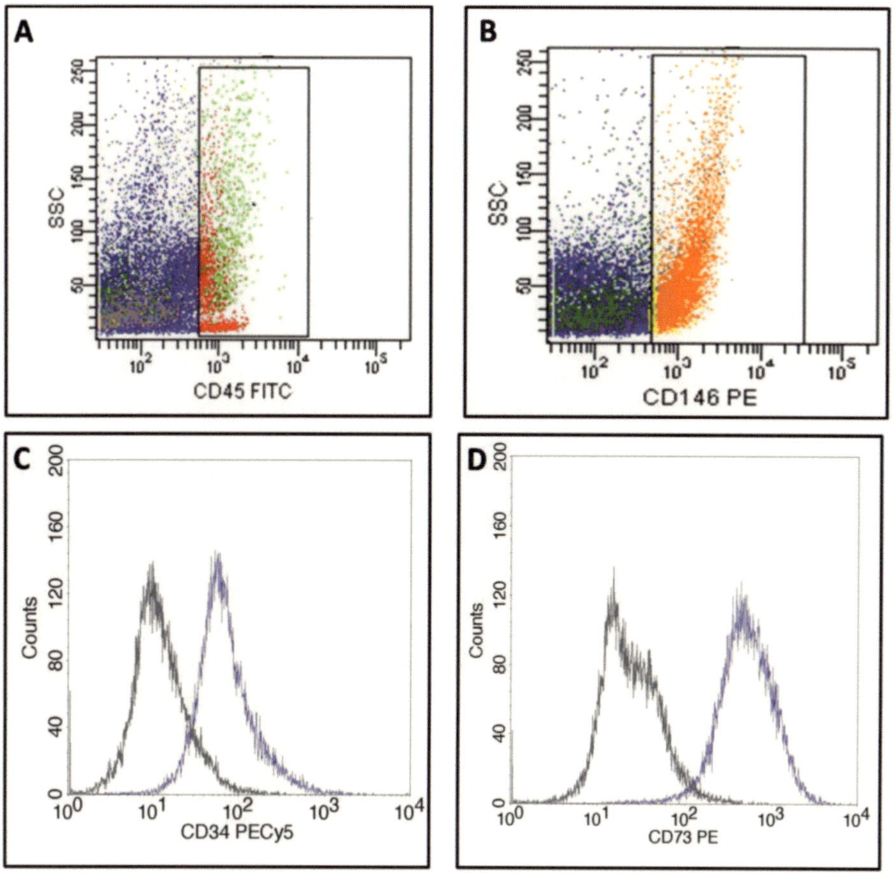

Fig. 8. Phenotypic characterization of subcutaneous adipose tissue cells. Cells isolated by the mechanic method were monitored for surface marker expression at the moment they were isolated (A, B) and at first passage *in vitro* (C, D) using flow cytometry. Cells were stained with monoclonal antibodies conjugated with fluorescent dies: CD45–fluorescein isothiocyanate (FITC), CD146–phycoerythrin (PE), CD73-PE and CD34– PECy5 (PECyanin-5) . For each profile, 200.000 events were acquired in freshly isolated samples and 50.000 events for cultured cells. Flow cytometry analysis were performed using a FACSCanto (A, B) or FACSCalibur (C, D) - BD Biosciences. (A, B) Dot-plots graphs. (A) Hematopoietic cells (CD45 positive) are gated (box). Cells outside the box (non-hematopoietic cells) in (A) are distributed in (B) and positive for the perivascular stem cell marker - CD146 (box). At first passage, cultured mesenchymal stem cells maintained the pre-adipocyte (C) and the mesensenchymal stem cell marker (D), CD34 and CD73, respectively. (C, D) Gray lines on histograms graphs represents isotype controls.

No unique single marker has been described yet to distinguish MSC from other cells in the tissue of origin (Mosna et al, 2010). Instead of it, a combination of markers is used for an adequate detection of these cells. Thereby, flow cytometry represents an important tool to make a detailed immunophenotypic analysis of these cells, providing information of many fluorescent markers in the same cell, reading millions of cells in few minutes (Perfetto et al., 2004). It allows a rapid qualitative and quantitative multiparametric analysis of cells, making measurements on single cells as they travel in suspension one by one.

With this understanding, we propose the use of flow cytometry to characterize the cell preparation obtained after the isolation procedure and after *in vitro* cell expansion, as an efficient standard method to identify the presence and viability of adipose-derived MSC in these preparations, to assure the quality of cells that will be used in therapeutic approaches.

4.2.3 Differentiation assays

To assure the multilineage differentiation capacity of expanded MSC, standard methods of *in vitro* cell differentiation are used. These functional assays allow testing the ability of MSC to differentiate to the adipogenic, osteogenic and condrogenic lineages. To test this capacity, specific stimuli are used for each lineage diferentiation, like growth factors, hormones and drugs. These molecules can act in specific cell receptors, which transduce signals of growth and differentiation through cascades of intracellular events (Gregoire et al., 1998).

For induction to the adipogenic lineage, cells are cultivated in monolayer and incubated for at least two weeks with culture medium containing 10% of fetal bovine serum, insulin 10μM, IBMX (isobutilmethilxantine) 0,5mM, dexamethasone 10^{-6}M and indomethacin 200μM. To test the osteogenic differentiation capacity, cells are cultivated in monolayer and incubated for three weeks with medium containing 10% fetal bovine serum, ascorbic acid 5 x 10^{-6}M, dexametasone 10^{-8}M and β-glicerophosphate 10^{-2}M.

To promote chondrogenic differentiation, we used three-dimensional cell culture methodology. Cells, expanded until third passage, were enzymatically detached from culture dishes and cell suspension was centrifuged 400g for 7 min. Pellet was resuspended in chondrogenic medium containing insulin 6,25μg/mL, transferrin 6,25μg/mL, ascorbic acid 50μg/mL, albumin 1,25μg/mL, dexamethasone 10^{-7}M and TGF-β3 (*Transforming Growth Factor- β3*).

Cell suspension containing 2x 10^5 cells were distributed in polypropylene conical tubes with capacity of 15ml, centrifuged 300g for 10 min and maintained at 37°C in a humid atmosphere with 5% CO_2 for four weeks. Chondrogenic medium was renewed every 3 or 4 days, taking care not to damage the cell pellet. After 4 days, the pellet appeared like a sphere, with around 0,9 mm of diameter.

The inductive media must be renewed twice in a week and after the appropriate time period, cells are fixed and evaluated for lipid accumulation, extracellular calcium deposition and cartilage tissue extracellular matrix (ECM) production, to assess adipogenic, osteogenic and condrogenic differentiation respectively (Baptista et al., 2009). The presence of lipid droplets can be detected by staining induced cells with specific hydrophobic stains, being Oil Red O the most used (Figure 9A, B). Mineral depots are revealed by Alizarin Red staining (Figure 9C, D). Both stains can be eluted from cells and quantified by spectrophotometry, giving a quantitative analysis about the level of differentiation. Production of sulfated glycosaminoglycans (GAGs) and type II collagen - the main molecules of cartilaginous tissue ECM - can be assessed by Alcian Blue (pH 1.0) and Safranin O-Fast Green (Figure 9E, F) stainings or by imunnofluorescence techniques, respectively.

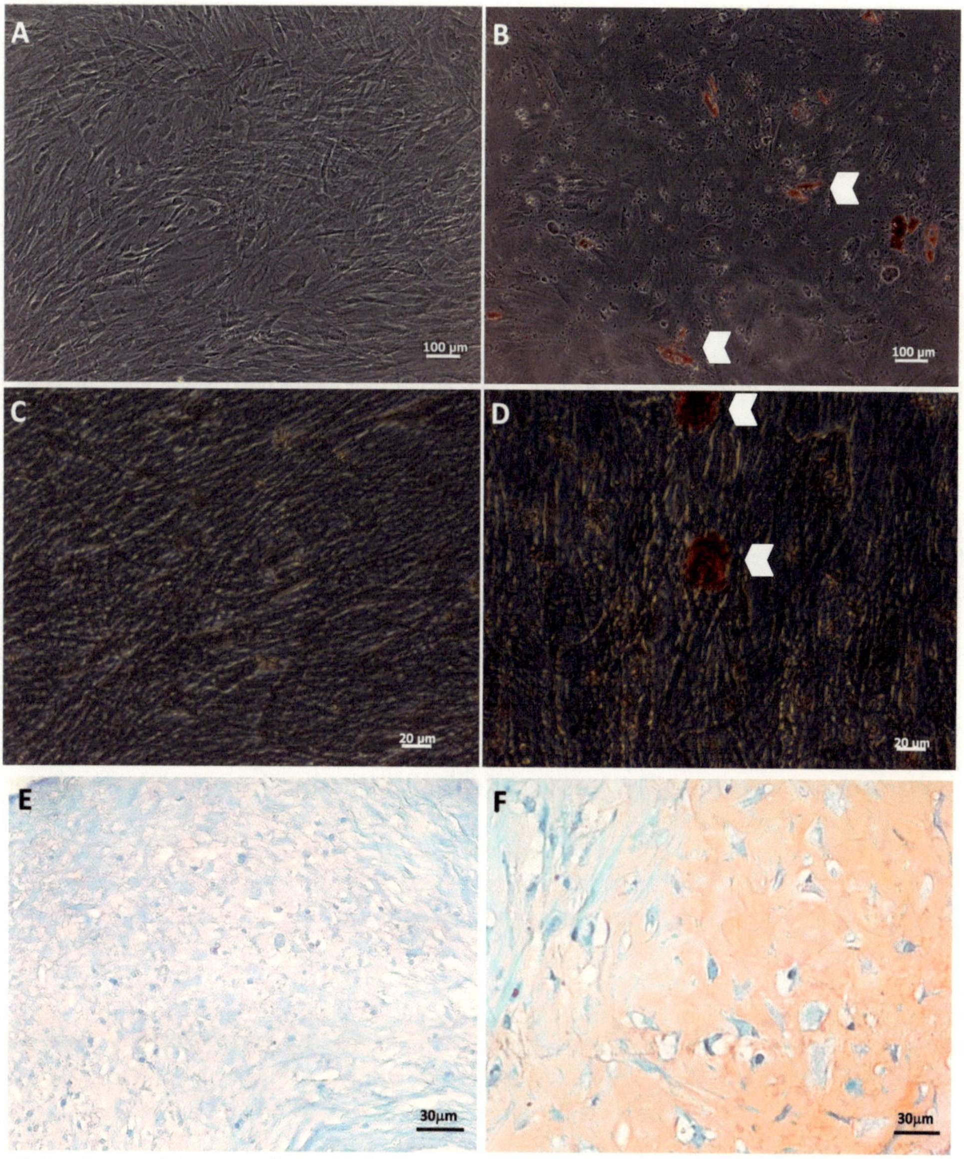

Fig. 9. *In vitro* multipotentiality of adipose tissue mesenchymal stem cells.Cultured mesenchymal stem cells were are able to differentiate into the three mesodermic lineages (adipogenic, osteogenic and chondrogenic). Cultures of cells were maintained under adipogenic (B) or osteogenic (D) inducing media for 14 days. After this period, they were fixed and stained with Oil Red O to identify the lipid droplets (B - arrowheads), and with Alizarin Red to reveal extracellular calcium deposits (D - arrowheads). Media without (A, C) and with (B, D) appropriate inducing factors. (A, B) Bar size, 100 µm. (C, D) Bar size, 20 µm. Pellet cultures formed by mesenchymal stem cells under media without (E), and with (F) chondrogenic inducing factors for 28 days. (E, F) Safranin O staining. Matrix accumulation is typical of cartilage only in induced cells (F). Bar size, 30 µm.

5. Future research

The use of adipocytes and MSC for tissue repair and regeneration can follow two different procedures. The liposculpture uses the freshly harvested adipose tissue, generally obtained by liposuction. The tissue is frequently harvested, processed and reinjected during the same surgical procedure. MSC can be introduced simultaneously, and the tissue processing should be concerned by their viability and their capacity to functionally integrate into the tissue where they are implanted.

Alternatively, MSC can be harvested and expanded *in vitro*, in order to reach the required cell number, and used subsequently for filling or repair of different tissues such as dermis, connective tissue, bone and associated tissues, as well as blood vessels in repair of both peripheral or cardiac tissue ischemia (Hicok et al., 2004; Casteilla et al., 2005; Hanson et al., 2010). In these cell therapies, the implantation of cells lags behind the harvesting for several days or weeks. The viability of harvested cells and their proliferative capacity *in vitro* are critical for such therapeutic approaches.

5.1 Mesenchymal stem cell bank

Autologous MSC, such as those derived from bone marrow or adipose tissue, can be used clinically for regenerative cell therapy or for tissue engineering only when isolated in a reproducible manner and in sufficient quantities. The expansion and differentiation steps may provide increased cell number, purity, and maturity, but they do so at a cost. This cost can include one or more of: loss of cell function due to cell aging, increased monetary cost, and increased risk of contamination of cells with environmental microorganisms during culture.

Liposuction surgery often generates large volumes of samples to be processed, so it is important not to waste them. There is need for alternative methods in which a population of active cells with increased yield can be prepared rapidly and reliably, and whereby the need for post-extraction manipulation of the cells can be reduced or eliminated. We developed an innovative method based on mechanic dissociation of adipose tissue in order to release MSC population from it and that attends all these needs described (Baptista et al., 2009). MSC population can be isolated in a manner that is suitable for their direct placement into a recipient or for their direct cryopreservation in a laboratory.

The possibility of cryopreservation of freshly isolated MSC abrogates culture-associated changes found in cells after prolonged expansion, and provides the possibility of generating extemporaneously a large stock of cells (MSC bank) using a relatively simple method. Once cryopreserved, MSC can be thawed as the need of use, without loss of cell viability and functionality.

5.2 Autologous fat grafts

Autologous fat grafts are becoming a major procedure for soft-tissue filling. However, resorption of fat transplanted has been reported (Sommer & Sattler, 2000; Masuda et al., 2004; Kaufman et al., 2007) and current efforts focus on identifying methods that may minimize this undesirable result. There is no universal agreement on what constitutes an ideal methodology to obtain better graft takes and results.

Our results showed that centrifugation, although cleaning adipose tissue of potentially harmful substances yields adipose tissue which is not only devoid of viable adipocytes but also has a diminished percentage of MSC (Condé-Green et al., 2010). Taken together, the long term graft of the implanted centrifuged adipose tissue is less probable, and the implant resorption naturally occurs with clearance of non-viable organic components introduced into the receptor site. In contrast, decantation acceptably separated the supranatant layer of adipose tissue from the oily and sero-sanguinous liquids (infranatant layer), besides preserving the integrity of adipose tissue, number and viability of adipocytes and MSC.

5.3 Fat graft enriched with mesenchymal stem cell

Adipose tissue harvesting and processing techniques employed in the surgery room play an important role on the viability and integrity of adipose tissue, and according our study, also on the percentage of MSC (Condé-Green et al., 2010). A long-term graft is reached mainly by angiogenesis and MSC enhance local angiogenesis by differentiation events, and secretion of angiogenic factors (Hanson et al., 2010).
To overcome drawbacks of autologous lipoinjection, Yoshimura et al., have developed a novel strategy which is based on MSC association with autologous fat working as scaffold. This novel strategy resulted on long-term retention of fat graft (Yoshimura et al., 2008). Recently, our group was responsible for the development of an innovative method to isolate adipose tissue MSC on lipoaspirate samples (Baptista et al., 2009). Our method is based on mechanic dissociation of adipose tissue instead of enzymatic, and generates a cell suspension devoid of both: tissue debris and enzyme waste. It is possible performed mechanical dissociation on operating room then, cell suspension enriched with MSC can be injected simultaneously with fresh adipose tissue scaffold. This association (cell suspension enriched with MSC and fresh adipose tissue from decanted lipoaspirate sample) could be used to volume restoration of facial depressions caused by sequelae of trauma and tumors.

6. Conclusion

The scientific community is working on ways to standardize processes so that it is safe and effective, no matter what the application. The major advantages of adipose tissue as a source of regenerative cells, which distinguish it from other alternative cell sources, include: 1) Yield: A therapeutic dose of regenerative cells can be isolated in approximately one hour without cell culture when using our mechanic method of isolation; 2) Safety: Patients receive their own cells (autologous-use) so there is no risk of immune rejection or disease transmission; 3) Versatility: Stem cells from adipose tissue impart benefit from multiple mechanisms of action.
The use of these cells as a product for cell therapies in humans implies the development of standard methods to ensure high cell quality. We described methods of harvesting and preparation of the human adipose tissue and isolation, cultivation, expansion and characterization of adipose derived MSC, developed to achieve this cell quality and to monitor MSC potential for clinical application.

7. Acknowledgments

This study was supported by the Brazilian Ministry of Science and Technology (CNPq) and the Rio de Janeiro State Government (FAPERJ) grants.
Excellion Biomedical Services SA, Petrópolis, is acknowledged for supplying facilities for tissue processing, cell manipulation and analyses.
Dr. Cesar Claudio-da-Silva and Dr. Marcelo Aniceto for providing the lipoaspirate samples.

8. References

Alberts, B., Johnson, A., Lewis, J., Raff, M., Roberts, K., and Walter, P. (2002). Manipulatingproteins, DNA, and RNA, In: *Molecular Biology of the Cell,* Bruce Alberts, AlexanderJohnson, Julian Lewis, Martin Raff, Keith Roberts, and Peter Walter, pp. (508509), Garland Science, ISBN-10: 0-8153-3218-1, New York

Ahmadbeigi, N., Shafiee, A., Seyedjafari, E., Gheisari, Y., Vassei, M., Amanpour, S., Amini,S., Bagherizadeh, I., Soleimani, M. Early spontaneous immortalization and loss ofplasticity of rabbit bone marrow mesenchymal stem cells. *Cell Proliferation.* Vol. 44,No. 1, (February 2011), pp. 67-74. ISSN 0960-7722

Bailey, AM., Kapur, S., & Katz, AJ. Characterization of adipose derived stem cells: anupdate. *Currently Stem Cell Research and Therapy,* Vol. 5, No. 2, (June 2010), pp. 95-102, ISSN 1574-888X

Baptista, LS., Pedrosa, CGS., Silva, KR., Otazu, MID. Bone marrow and adipose tissue derived mesenchymal stem cells: how close are they? *Journal of Stem Cell,* Vol. 2, (2007), pp. 73–89, ISSN 1556-8539

Baptista, LS., do Amaral, RJ., Carias, RB., Aniceto, M., Claudio-da-Silva, C., & Borojevic, R. An alternative method for the isolation of mesenchymal stromal cells derived from lipoaspirate samples. *Cytotherapy,* Vol. 11, No. 6, (2009), pp. 706–715, ISSN 1465-3249

Bernardo, ME., Locatelli, F., & Fibbe, WE. Mesenchymal stromal cells *Annals of the New York Academy of Science,* Vol. 1176, No.1, (September 2009), pp.101–117, ISSN 0077-8923

Bunnell, BA., Flaat, M., Gagliardi, C., Patel, B., & Ripoll, C. Adipose derived stem cells: isolation, expansion and differentiation. *Methods,* Vol. 45, No. 2, (June 2008), pp. 115-120, ISSN 1046-2023

Caplan, AL. Mesenchymal stem cells. *Journal of Orthopaedic Research,* Vol. 9, No. 5, (September 1991) pp- 641-650, ISSN0736-0266

Caplan, AI. Adult mesenchymal stem cells for tissue engineering versus regenerative medicine. *Journal of Cellular Physiology.* Vol., 213, No. 2, (November 2007), pp. 341 347. ISSN 0021-9541

Caspar-Bauguil, S.; Cousin, B., Galinier, A., Segafredo, C., Nibbelink, M., André, M., Casteilla, L., & Pénicaud, L. Adipose tissue as an ancestral immune organ: site specific change in obesity. *FEBS Letters,* Vol. 579, No. 17, (July 2005), pp.3487-3492, ISSN 0014-5793

Casteilla, L., Charrière, G., Laharrague, P., Cousin, B., Planat- Benard, V., Péricaud, L., & Chavoin, JP. Tissus adipeux, chirurgie plastique et reconstructrice: le retour aux sources. *Annales de Chirurgie Plastique et Esthétique.* Vol. 49, No. 5, (October 2004), pp. 409-418, ISSN 0294-1260

Casteilla, L., Planat-Bénard, V., Cousin, B., Silvestre, J.S., Laharrague, P., Charrière, G., Carrière, A., Pénicaud, L. Plasticity of adipose tissue: a promising therapeutic avenue in the treatment of cardiovascular and blood diseases? *Archives des maladies du coeur et des vaisseaux,* Vol. 98, No. 9, (September 2005), pp.922-926. ISSN 0003-9683

Chajchir, A., Benzaquen, I., & Moretti, E. Comparative experimental study of autologous adipose tissue processed by different techniques. *Aesthetic Plastic Surgery,* Vol. 17, No. 2, (1993), pp. 113-115. ISSN 0364-216X

Chamberlain, G., Fox, J., Ashton, B., Middleton, J. Mesenchymal stem cells: Their phenotype, differentiation capacity, immunological features, and potential for homing. *Stem Cells.* Vol. 25, No. 11 (November 2007), pp. 2739–2749. ISSN 1066-5099

Condé-Green, A., Baptista, LS., de Amorin, NF., de Oliveira, ED., da Silva, KR., Pedrosa, C da S., Borojevic R., Pitanguy I. Effects of centrifugation on cell composition and viability of aspirated adipose tissueprocessed for transplantation. *Aesthetic Surgery Journal*, Vol. 30, No. 2, (March 2010), pp. 249-55, ISSN 1090-820X

Crisan, M., Yap, S., Casteilla, L., Chen, C., Corselli, M., Park, TS., Andriollo, G., Sun, B., Zheng, B., Zhang, L., Norotte, C., Teng, P., Trass, J., Schugar, R., Deasy, BM., Badylak, S., Buhring, H., Giacobino, J., Lazzari, L. Huard, J., Péault, B. A perivascular origin for mesenchymal stem cells in multiple human organs. *CellStem Cell*. Vol. 3, No. 3, (September 2008), pp.301-313. ISSN 1934-5909

da Silva Meirelles, L., Caplan, AI., Nardi, NB. In search of the in vivo identity of mesenchymal stem cells. *Stem Cells*,Vol. 26, No. 9, (September 2008), pp. 2287-2299, ISSN 1066-5099

Dominici, M., Le Blanc, K., Mueller, I., Slaper-Cortenbach, I., Marini, F., Krause, D., Deans, R., Keating, A., Prockop, Dj., & Horwitz, E. Minimal criteria for defining multipotent mesenchymal stromal cells. The International Society for Cellular Therapy position statement. *Cytotherapy*. Vol. 8, No. 4, (2006), pp. 315–317. ISSN 1465-3249

Duckers, HJ., Pinkernell, K., Milstein, AM., & Hedrick, MH. The Bedside Celution TM system for isolation of adipose derived regenerative stem cells. *EuroIntervention*, Vol. 2, No. 3, (November 2006), pp. 395–398, ISSN 1774-024X

Fraser, JK., Zhu, M.,Wulur I., & Alfonso, Z. Adipose-derived stem cells. *Methods in Molecular Biology*, Vol. 449 (2008), pp. 59-67, ISSN 1064-3745

Ferrari, G., Cusella-de-angelis, G., Coletta, M., Paolucci, E., Stornaiuolo, A., Cossu, G., & Mavilio, F. Muscle regeneration by bone marrow-derived myogenic progenitors. *Science*. Vol. 279, No. 5356, (março 1998), pp.1528–1530. ISSN 0036-8075

Friedenstein, AJ., Petrakova, KV., Kurolesova, AI., & Frolova, GP. Heterotopic bone marrow. Analysis of precursor cells for osteogenic and hematopoietic tissues. *Transplantation*, Vol. 6, No. 2, (1968), pp.230-247, ISSN0041-1337

Friedenstein, AJ., Deriglasova, UF., Kulagina, NN., Panasuk, AF., Rudakowa, SF., Luriá, EA., & Ruadkow, IA. Precursors for fibroblasts in different populations of hematopoietic cells as detected by the *in vitro* colony assay method. *Experimental Hematology*, Vol. 2, (1974), pp. 83-92, ISSN 0301-472X

Garcia, S., Bernad, A., Martín, MC., Cigudosa, JC., Garcia-Castro, J., de la Fuente, R. Pitfalls in spontaneous in vitro transformation of human mesenchymal stem cells. *Experimental Cell Research*. Vol. 316, No. 9, (May 2010), pp. 1648-1650. ISSN 0014 4827.

Gimble, J., & Guilak, F. Adipose-derived adult stem cells: isolation, characterization and differentiation potential. *Cytotherapy*, Vol. 5, No. 5, (2003), pp. 362-369, ISSN 1465-3249

Gregoire, FM.; Smas, CM.; & Sul, HS. Understanding adipocyte differentiation. *Physiological Reviews*, Vol. 78, No. 3, (July 1998), pp. 783-809, ISSN 0031-9333

Gregoire, FM. Adipocyte differentiation: from fibroblast to endocrine cell. *Experimental Biology and Medicine*, Vol. 226, No. 11, (December 2001), pp. 997-1002, ISSN 1535-3702

Hanson, S.E., Bentz, M.L., & Hematti, P. Mesenchymal stem cell therapy for nonhealing cutaneous wounds. *Plastic and reconstructive surgery*, Vol. 125, No. 2, (February2010), pp. 510-516. ISSN 1529-4242

Hicok, K.C., Du Laney, T.V., Zhou, Y.S., Halvorsen, Y.D., Hitt, D.C., Cooper, L.F., & Gimble, J.M. Human adipose-derived adult stem cells produce osteoid *in vivo*. *Tissue Engeneering*, Vol. 10, No. 3-4, (March-April 2004), pp. 371-380, ISSN 1076-3279

Ishige, I., Nagamura-Inoue, T., Honda, MJ., Harnprasopvat, R., Kido, M., Sugimoto, M., Nakauchi, H., & Tojo, A. Comparison of mesenchymal stem cells derived from arterial, venous, and Wharton's jelly explants of human umbilical cord. *International Journal of Hematology*, Vol. 90, No. 2, (September 2009), pp. 261–269, ISSN 0925-5710

Jing, W., Lin, Y., Wu, L., Li, X., Nie, X., Niu, L., Tang, W., Zheng, X & Tian, W. Ectopic adipogenesis of preconditioned adipose-derived stromal cells in an alginate system. *Cell and Tissue Research*, Vol. 330, No. 3, (December 2007), pp. 567-72, ISSN 0302-766X

Jing, W., Xiao, J., Xiong, Z., Yang, X., Huang, Y., Zhou, M., Chen, S., Lin, Y., & Tian, W. Explant Culture: An Efficient Method to Isolate Adipose-Derived Stromal Cells for Tissue Engineering. *Artificial Organs*, Vol. 35, No. 2, (February 2010), pp. 105-112, ISSN 0160-564X

Kaufman, M.R., Miller, T.A., Huang, C., Roostaeian, J., Wasson, K.L., Ashley, R.K., Bradley, J.P. Autologous fat transfer for facial recontouring: Is there science behind the art? *Plastic and reconstructive surgery*, Vol. 119, No.7, (June 2007), pp. 2287 2296. ISSN 1529-4242

Karnoub AE, Dash AB, Vo AP, Sullivan A, Brooks MW, Bell GW, Richardson, AL., Polyak, K., Tubo, R., Weinberg, RA. Mesenchymal stem cells within tumour stroma promote breast cancer metastasis. *Nature*. Vol. 449, No. 7162 (October 2007), pp. 557-563. ISSN 0028-0836

Khoo, ML., Shen, B., Tao, H., Ma, DD. Long-term serial passage and neuronal differentiation capability of human bone marrow mesenchymal stem cells. *Stem Cells and Development*. Vol. 17, No. 5, (October 2008), pp. 883-96. ISSN 1557-8534.

Klingbeil, MF., Herson, MR., Cristo, EB., dos Santos Pinto D JR., Yoshito, D., & Mathor, MB. Comparison of two cellular harvesting methods for primary human oral culture of keratinocytes. *Cell and Tissue Banking*, Vol. 10, No. 3, (August 2009), pp. 197–204, ISSN 1389-9333

Klopp, AH., Gupta, A., Spaeth, E., Andreeff, M., & Marini, F3rd. Dissecting a discrepancy in the literature: do mesenchymal stem cells support or suppress tumor growth? *Stem Cells*. Vol. 29, No. 1, (Janueary 2011), pp. 11-19. ISSN 1066-5099

Kurita, M., Matsumoto, D., Shigeura, T., Sato, K., Gonda, K., Harii, K., & Yoshimura, K. Influences of centrifugation on cells and tissues in liposuction aspirates: optimizedcentrifugation for lipotransfer and cell isolation. *Plastic and reconstructive surgery*, Vol. 121, No. 3, (March 2008), pp. 1033-1041. ISSN 1529-4242

Liu, G., Zhou, H., Li, Y., Li, G., Cui, L., Liu, W., & Cao, Y. Evaluation of the viability and osteogenic differentiation of cryopreserved human adipose-derived stem cells. *Cryobiology*, Vol. 57, No.1, (August 2008), pp. 18-24. ISSN 1090-2392

Masuda, T., Furue, M., & Matsuda, T. Novel strategy for soft tissue augmentation based on transplantation of fragmented omentum and preadipocytes. *Tissue Engeneering*, Vol. 10, No. 11-12, (November-December 2004, pp.1672–1683. ISSN 1076-3279

May, SG., Savell, JW., Lunt, DK., Wilson, JJ., Laurenz, JC., & Smith, SB. Evidence for preadipocyte proliferation during culture of subcutaneous and intramuscular adipose tissues from Angus and Wagyu crossbred steers. *Journal of Animal Science*, Vol. 72, No. 12, (December 1994), pp. 3110-3117, ISSN 0021-8812

McIntosh K, Zvonic, S., Garrett, S., Mitchell, JB., Floyd, ZE., Hammill, L., Kloster, A., Halvorsen, YD., Ting, JP., Storms, RW., Goh, B., Kilroy, G., Wu, X., & Gimble, JM. The immunogenicity of human adipose-derived cells: temporal changes in vitro. *Stem Cells*, Vol. 24, (May 2006), pp. 1246–1253, ISSN 1066-5099

Midgley, M. An efflux system for cationic dyes and related compounds in E.coli. *Microbiological Sciences,* Vol. 4, No. 4, (April 1987), pp. 125-128, ISSN 0265-1351

Mitchell, JB., McIntosh, K., Zvonic, S., Garrett, S., Floyd, ZE., Kloster, A., Halvorsen, YD., Storms, RW., Goh, B., Kilroy, G., Wu, X., & Gimble, JM. Immunophenotype of human adipose derived cells: temporal changes in stromal-associated and stem cell-associated markers. *Stem Cells,* Vol. 24, No. 2, (February 2006), pp. 376-385, ISSN 1066-5099

Miura, M., Miura, Y., Padilla-Nash, HM., Molinolo, AA., Fu, B., Patel, V., Seo, BM., Sonoyama, W., Zheng, JJ., Baker, CC., Chen, W., Ried, T., Shi, S. Accumulated chromosomal instability in murine bone marrow mesenchymal stem cells leads to malignant transformation. *Stem Cells*. Vol. 24, No. 4, (April 2006), pp. 1095-1103. ISSN 1066-5099

Mizuno, H., Zuk, PA., Zhu, M., Lorenz, HP., benhaim, P., Hedrick, MH. Myogenic differentiation by human processed lipoaspirate cells. *Plastic and Reconstructive Surgery*. Vol. 109, No. 1, (January 2002), pp.199-209. ISSN 0032-1052

Mosna, F., Sensebé L., & Krampera, M. Human bone marrow and adipose tissue mesenchymal stem cells: a user's guide. *Stem Cells Development,* Vol. 19, No. 10, (October 2010), pp. 1449-1470, ISSN 1547-3287

Muehlberg, FL., Song, YH., Krohn, A., Pinilla, SP., Droll, LH., Leng, X., Seidensticker, M., Ricke, J., Altman, AM., Devarajan, E., Liu, W., Arlinghaus, RB., Alt, EU. Tissue resident stem cells promote breast cancer growth and metastasis. *Carcinogenesis*. Vol. 30, No. 4 (April 2009), pp. 589-97. ISSN 0143-3334

Perfetto, SP., Chattopadhyay, PK., & Roederer, M. Seventeen-colour flow cytometry: unravelling the immune system. *Nature Reviews. Immunology,* Vol. 4, No. 8, (August 2004), pp. 648-655, ISSN 1474-1733

Poloni, A., Maurizi, G., Babini, L., Serrani, F., Berardinelli, E., Mancini, S., Costantini, B., Discepoli, G., Leoni, P. Human Mesenchymal Stem Cells from chorionic villi and amniotic fluid are not susceptible to transformation after extensive in vitro expansion. *Cell Transplantantion*. (November 2010), Epub ahead of print. ISSN 0963-8791

Planat-Benard, V., Silvestre, JS., Cousin, B., André M., Nibbelink M., Tamarat R., Clergue M., Manneville C., Saillan-Barreau C., Duriez M., Tedgui A., Levy B., Pénicaud L., & Casteilla L. Plasticity of human adipose lineage cells toward endothelial cells: physiological and therapeutic perspectives. *Circulation,* Vol. 109, No. 5, (February 2004), pp.656-663, ISSN 0009-7322

Qin, Y., Ji, H., Wu, Y., Liu, H. Chromosomal instability of murine adipose tissue-derived mesenchymal stem cells in long-term culture and development of cloned embryos. *Cloning and Stem Cells*. Vol. 11, No. 3, (September 2009), pp. 445-52. ISSN 1536-2302

Rigotti, G., Marchi, A., & Sbarbati, A. Adipose-derived mesenchymal stem cells: past, present, and future. *Aesthetic Plastic Surgery,* Vol. 33, No. 3, (May 2009), pp. 271-273, ISSN 0364-216X

Rose, J.G. Jr., Lucarelli, M.J., Lemke, B.N., Dortzbach, R.K., Boxrud, C.A., Obagi, S., & Patel, S. Histologic comparison of autologous fat processing methods. *Ophthalmic plastic and reconstructive surgery,* Vol. 22, No. 3, (May-June 2006), pp. 195-200, ISSN1537-2677

Rubio, D., Garcia-Castro, J., Martín, M.C., de la Fuente, R., Cigudosa, J.C., Lloyd, A.C., Bernad, A. Spontaneous human adult stem cell transformation. *Cancer Research,* Vol. 65, No.8, (April 2005), pp. 3035-3039. ISSN 1538- 7445

Serakinci, N., Guldberg, P., Burns, J.S., Abdallah, B., Schrødder, H., Jensen, T., & Kassem, M. Adult human mesenchymal stem cell as a target for neoplastic transformation. *Oncogene,* Vol. 23, No. 29, (June 2004), pp. 5095–5098, ISSN 1476-5594.

Smith, U. Studies of human adipose tissue in culture. 3. Influence of insulin and medium glucose concentration on cellular metabolism. *The Journal of Clinical Investigation,* Vol. 53, No. 1, (January 1974), pp. 91-98, ISSN 0021-9738

Sommer, B., & Sattler, G. Current concepts of fat graft survival: Histology of aspirated adipose tissue and review of the literature. *Dermatologic surgery: official publication for American Society for Dermatologic Surgery, Vol.* 26, No. 12, (December 2000), pp. 1159–1166, ISSN 1524-4725

Spees, J.L., Gregory, C.A., Singh, H., Tucker, H.A., Peister, A., Lynch, P.J., Hsu, S.C., Smith, J., & Prockop, D.J. Internalized antigens must be removed to prepare hypoimmunogenic mesenchymal stem cells for cell and gene therapy. *Molecular therapy: the journal of the American Society of Gene Therapy,* Vol. 9, No. 5, (May 2004), pp. 747-756. ISSN 1525-0024

Suga., H., Matsumoto, D., Inoue, K., Shigeura, T., Eto, H., Aoi, N., Kato., H., Abe, H., & Yoshimura, K. Numerical measurement of viable and nonviable adipocytes and other cellular components in aspirated fat tissue. *Plastic and reconstructive surgery,* Vol. 122, No 1, (July 2008), pp. 103-114, ISSN 1529-4242

Trayhurn, P. The biology of obesity. *The Proceedings of the Nutrition Society,* Vol. 64, No. 1, (February 2005), pp. 31-38,ISSN 0029-6651

Viterbo, F., & Ochoa, JS. Vibroliposuction: a study of rate of aspiration. *Aesthetic Plastic Surgery,* Vol. 26, No. 2, (March-April 2002), pp. 118-122, ISSN 0364-216X

Vunjak-Novakovic, G. (2006) Tissue Engineering: Basic Considerations, in Culture of Cells for Tissue Engineering (eds G. Vunjak-Novakovic and R. I. Freshney), John Wiley & Sons, Inc., Hoboken, NJ, USA. doi: 10.1002/0471741817.ch6

Wajchenberg, BL. Subcutaneous and visceral adipose tissue: their relation to the metabolic syndrome. *Endocrine Reviews.* Vol. 21, No. 6, (December 2000), pp. 697–738, ISSN 0163-769X

Wakitani, S., Saito, T., & Caplan, AI. Myogenic cells derived from rat bone marrow mesenchymal stem cells exposed to 5-azacytidine. *Muscle & Nerve.* Vol. 18, No. 12, (December 1995), pp. 1417–1426, ISSN 0148-639X

Yoshimura, K., Sato, K., Aoi, N., Kurita, M., Hirohi, T., Harii, K. Cell-assisted lipotransfer for cosmetic breast augmentation: supportive use of adipose-derived stem/stromal cells. *Aesthetic Plastic Surgery.* Vol. 32, No.1, (January 2008), pp. 48-55. ISSN 0364-216X

Zimmerlin, L., Donnenberg, AD., Rubin, JP., Basse, P., Landreneau, RJ., Donnenberg, VS. Regenerative therapy and cancer: in vitro and in vivo studies of the interaction between adipose-derived stem cells and breast cancer cells from clinical isolates. *Tissue Engineering Part A.* Vol. 17, No. 1-2, (January 2011), pp. 93-106. ISSN 1937-3341

Zhang, X., Sun, H., Tang, X., Ji, J., Li, X., Sun, J., Ma, Z., Huan, J., & Han, ZC. Comparison of cell-suspension and explant culture of rabbit limbal epithelial cells. *Experimental Eye Research,* Vol. 80, No. 2, (February 2005), pp. 227–233, ISSN 0014-4835

Zuk, PA., Zhu, M., Mizuno, H., Huang, J., Futrell, JW., Katz, AJ., Benhaim, P., Lorenz, HP., & Hedrick, MH. Multilineage cells from human adipose tissue: implications for cell-based therapies. *Tissue Engeneering.* Vol. 7, No. 2, (April 2001) , pp. 211-228, ISSN 1076-3279

12

Stem Cell Enriched Fat Transfer

Maurizio Ceccarelli[1] and J. Víctor García[2]
[1]International Centre for Study and Research in Aesthetic and Physiological Medicine, Roma
[2]Sociedad Española de Medicina y Cirugía Cosmética, Barcelona
[1]Italy
[2]Spain

1. Introduction

Recently, medical techniques have been proposed for tissue regeneration using autologous adult fat stem cells obtained with liposuction to restore the regular volumes of adipose tissue in the body and especially in the face.
The regeneration of the face adipose tissue follows the outline of a technique already in use: the lipofilling. This process is based on fat cells obtained with low-pressure suction and further centrifugation to separate fat cells from the stroma-vascular connective tissue.. The aim is to infiltrate only intact cells, able to survive in their new home [1].
For the technique of regeneration we basically do not use only normal fat cells but mainly **fat stem cells**. These are sown in small amounts to stimulate the formation of new adipose tissue (**liposowing**) [2]
The fat is rich of stem cells [3]. An average rate of fat stem cells in adipose tissue is one of every 50 normal fat cells (compared to bone marrow that contains 1 for 10000).
Today there is a huge discussion about the use of stem cells present in adipose tissue. [4] The large numbers of stem cells in adipose tissue means that clinically relevant stem cell numbers could be extracted from the tissue, potentially eliminating the need for in vitro expansion. To utilize these characteristics of adipose tissue fully, Cytori Therapeutics Inc. has developed a closed system called Celution to isolate and concentrate stem cells and regenerative cells automatically from adipose tissue. [5]
J. Victor Garcia and Maurizio Ceccarelli have developed a simple technique to enrich stem cells in the area of collection for Liposowing. This technique has been presented for the first time at BioBridge Event of 2008 in Geneva Palais des Nations and you can find references about it on *www.ijcs.org* and on *www.aephymed.org*. [49] [2]
The explanation of why fat is so rich in adult stem cells, can be sought in the biological function of this tissue: the energy storage. The adipocyte is able to significantly increase its volume to collect energy in the triglycerides form. [6] But when its volume is very high (higher than 170% of normal volume) the adipocyte stimulates the formation of new adipose tissue by activating the differentiation of stem cells in the stroma-vascular connective tissue. [7] The liposintetic stimulus leads to adipocyte hypertrophy that, at a certain volume, stimulates perivascular stem cell propagation and differentiation. The stimulus for preadipocytes mitosis and differentiation, follows mainly the increase of the insulin rate for the receptor down regulation and the liberation IGF-1 in the hypertrophic adipocyte. [8]

The insulin receptor down regulation (internalization of the insulin receptor for excess of adipocyte volume) creates insulin resistance. [9](*Kim E*). The insulin concentration increasing leads to stem cells proliferation with the new pre-adipocytes formation. [10]. The volume increase of adipocytes activates, also, paracrine secretion of IGF-1 and stimulates the preadipocytes formation. [11]

The liposowing differs therefore from lipofilling mainly because we implant fresh fat stem cells to prevent stem cell eventual differentiation and transformation when cultured.

Based on the foregoing, the Liposowing uses the following protocol:

1. Stimulation of the fat donation area in the body with a ready insulin and glucose solution to increase the adipocyte volume.
2. Insulin, the main lipogenetic hormone, stimulates the function of lipoproteinlipase allowing the fatty acids uptake from the circulating lipoprotein and the glucose entry in the adipocyte. Glucose is the precursor of glycerol phosphate. [12] The latter binds fatty acids to form triglycerides. [13] We use an amount corresponding to 1 IU of insulin per kilo of fat to stimulate. [14]
3. 100 units of insulin are diluted in 250 cc of saline solution or glucose 5%. The resultant solution contains insulin 0.4 U.I. per milliliter.
4. We use one milliliter of this solution diluted in 200 ml of 5% glucose to inject it and stimulate a body area containing about 400 cubic centimeters fat. Usually, we use the abdominal area ease to handle.
5. We inject 0.5 milliliters of the prepared solution per one square centimeter in an area of stimulation.
6. 4 hours after the infiltration we do an infiltration with local anesthetic (1% lidocaine and adrenaline) to the same area.
7. When bleaching of the tissue is visible (bleaching is a sign of vasoconstriction and anesthesia), we aspirate fat from the area with 14 G needle which allowes to collect rich stromal fraction of stem cells. The collection of stromal-vascular fraction is important because it is rich on stem cells.
8. To transfer and replant the fat rich on stem cells we use a small cannula with a diameter of 2.1 mm. The fat cells are inserted into the face fatty tissue in small amounts (rice grain technic - Fischer). We can use an automatic gun to maintain constant low volumes.

The liposowing, using amplified fat rich on stem cells, allow regeneration of the adipose tissue. Moreover, the presence of CD31 and CD34 positive cells could also induce a regeneration of skin tissues. [15]

2. Methods

The first clinical work and basic research of skin bio-stimulation with PDGF, made by Prof. J. Victor Garcia and Dr. Antonio González-Nicolás gives us important histological information. [16]

- After 7 days of biostimulation with PDGF we have a maximum of angiogenesis. [16] The improvement of vascularization allows for better engraftment of fat cells that we will insert.

To increase the concentration of adipose stem cells we must induce the proliferation of these in the donor area. Insulin and IGF-1 have this feature and act when the adipocyte volume exceeds 170%.

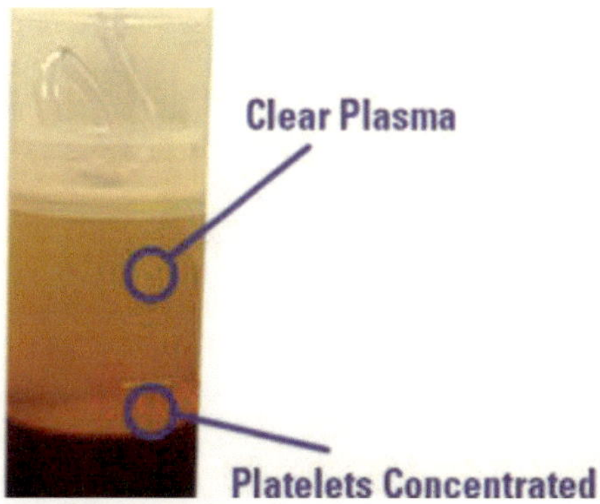

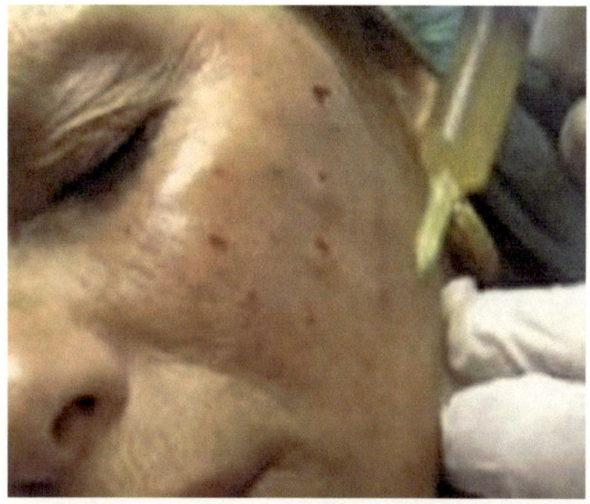

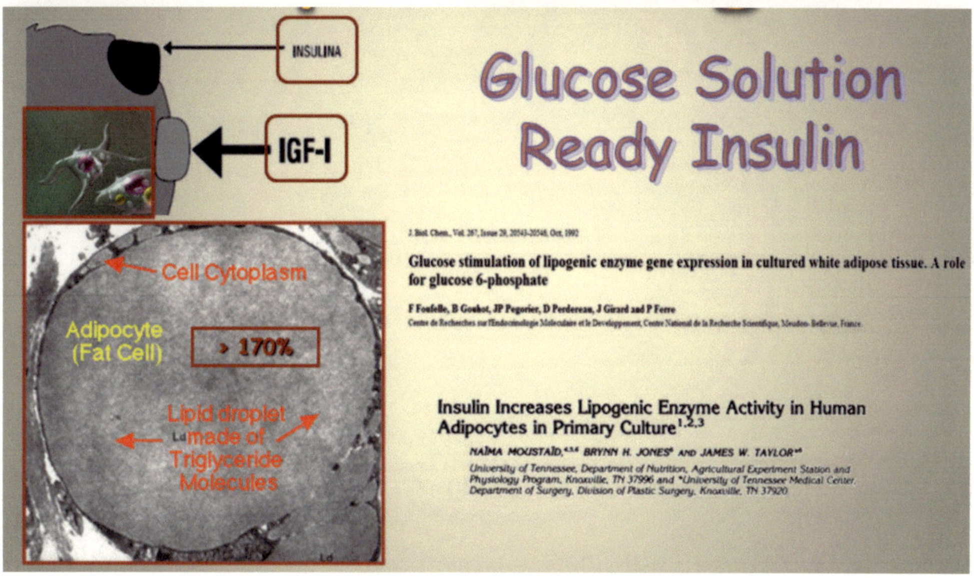

To stimulate the increase in adipocyte volume that stimulates the new formation of triglycerides we infiltrate the donor area with Ready Insulin and Glucose Solution.

We perform an initial dilution using 100 IU of Insulin Ready in 250 cc of glucose solution 5% to get a concentration of 0.4 IU of insulin per milliliter.

Considering that the normal amount of insulin used for stimulation is 1 IU per kg, if we want to stimulate an drawing area of 20 cm for 20 cm corresponding to a total area of 400 square centimeters, we use 0.4 IU i.e. 1 ml of solution that we have prepared.

Solution for infiltration and stimulation of 400 cc fat:

We prepare the solution to infiltrate in 400 cc of fat, like this:

- We take 1 ml from the solution already prepared (containing 0.4 IU of insulin per milliliter),
- Than we dilute the same one milliliter with 0.4 IU insulin in 200 ml of glucose 5%.
- The new solution (200 ml sol. Glucose 5% + 0.4 IU of insulin) we use to infiltrate the donor area of 400 square centimeters. This is equivalent to a volume of 0.5 cc of the new solution per cubic centimeter of fat.

- We wait for four hours to allow the formation of new triglycerides intraadipocyte and the resulting proliferation of stem cells by insulin and IGF-1. [17]

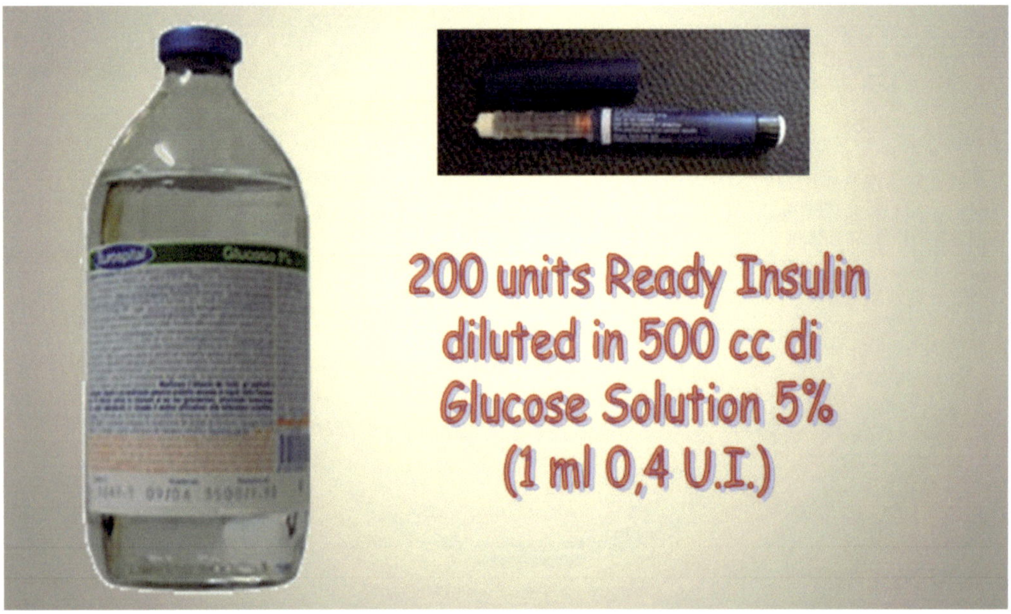

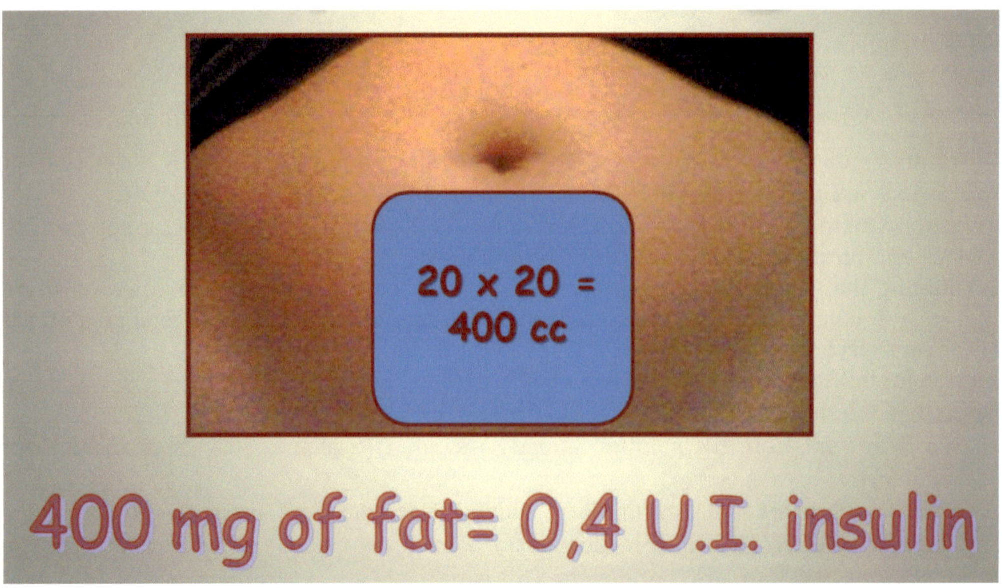

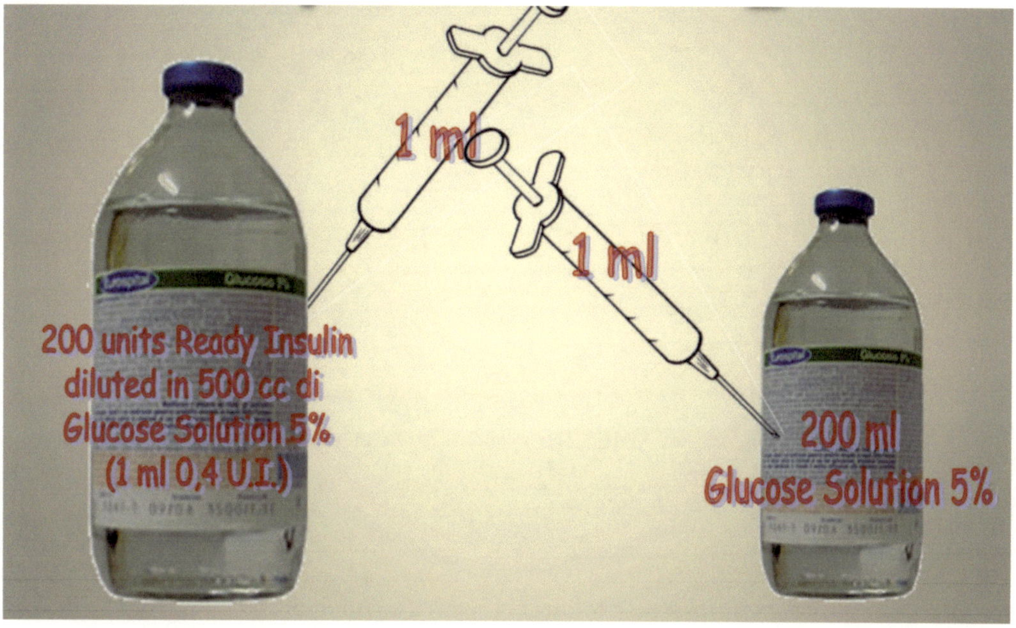
1 ml
1 ml
200 units Ready Insulin
diluted in 500 cc di
Glucose Solution 5%
(1 ml 0,4 U.I.)
200 ml
Glucose Solution 5%

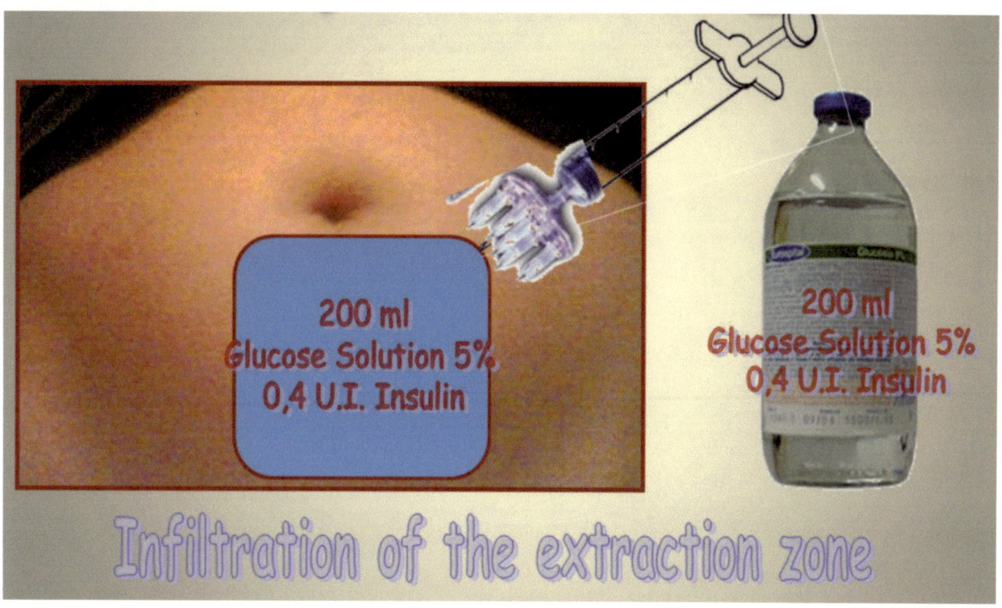
200 ml
Glucose Solution 5%
0,4 U.I. Insulin
200 ml
Glucose Solution 5%
0,4 U.I. Insulin
Infiltration of the extraction zone

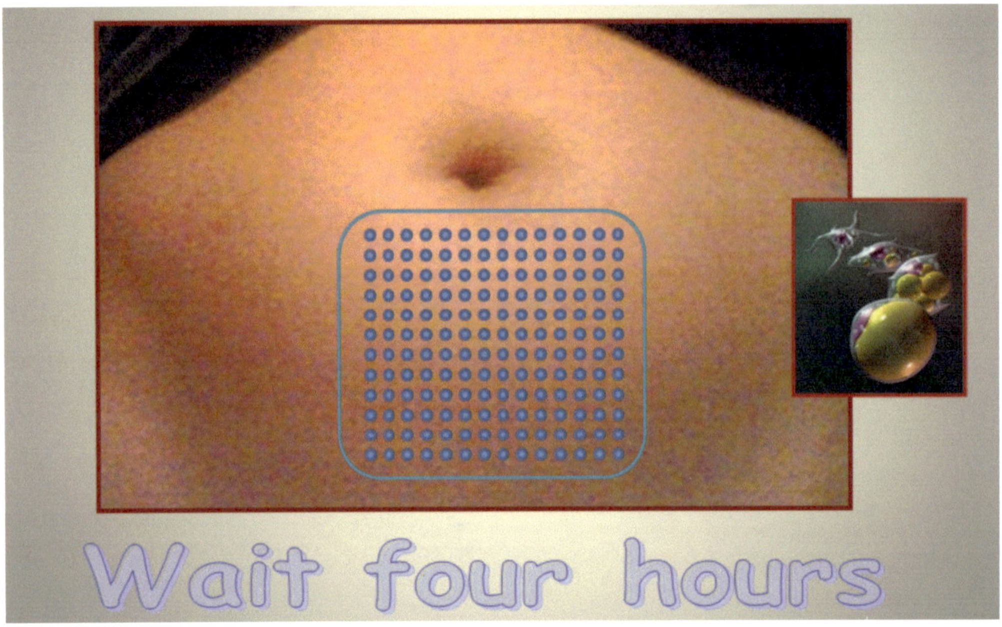

- After 4 hours we perform a new infiltration with a solution of 200 ml of Sol 5% glucose with 0.4 IU insulin and adding 5 ml of 1% lidocaine with 1:50,000 Adrenalin.

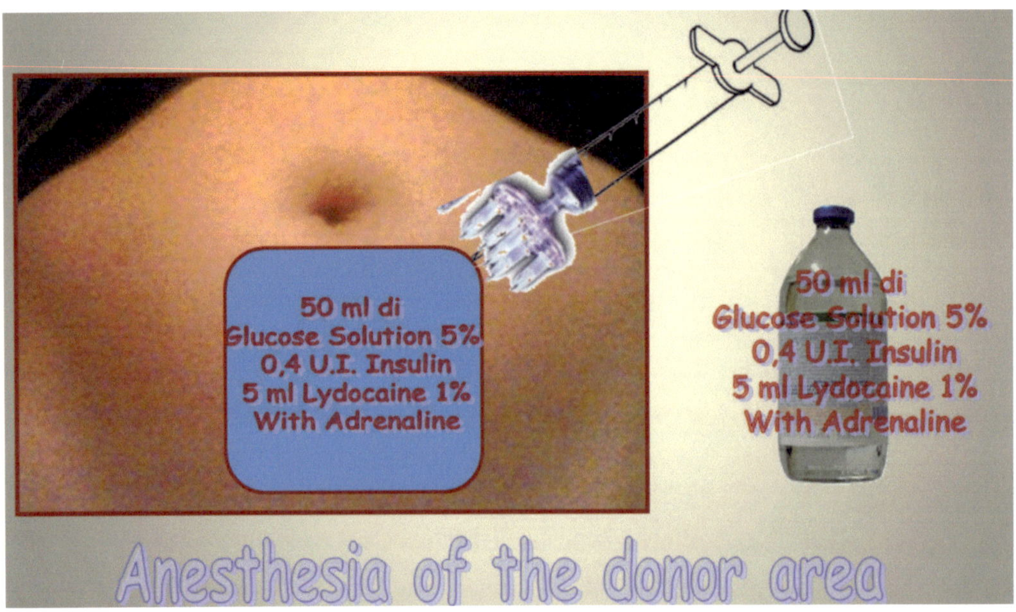

- We wait for the sign of complete bleaching of the zone confirming the action of the anesthetic and vasoconstrictor.

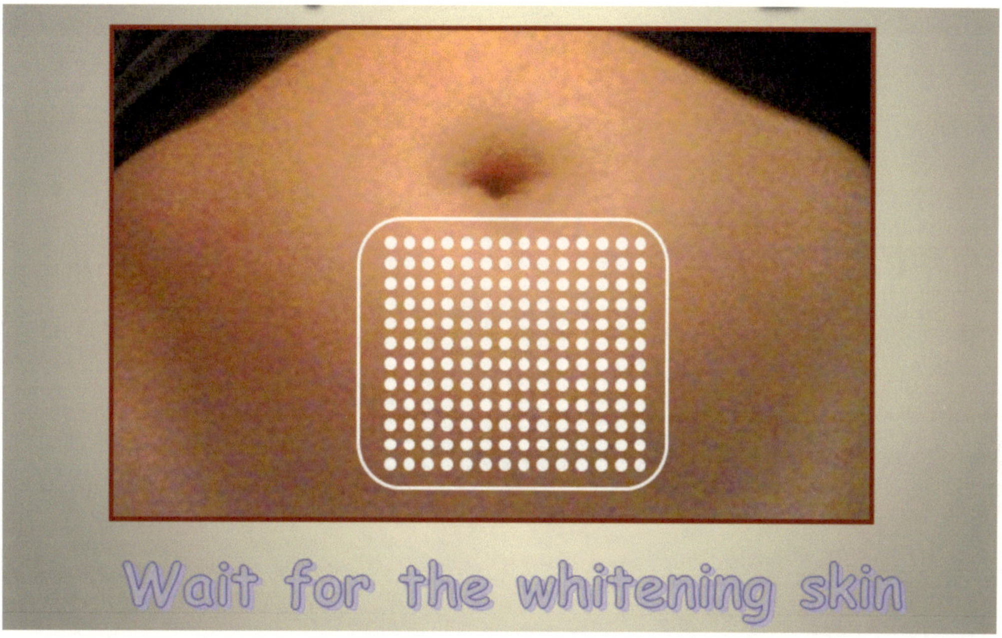

- We perform the aspiration of fat stem cells using 14 G needle mounted on a 5 ml syringe.

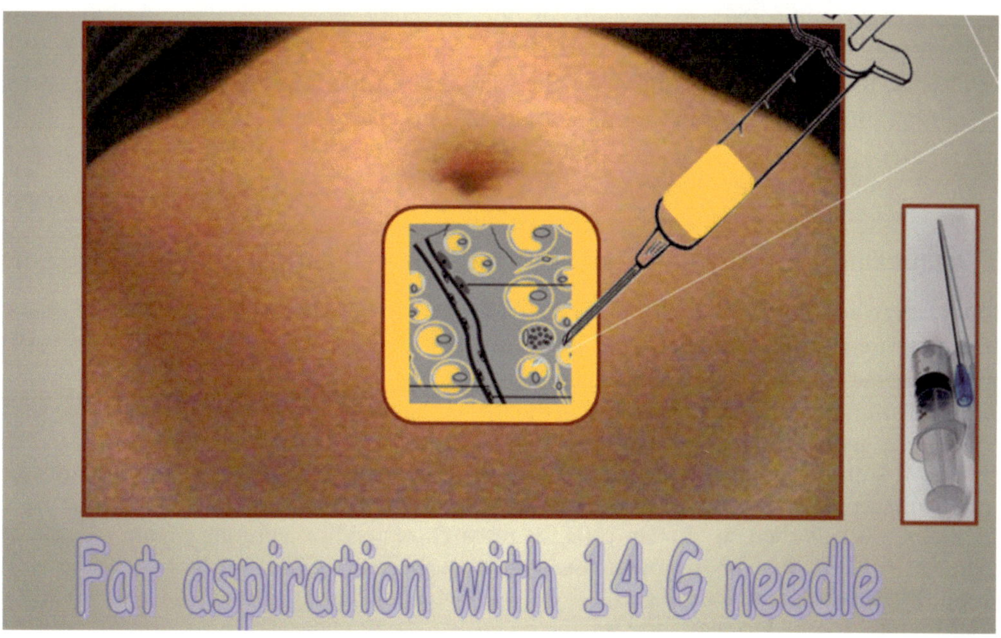

This is to collect the stromal-vascular fraction, where stem cells are located, [18] and to avoid injury to these very sensitive cells. The needle picks up real small fraction-vascular stromal cores. Stem cells (CD34 +/CD31-) differ into adipoblast (CD34+/CD31+) [19] that are implanted more easily, and with their propagation give rise to the formation of a new fat. [20] [21]

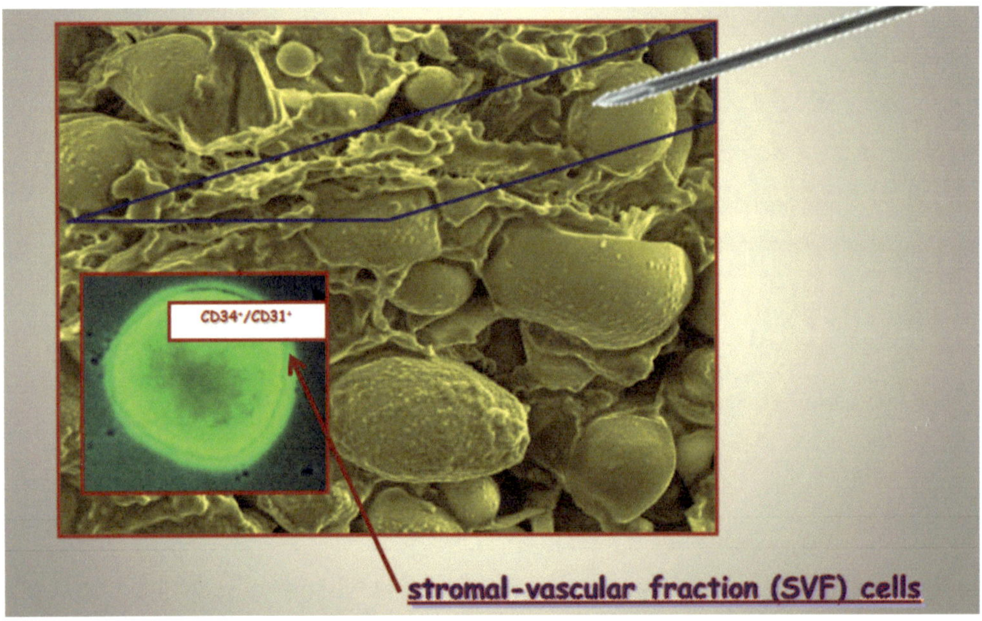

- The fat obtained with stem cells is retained in the syringe with glucose and insulin solution during the preparation of the recipient area (cleaning, desinfect and anesthesia).
- Lastly, the syringes are emptied of the solution and the fat with stem cells is injected with a cannula of 2.1 mm into the donor area. In areas where fat tissue is hypotrophic (Bichat fat pad area, nasolabial fold)., the fat transplant is injected in small amounts (rice grain technique - Fischer).

3. Discussion on safety in use of adult fat stem cells in regenerative medicine

Today, more and more, we talk about stem cells and their possible use to regenerate tissues or organs. Even in physiological medicine, recently, treatments have been proposed based on cells defined as stem cell (**liposowing**).

In the light of any legislative issues, we should, make a clarification in this scientific field. Indeed, the generalization of the term stem cell can lead to include useful treatments and therapies, without biological damage, including treatments that must be rightly adjusted and maintained in appropriate environment.

Attitudes towards the use of stem cells for research or medical care vary from country to country. In Germany, for example, the extraction of stem cells from human embryos is illegal. In Britain is perfectly legal, but laws are strict. In many countries there is still no explicit laws designed to regulate research on human stem cells.

Since the use of embryos is a matter of great controversy in ethical terms, scientists around the world are looking for other sources of stem cells. The type of stem cells found in bone marrow of adults seems to be one possibility. Today, the discovery of the high numbers of adult stem cells present in adipose tissue resulted in vogue for conservation of this cell type. Moreover, scientists have begun to manipulate these adult mesenchymal stem cells so that instead of producing only one type of tissue, it became possible to give rise to cells of other tissues.

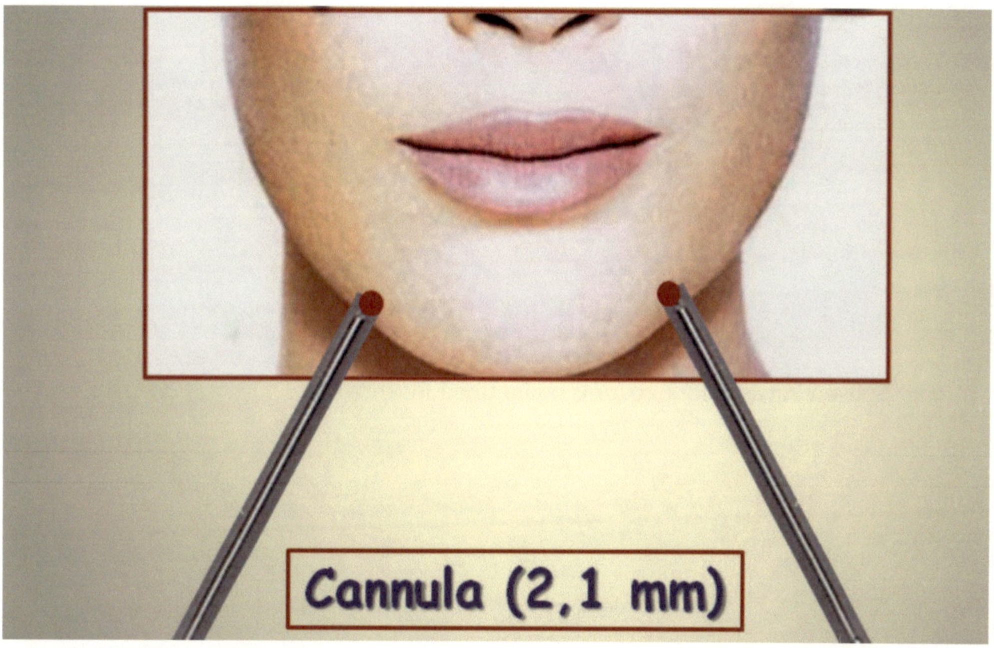

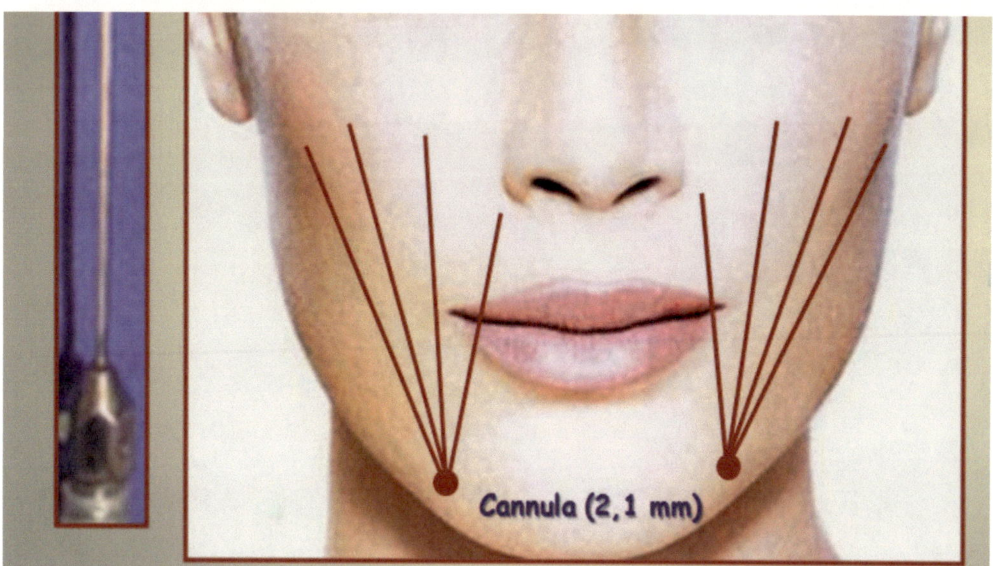

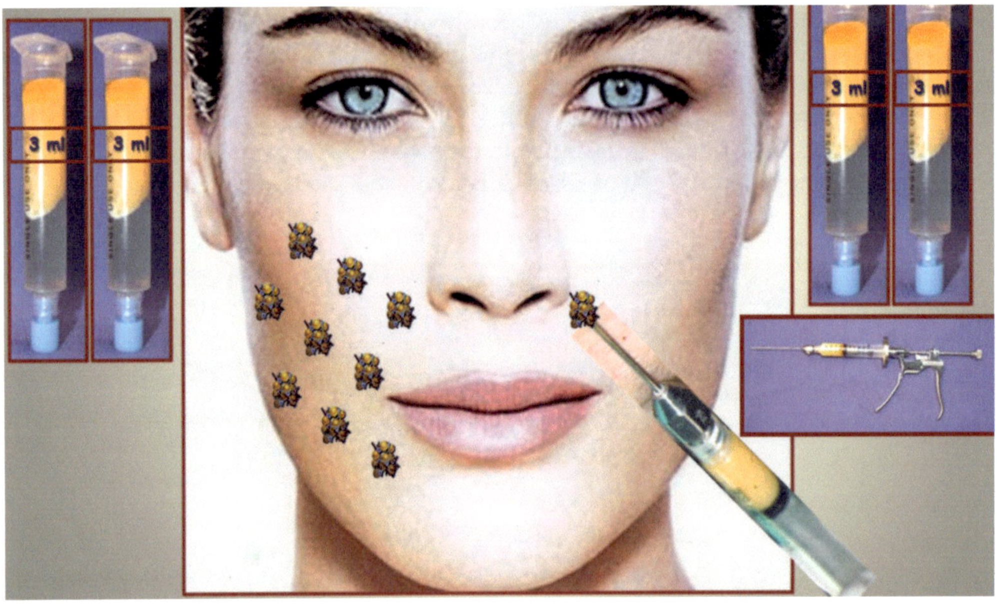

- After liposowing antibiotic cover is maintained for three days.

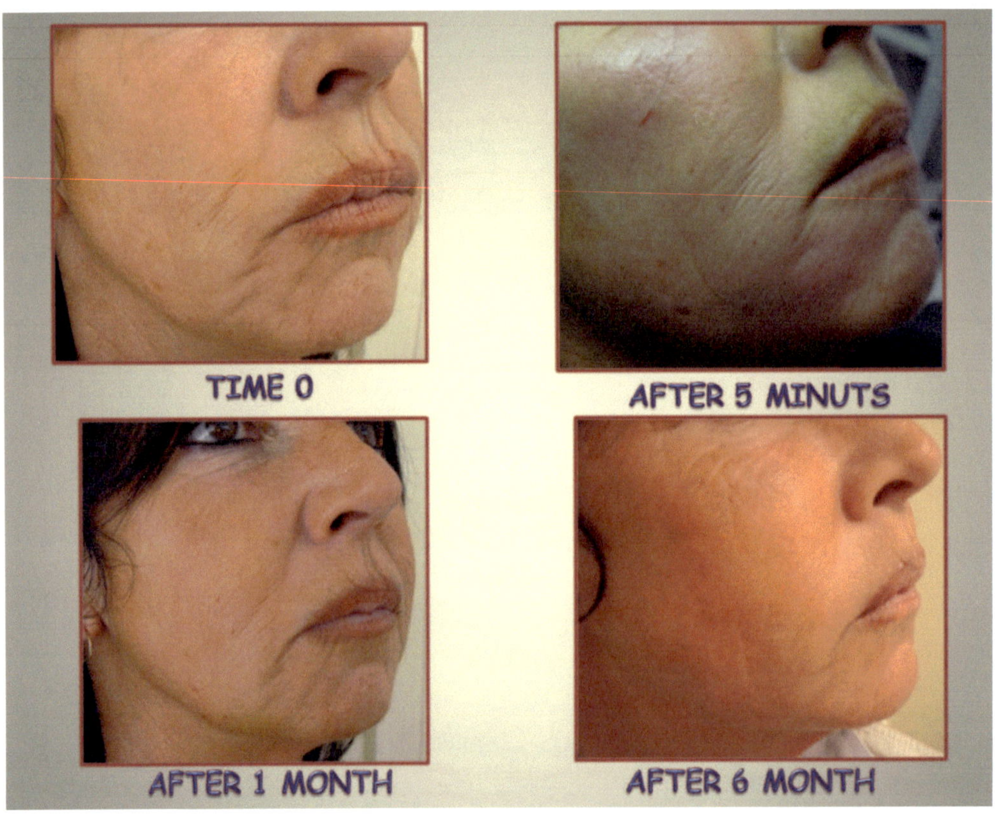

3.1 Stem cells

With the term *stem cells* are defined primitive cells and non-specialized capable subsequently to differentiate into many different cell types. A stem cell must have the ability to run an unlimited number of replication cycles, without differentiation.
Depending on the capabilities we can distinguish four types of stem cells:

- The **totipotent stem** cells capable to develop into a complete organism. [22]
- The **pluripotent stem** cells able to specialize in all types of cells that can be found in an individual. [23]
- The **multipotent stem** cells able to specialize only in certain cell types. [24]
- The **unipotent stem** cells that generate only one type of specialized cell. [25]

Stem cells are also classified according to the source of derivation, as embryonic, fetal, amniotic, and adult.
The **pluripotent stem cells** are induced, obtained in the laboratory to the regression of adult cells (already determined, for example, skin) in a state stem cell (pluripotent), using a pool of specific genes, placed via a viral vector. Therefore, in future these cells may be used to obtain adult stem cells already established, belonging to any tissue or organ.
The bulk of the regenerative work leading to the repair and/or to proliferation of tissues, is played by cells no-stem defined **progenitors** or **transit amplifying cells (TACs)**, [26] directly derived from stem cells, but partially differentiated with lack of ability to self-renewal [27] This replicative strategy, which limits the number of replication events that a stem cell can do, is based on the need to keep checking the number of stem cells and maintain the integrity of the genome of stem cells by reducing the risk of damage to DNA (i.e. mutations). [28] Mutations in stem cells are extremely harmful and dangerous, because are transmitted to all generations of daughter cells derived from stem cells. Unlike, a mutation in a TAC affects only a single generation of cells that after some time will be replaced, or may induce stem cells to develop into cancer, becoming a stem cell tumor, a type of cell that is probably responsible for the continuous supply of new cells that characterizes the development and especially the recurrence of cancer. [29]

3.2 The transit amplifying cells

Adult stem cells or transit amplifying cells are unspecialized cells that reproduce daily to provide certain specific cells, e.g. red blood cells are generated daily in the body from hematopoietic stem cells. [30] Until recently it was thought that each of these cells can produce only one type cell. [31] Today there is evidence that adult stem cells can become many different forms: it is known that stem cells in the stroma of the bone marrow can become liver cells, neural, muscle, kidney, and follicular. [32] Transformation of one type stem cell into another is called **transdifferentiation**. . [33] Useful sources of adult stem cells are actually detectable in all organs of the body.

3.3 Cell differentiation

This is the process by which a less specialized cell becomes more specialized. Cell differentiation occurs during the development of a multicellular organism, but also common in adult stem cells during tissue repair and during normal cell turnover. [34] The differentiation changes dramatically the size of shape cell the membrane potential, activities and metabolic response to signals. [35]
The main types of molecular processes that control the cell differentiation, involve the cellular signals. Many of the signaling molecules used to transmit information from one cell

to another are called **growth factors**. Typically, a ligand produced by a cell binds to a receptor of another cell, inducing a conformational change of the receptor. The receptor then catalyzes a cascade of phosphorylation reactions that eventually trigger a transcription factor or cytoskeleton proteins, activating the differentiation process of the target cell. [36]
Other important mechanisms fall into the category of the **asymmetric cell divisions**, divisions which give rise to daughter cells with distinct developmental fates. Asymmetric division is a fundamental step for the development of the embryo and also for storage of stem cells. Normally when a cell divides, produces two identical daughter cells but in some cases the daughter cells have different properties. Scientists have found that for the occurence of the asymmetric division, it is necessary that the mitotic fuse is positioned towards the rear of the cell (not centrally). This positioning of the fuse occurs through the interaction of the microtubules forming the mitotic fuse and the network of actin filaments adhering to the plasma membrane. This leads us to investigate the molecular interactions of cells with other cells based on the accession process . [37]

3.4 The cell adhesion

Adhesion is a system of communication between cells based on the interaction of pairs of receptors expressed by cells adhering to each other. This system is an alternative to communication related to the release of cellular soluble messengers (hormones, neurotransmitters, cytokines, etc.). The cell adhesion is involved in a variety of physiological and pathological mechanisms. The adhesion between cells happens when a plasma membrane receptor form a bond with one molecule that is located in the extracellular matrix, or in the neighboring cell. The receptor binding then establishes a connection with the cell cytoskeleton. From this, adult stem cells have a state of differentiation that implies cell junctions. These are a specialization of the membrane strip that enables and controls the processes of adhesion between cells. Among the various types of cell junctions, the junction's members provide to structural support to tissues using binding to actin filaments. We can differentiate groups of **adhesion and focal contacts**.
The adhesion contacts are links established, between a cell and other adjacent, thanks to cadherins. The focal contacts, however, are joints that connect the cell to the matrix, except that instead of cadherins they use integrins, associates with actin filaments via transmembrane proteins such as the alfa-actina, talina, vinculina and filamina . Therefore, this type of cells may express a regulation of inhibition contact with other cells following the accession which induces a block to the anarchic proliferation. In the normal process of contact inhibition is mainly the accumulation of p27Kip1 . protein to trigger the inhibition of Cyclin E/CDK2 complex, which in turn inhibits the phosphorylation of Rb protein, leading to cell cycle block. [38] [39]
We can now reach the ultimate explanation and that the absence risk of neoplastic transformation of adult stem cells.

3.5 Carcinogenesis

Cancer is characterized by the uncontrolled reproduction of some body cells that stop responding to physiological mechanisms of cell control after damage to their genetic heritage.
A cell to become cancerous, it must accumulate a series of damage to its system of control of reproduction. To all cancer and precancerous cells changes have occurred, often very large,

in their chromosome structure (karyotype). Underlying the pathogenesis of cancer is therefore the mutation of certain genes

- proto-oncogenes,
- tumor suppressor genes,
- genes involved in DNA repair.

The latter are those that ensure genetic stability because if other genes are mutated by the carcinogens actions, these repair the DNA before the replication, which was before these changes become permanent.

Mutations necessary that a given cell must accumulate to give rise to cancer are as follows, and are common to all types of cancer:

1. acquisition of autonomy multiplicative for incapacity to submit to the regulatory mechanisms of cell proliferation;
2. absence of density-dependent inhibition (the normal cells multiply up to a certain cell density, reached by which they become quiescent);
3. reduced adhesion with other cells or tissue components;
4. absence of extracellular matrix (usually digested by proteases), which promotes the invasion of adjacent normal tissues;
5. angiogenesis: formation of new blood vessels to deliver oxygen and nutritional factors to cancer cells;
6. reduction or loss of ability to differentiate;
7. acquisition of the capacity for unlimited replication effect of the expression of telomerase;
8. reduction or loss of the possibility of getting programmed cell death (apoptosis).
9. loss of so-called contact inhibition.

These events require more than one mutation, in general, the most mutations of certain classes of genes. The loss of proliferation control will take place only in response to mutations in genes that control cell division, cell death and DNA repair processes.

Because the cells begin a uncontrollably division must be damaged the genes that regulate growth. The proto-oncogenes are genes that promote cell growth and mitosis that is the process of cell division, the tumor suppressor genes discourage cell growth or prevent cell division to allow DNA repair. Typically requires a series of several mutations in these genes before a normal cell turns into a cancer cell.

So, various types of gene mutations are required to form cancer. A mutation limited to one oncogene would be removed from the normal control processes of mitosis and tumor suppressor genes. A mutation of a single tumor suppressor gene, would also be insufficient to cause cancer by the presence of numerous copies of "backup" genes that duplicate its function. It is only when a sufficient number of proto-oncogene is mutated in oncogenes and a sufficient quantity of tumor suppressor genes have been turned off that the signals to cell growth are superior to the inhibitors signals that this increases rapidly and out of control. [40] [41] [42] [43] [44] [45] [46] [47] [48]

4. Conclusions

From the above, we can conclude that the use of adult stem cells or transit amplifying cells adipose tissue derived (Liposowing) is devoid of possible side effects and does not require control laws. The proposed treatment, in fact, does not include cell handling. The proliferation of adult stem cells is done by physiological means and the new stem cells produced are returned to the same tissue (adipose) allowing the multiplication adjustment by contact inhibition.

5. References

[1] Coleman SR. Structural fat grafts: the ideal filler? Clin Plast Surg. 2001 Jan;28(1):111-9.
[2] Ceccarelli M., García J. V., The Medical Face Lift: Face Tissue Regeneration, The Medical Letter Physiological Vol I, No. 1, January 2010
[3] Witkowska-Zimny M, Walenko K. Stem cells from adipose tissue. Cell Mol Biol Lett. 2011 Jun;16(2):236-57
[4] Jezierska-Woźniak K, Nosarzewska D, Tutas A, Mikołajczyk A, Okliński M, Jurkowski MK. Use of adipose tissue as a source of mesenchymal stem cells. Postepy Hig Med Dosw 2010 Jul 27;64:326-32.
[5] Lin K, Matsubara Y, Masuda Y, Togashi K, Ohno T, Tamura T, Toyoshima Y, Sugimachi K, Toyoda M, Marc H, Douglas A. Characterization of adipose tissue-derived cells isolated with the Celution system. Cytotherapy. 2008;10(4):417-26
[6] Avram MM, Avram AS, James WD Subcutaneous fat in normal and diseased states 3. Adipogenesis: from stem cell to fat cell. J Am Acad Dermatol. 2007 Mar;56(3):472-92
[7] Butterwith SC. Regulators of adipocyte precursor cells. Poult Sci. 1997 Jan;76(1):118-23
[8] Sorisky A. From preadipocyte to adipocyte: differentiation-directed signals of insulin from the cell surface to the nucleus. Crit Rev Clin Lab Sci. 1999 Feb;36(1):1-34.
[9] Kim E. Insulin resistance at the crossroads of metabolic syndrome: systemic analysis using microarrays. Biotechnol J. 2010 Sep;5(9):919-29.
[10] Zhang HH, Huang J, Düvel K, Boback B, Wu S, Squillace RM, Wu CL, Manning BD. Insulin stimulates adipogenesis through the Akt-TSC2-mTORC1 pathway. PLoS One. 2009 Jul 10;4(7):e6189
[11] Sul HS, Smas CM, Wang D, Chen L. Regulation of fat synthesis and adipose differentiation. Prog Nucleic Acid Res Mol Biol. 1998;60:317-45.
[12] Landau BR. Glycerol production and utilization measured using stable isotopes. Proc Nutr Soc. 1999 Nov;58(4):973-8
[13] Dallinga-Thie GM, Franssen R, Mooij HL, Visser ME, Hassing HC, Peelman F, Kastelein JJ, Péterfy M, Nieuwdorp M. The metabolism of triglyceride-rich lipoproteins revisited: new players, new insight. Atherosclerosis. 2010 Jul;211(1):1-8
[14] Quinn SM, Baur LA, Garnett SP, Cowell CT. Treatment of clinical insulin resistance in children: a systematic review. Obes Rev. 2010 Oct;11(10):722-30
[15] Lin CS, Xin ZC, Deng CH, Ning H, Lin G, Lue TF. Defining adipose tissue-derived stem cells in tissue and in culture. Histol Histopathol. 2010 Jun;25(6):807-15
[16] García J. Víctor Giménez, González Nicolás Albandea J. Antonio Tratamiento Del Envejecimiento Cutaneo Mediante Bioestimulación Con Factores De Crecimiento Autógenos International Journal Of Cosmetic Medicine And Surgery Volume 7 - Numero 2 – 2005
[17] Herodek S. Formation of diglycerides of long turnover time from labeled acetate and glucose in rat tissues. Lipids. 1972 Sep;7(9):572-5
[18] Almeida, K. A., Campa, A., Alonso-Vale, M. I. C. , Lima, F. B., Daud, E. D., Stocchero, I. N. Fracción vascular estromal de tejido adiposo: cómo obtener células madre y su rendimiento de acuerdo a la topografía de las áreas donantes: estudio preliminary Cir.plást. iberolatinoam. - Vol. 34 - N° 1 Enero - Febrero - Marzo 2008 / Pag. 71-79)

[19] Zhu M, Gao JH, Lu F, Li H.Cell biological study of adipose-derived stem cells Nan Fang Yi Ke Da Xue Xue Bao. 2007 Apr;27(4):518-23
[20] Poulos SP, Dodson MV, Hausman GJ. Cell line models for differentiation: preadipocytes and adipocytes. Exp Biol Med (Maywood). 2010 Oct;235(10):1185-93
[21] Zhu M, Gao JH, Lu F.Cell biological study of cultured cells derived from the fatty of fluid portions of liposuction aspirates. Zhonghua Zheng Xing Wai Ke Za Zhi. 2008 Mar;24(2):138-44
[22] Hemmat S, Lieberman DM, Most SP. An introduction to stem cell biology. Facial Plast Surg. 2010 Oct;26(5):343-9
[23] Mitalipov S, Wolf D "Totipotency, pluripotency and nuclear reprogramming.". Adv Biochem Eng Biotechnol 114: 185–99 2009
[24] Panagiotis A. Tsonis; Stem Cells from Differentiated Cells; Molecular Interventions 4:81-83, 2004
[25] Raewyn M. Seaberg and Derek van der Kooy(2003). Stem and progenitor cells: the premature desertion of rigorous definitions. Trends in Neurosciences 26, 125-131
[26] StemBook Cambridge (MA): Harvard Stem Cell Institute; 2008
[27] Alberts B, Johnson A, Lewis J, et al.Molecular Biology of the Cell. 4th edition. New York: Garland Science; 2002
[28] Sarasin A, An overview of the mechanisms of mutagenesis and carcinogenesis., Mutat Res, 2003
[29] Stewart Sell; Cellular Origin of Cancer - Dedifferentiation or Stem Cell Maturation Arrest?; Environmental Health Perspectives, 1993
[30] Raff, M "Adult stem cell plasticity: Fact or Artifact?". Annual Review of Cell and Developmental Biology 19: 1–22 2003
[31] Barrilleaux B, Phinney DG, Prockop DJ, O'Connor KC "Review: ex vivo engineering of living tissues with adult stem cells". Tissue Eng. 12 (11): 3007–19 2006
[32] Kruger GM, Mosher JT, Bixby S, Joseph N, Iwashita T, Morrison SJ "Neural crest stem cells persist in the adult gut but undergo changes in self-renewal, neuronal subtype potential, and factor responsiveness". Neuron 35 (4): 657–69 August 2002
[33] Okada, T. S. Transdifferentiation. Clarendon Press, Oxford 1991
[34] Tsonis PA "Stem cells from differentiated cells". Mol. Interv. 4 (2): 81–3 April 2004)
[35] Knisely, Karen; Gilbert, Scott F. Developmental Biology (8th ed.). Sunderland, Mass: Sinauer Associates. p. 147 2009
[36] Rana Anjum John Blenis The RSK family of kinases: emerging roles in cellular signaling Nature Reviews Molecular Cell Biology 9, 747-758 October 2008
[37] Pierre Gönczy Mechanisms of asymmetric cell division: flies and worms pave the way Nature Reviews Molecular Cell Biology 9, 355-366 May 2008
[38] Martin J. Humphries Cell Adhesion Assays Methods in Molecular Biology, 2009, Volume 522, 2, 203-210
[39] Timothy Craig Allen and Philip T. Cagle Cell Adhesion Molecules Molecular Pathology Library, 2008, Volume 1, Section 1, 22-39
[40] Baker, Monya "Adult cells reprogrammed to pluripotency, without tumors". Nature Reports Stem Cells. Retrieved 2007-12-11
[41] Ben-Tabou De-Leon, S.; Davidson, E. "Gene regulation: gene control network in development". Annual review of biophysics and biomolecular structure 36: 191. 2007

[42] CM Casimir, PB Gates, RK Patient and JP Brockes; Evidence for dedifferentiation and metaplasia in amphibian limb regeneration from inheritance of DNA methylation; Development, Vol 104, Issue 4 657-668
[43] DeLeon SBT, EH Davidson; Gene regulation: Gene control network in development. Annual Review of Biophysics and Biomolecular Structure 36:191-212, 2007
[44] Dixon K, Kopras E, Genetic alterations and DNA repair in human carcinogenesis., Semin Cancer Biol, 2004
[45] Fearon ER, Vogelstein B, A genetic model for colorectal tumorigenesis, Cell, 1990
[46] Kleinsmith, LJ. Pearson Benjamin Cummings Principles of Cancer Biology. 2006
[47] Knudson AG, Two genetic hits (more or less) to cancer, Nat Rev Cancer, 2001, 157-62
[48] Schottenfeld D, Beebe-Dimmer JL, Advances in cancer epidemiology: understanding causal mechanisms and the evidence for implementing interventions., Annu Rev Public Health, 2005
[49] Maurizio Ceccarelli, J. Victor Garcia The Medical Face Lifting - Regeneration Of The Face Tissues - International Journal Of Cosmetic Surgery Vol 11 Num 1 2010

Part 3

Complications of Liposuction

13

Complications of Liposuction

Francisco J. Agullo[1,2], Humberto Palladino[3] and Sadri O. Sozer[1,2]
[1]*Texas Tech University Health Sciences Center – El Paso, TX*
[2]*El Paso Cosmetic Surgery Center – El Paso, TX*
[3]*Mayo Clinic – Rochester, MN*
USA

1. Introduction

Liposuction, a surgical intervention designed to treat superficial and deep deposits of subcutaneous fat distributed in aesthetically unpleasing proportions, has proven to be a successful method of improving body contour. Liposuction is so successful, in fact, that it is commonly performed in the office-based surgery setting. Liposuction is one of the most common surgical interventions carried out by physicians around the world and within the top five surgical procedures in the United States. [1] The procedure is of moderate complexity with a death rate of 1/5000 over all. [2] It is performed by multiple specialties within the aesthetic arena, expanding the possibilities for adverse outcomes.

2. Evolution of liposuction

Since the introduction of liposuction techniques in 1982 the management of adipose tissue for aesthetic and reconstructive purposes had undergone a significant change. [3] The introduction of new techniques such as wet, superwet and tumescent suction assisted liposuction (SAL), [4, 5] as well as the development of new technologies such as power assisted liposuction (PAL), ultrasound assisted liposuction (UAL) and laser assisted liposuction (LAL), broaden the possibilities within the field. The advent of new techniques and technologies is not free of complications and each of these developments has been associated with a subgroup of problems that should not be overlooked.

Over the past decades the safety standards have also developed along with the innovations in the field of liposuction. In the year 2010 over 200,000 liposuction cases have been recorded in the United States alone. [1] In the most recent survey published by Dr. Jamil Ahmad, et al. the vast majority of complications were related to UAL (35.2%), LAL (22.9%), and SAL (22.1%). [6] Another important point of this review is the new trends in the market, which create an indirect pressure on the physician through the patient (consumer). The marketing of new products is poorly regulated and the early release of new technology to the public creates an added risk to the population undergoing these procedures perhaps due to the lack of experience with the product.

The complications can be subdivided in local or systemic. Local complications include contour deformities (irregularities, depressions, undercorrection and overcorrection), hematomas, seromas, alterations of skin color and sensitivity, infection, skin necrosis, *cutis mamorata*, etc. The systemic complications are in general of greater severity and include:

deep venous thrombosis, pulmonary embolism, fat emboli, hypovolemia, edema, toxicity or medication interaction, perforation of abdominal wall or viscera, sepsis as well as the usual complications associated with any other surgical procedures.

3. Prevention

As we experienced and rapid expansion in technology and developments of new techniques over the last two decades the emphasis now has shifted to an essential component of our practice: patient safety. Several meetings with emphasis on patient safety have taken place over the last decade around the world. As in any other portion of the medical field, patient safety is mainly focused on prevention although many times adds recommendations on how to deal with complications when necessary. On the topic of prevention we should outline some of the main resources in the literature and its recommendations for further reference. No strict rules have been set to regulate every specific aspect of the practice of liposuction although several guidelines have been issued to avoid complications. Failure to comply with this guidelines could result in legal actions against practitioners since this have been set over evidence based medicine and are held as the most relevant safety measures in the literature today.

We would like to start by citing the recommendations included in Fatal Outcomes from Liposuction: Census Survey of Cosmetic Surgeons published in the Plastic and Reconstructive Surgery Journal. [7] In this paper the following guidelines are outlined: 1. Appropriate patient selection (ASA class I, within 30 percent of ideal body weight) 2. Use of superwet techniques of infiltration 3. Meticulous monitoring of volume status (urinary catheterization, noninvasive hemodynamic monitoring, communication with anesthesiologist) 4. Judicious fluid resuscitation a. For aspirate less than 5 liters: maintenance fluid plus subcutaneous infiltrate b. For aspirate over 5 liters: maintenance fluid plus subcutaneous infiltrate plus 0.25 ml of intravenous crystalloid per milliliter of aspirate over 5 liters 5. Overnight monitoring of large-volume (over 5-liter total aspirate) liposuction patients in an appropriate healthcare facility 6. Use of pneumatic compression devices in cases performed under general anesthesia or lasting longer than 1 hour 7. Maintaining total lidocaine doses below 35 mg/kg (wetting solution).

1	Quantity of tumescent fluid infused
2	Total dosages and drugs utilized
3	Total volume of fat and fluid extracted
4	Technique utilized
5	Type of anesthesia
6	Volume of supranatant fat
7	Anatomical sites treated
8	Use of ultra-assisted technique (internal of external)
9	Drains (if placed)
10	Complications should be noted
11	Post-operative garments utilized

*From AACS 2006 Update in Guidelines for Liposuction

Table 1. Operative Record for Liposuction

Another important document issued in 2006 by the American Academy of Cosmetic Surgery was an update on the Guidelines for Liposuction, which includes a series of recommendations for the pre, intra and post operative management of the patient undergoing liposuction. [8] Among other suggestions a good systematic approach at data gathering is provided including the information presented in Table 1.

Finally, we would like to conclude the prevention section with one of the latest evidence based medicine documents in the literature published in 2009. [9] This document provides the most up to date information regarding patient safety related to liposuction in an heavily referenced evidence-based structure and is a key paper of the current literature. The paper is a well organized overview of the field of liposuctions that correlates well with the information presented in this Chapter.

4. Complications

4.1 Systemic complications

4.1.1 Deep venous thrombosis and pulmonary embolism

Deep venous thrombosis (DVT) is one of the most feared complications due to its relation to pulmonary embolism (PE) and its fatal consequences. PE is been the main cause of death among patients undergoing cosmetic surgery claiming one forth of the deaths. [10] A thorough preoperative evaluation to identify risk factors of thrombosis and the use of preventive measures (stockings, pneumatic intermittent compression systems, etc) together with early mobilization, appropriate hydration and anticoagulation when indicated are sufficient to prevent venous thrombosis in healthy individuals. During the immediate postoperative period (first 24 hours) is imperative to carry out early mobilization (6-8 hours after surgery) as well as the use of compressive garments. Lymphatic drainage and massage could be considered as adjuvant therapies as well. The symptoms of pulmonary embolism include sharp hest pain, shortness of breath, chest pain that worsens with deep breathing or coughing, coughing up blood, tachycardia, sweating and anxiety.

4.1.2 Hypothermia

Hypothermia has been recognized as a significant factor associated with a broad arrange of complications in the last two decades. It has influence not only in the coagulation system but also affects the immune system as well. Because of this proper precautions have to be taken to prevent excessive heat loss. The use of warming devices, warm fluids and attention to room temperature are the basic steps to prevent hypothermia.

4.1.3 Lidocaine and epinephrine toxicity

Accepted doses of lidocaine are 7mg/kg for lidocaine with epinephrine and 4-5 mg/kg of lidocaine alone. Doses up to 33-35 mg/kg have been reported as safe in the literature when utilized in large volume infiltration as a tumescent solution. [5] The next important factor to consider is the pharmacokinetics of the drug with a peak concentration between 8-12 hours from infiltration. Liver metabolism should be assessed prior to liposuction procedures with lidocaine infiltration since its impairment of drug interference may affect the usual lidocaine clearance with detrimental effects for the patient.

Epinephrine effect also should be considered as an added factor to the overall stress in the procedures. Cardiac function should be interrogated during the history and physical and appropriately evaluated if necessary. Epinephrine use should be avoided in patients who present with pheochromocytoma, hyperthyroidism, severe hypertension, cardiac disease, or peripheral vascular disease. In addition, cardiac arrhythmias can occur in predisposed individuals or when epinephrine is used with halothane anesthesia. Alterations in the rate and force of contraction or cardiac irritability and hypertension can occur, particularly in hyperthyroid patients. [11]

4.1.4 Cardiopulmonary arrest & fluid shifts

Proper pre-operative, intra-operative and post-operative fluid management is essential to optimize the good perfusion and minimize the risk of cardiopulmonary complications and death.

Fluid aspirations should be limited to 5 L per session to avoid the excessive third spacing that could jeopardized the ability to compensate the fluid shifts on the average patient. Other rules are to limit the aspirate to less than 5% of the body weight and treat less than 30% of the body surface

4.1.5 Infection and sepsis

Erythema, drainage or even swelling should not be taken lightly. Local sings of infections should be promptly investigated and treated. Unrecognized or untreated infections could lead to compromise of a large surface area or even to necrotizing fasciitis and other more severe systemic manifestations. Also systemic symptoms without local evidence should be addressed since the risk of perforation of an intra-abdominal organ is always a risk. Carful aseptic technique is essential including skin prep and proper instrument management. Perioperative antibiotics play a significant role in liposuction. Although the procedure may be considered of moderate complexity the total areas treated are usually broad and proper antibiotic delivery during the operations is essential.

4.1.6 Fat emboli

Although of rare occurrence, fat emboli could lead to fatal outcomes. The syndrome presents with a triad of petechial rash, respiratory distress and cerebral dysfunction. The diagnosis is difficult and the treatment is supportive. Corticosteroids may play a role in the management of this rare entity.

4.1.7 Perforation of abdomen and viscera

These complications are frequently related to the lack of proper training. Although it may occur to well-trained professionals, usually undertrained physicians or even non-physicians performing the procedure lack proper anatomical knowledge and soft tissue handling experience. This combination can lead to a catastrophic outcome requiring more aggressive interventions with increase morbidity and even the risk of death. Care should be taken when using power assisted cannulas and even ultrasonic or laser technologies since the tissue resistance changes making easier the penetration of undesired structures. Patient positioning is another important point since might expose areas to undesired trauma during suction lipectomy. The type of cannula is another important considerations since blunt cannulas are safer than small sharp ones.

4.2 Local complications

4.2.1 Hematoma and seroma

Hematoma may result from inappropriate technique or increase-bleeding diathesis from congenital vs. acquired reasons. A carful history and physical will, most of the time, give away any increase bleeding tendencies in a particular patient. The use of wet, superwet or tumescent liposuction has decrease significantly the risk of bleeding after suction lipectomy.
Seromas are related to an excessive liposuction with inappropriate postoperative management. The use of compressive garments may provide comfort and at the same time decrease the death space suitable for fluid accumulation. Lymphatic drainage is usually unaffected with proper SAL although other techniques such as UAL have been associated with an increase risk of seroma formation. Some advocate the use of drains over the first 24 hours incases on large volume liposuction as well as manual drainage.

4.2.2 Surface irregularities

This complication is related to a poor technique in most cases. The violation of anatomical structures and the incorrect level of treatment may result in undesirable outcome. The type and orientation of the cannulas is key as well as the level of suction. With the increase in understanding of the tissue anatomy we can perform a safe procedure removing the reserve fat in the adequate plane.
The treatment of the skin irregularities is challenging and entails the release of the scarred tissue with or without interposition of autologous tissue, such as fat injections, etc. (liposculpture). Preexisting cellulite deformities should be pointed out since these types of deformities are likely to persist after suction lipectomy. Continuous assessment of the tissues by pinch maneuvers or similar is essential to avoid surface irregularities, undercorrection or overcorrection.
Finally the inappropriate use of postoperative garment can result in skin irregularities. Close attention should be given to the post-operative dressings. (Figure 1)

4.2.3 Skin excess

If a large amount of skin excess is expected the procedure should be combined with skin resection. The retractile properties of skin will compensate for a mild to moderate amount of skin excess after suction lipectomy. In most cases the distinction between a poor and a good result comes with experience.

4.2.4 Cutaneous hyperpigmentation

This complication is related to the deposition of hemosiderin derived from degradation of hemoglobin to ultraviolet light. This process causes fixation of the pigments to the superficial layers of the skin. Prevention entails avoidance of sun exposure until ecchymosis is resolved. Often the cases of hyperpigmentation are related to vasculopathies. The use of newer technologies such as LAL has decreased the amount of ecchymosis and hyperpigmentation.

4.2.5 Skin necrosis

If the subdermal plexus is violated or traumatized the overlying skin is prone to necrosis. The more invasive technologies such as UAL and LAL are also at risk of skin burning which will ultimately result in skin necrosis and scarring. Excessive compression from garments can also jeopardize the viability of the treated area. (Figure 2)

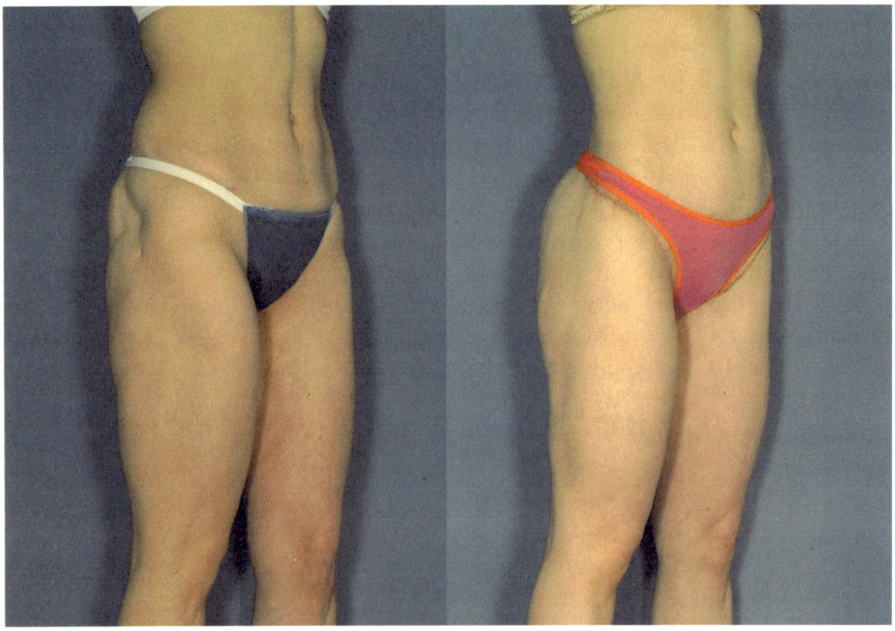

Fig. 1. Skin surface irregularities corrected by spiral lift and rotational dermal-fat flap with fat injection

4.2.6 Skin sensation

Anesthesia, hypersesthesia and dystesthesia are usual manifestation of the procedures. In most cases are temporary with return of normal sensory function within few months.

4.2.7 Cutis marmorata

It is believed that *cutis marmorata* after liposuction is related to trauma to the subdermal plexus resulting in a skin pattern resembling cutis marmorata. These patterns can persist after the operation up to one year.

5. Discussion

A brief historical note and a review of the literature of the last five years are presented in our discussion.

When addressing complications in liposuction is impossible not to mention the earliest and, perhaps one of the worst complications cited in the literature. The concept of removing excess fat from localized body sites to achieve similar gains is credited to Charles Dujarrier, who in France [12-14] attempted to remove subcutaneous fat using a uterine curette on calves and knees of a ballerina in 1921. An inadvertent injury of the femoral artery led to amputation of the dancer's leg. This unfortunate complication arrested further progress in this field and but it was a valiant attempt at the time. [15]

Schrudde in 1964 [14] revived interest in this procedure and extracted fat from the leg, gaining access through a small incision with a curette, but was faced with a daunting task of managing the difficult hematoma and seroma that resulted from this technique. Subsequently, Pitanguy [16] favored an en bloc removal of both fat and skin to remove excess thigh adiposities, but the extensively noticeable incisions did not allow the technique to become popular.

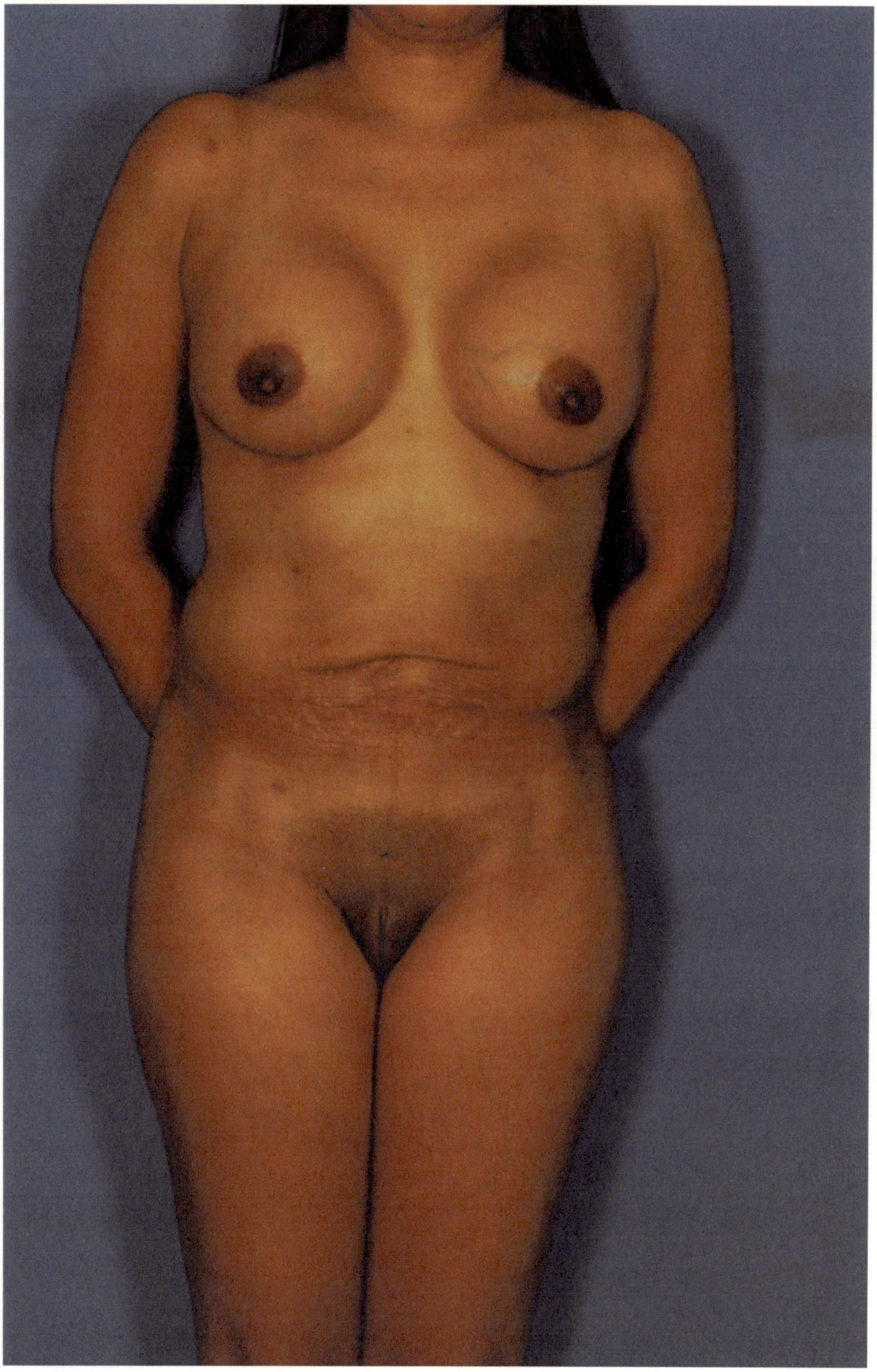

Fig. 2. Periumbilical skin excess, necrosis, and surface irregularities.

Some recommendations to avoid complications related to the different techniques and technologies available are: to prevent thermal injuries while performing ultrasound-assisted liposuction, two technique rules are of critical importance. First, the ultrasound probe or cannula must be kept in motion; second, the infiltrate solution is a required component of ultrasound-assisted liposuction as it plays a crucial role in the process of fat emulsification. Due to the amount of blood loss associated with the dry technique, its use is not recommended except in limited applications with a volume of 100 cc of total aspirate or less. The dry technique should never be used in conjunction with ultrasound-assisted liposuction. No one single liposuction technique is best suited for all patients in all circumstances. Factors such as the patient's overall health, the patient's body mass index, the estimated volume of aspirate to be removed, the number of sites to be addressed, and any other concomitant procedures to be performed should be considered by the surgeon to determine the best technique for the individual patient. Multiple openings facilitate extraction of fat and traumatize the tissue less because repeated movement over a given area is minimized [5, 17] The selection of the appropriate cannulas is key to avoid adverse outcomes. The design, size, and length of the liposuction cannula vary greatly depending on the area(s) to be suctioned, the type of liposuction performed, and the physician's preference. The diameters of cannulas typically range from 2 to 6 mm and are available in a variety of lengths. [18-21] No one cannula is appropriate for all procedures, patients, or surgeons. PAL is effective for large-volume removals, fibrous areas, and revisions. It is typically used in conjunction with the tumescent or superwet technique. Care should be exercise since the added vibration could result in further complications such us skin trauma and necrosis. The recent introduction of newer technologies such as LAL facilitates the extraction of adipose tissue at the expense of a carful technique since the heat dispersion is higher and a different technical skill needs to be developed to avoid complications. In a recent study LAL showed to be an effective adjunct to liposuction with low complication rate. [22]

Among other rare complications ischemic optic neuropathy [23] as well as self inflicted postoperative injuries [24] show that even undertaken all safety precautions, patients and physicians are exposed to complications. Preventive measures, proper patient selection, accurate documentation, and respect for current standards of practice are the minimum requirement for a safe practice.

6. Conclusion

Liposuction is one of the most common surgically performed procedures, and its low complication rate supports the procedure's popularity. A complete preoperative assessment along with a proper training and respect of industry standards is essential to avoid unwanted occurrences. The constant evolution of techniques and technology calls to a dynamic reassessment of the safety standards to keep the patient and physician safe. As physicians we should educate our patients to avoid dissatisfaction and more important, complications.

7. References

[1] Top 5 Cosmetic Surgical Procedures 2010 [http://www.plasticsurgery.org/Documents/news-resources/statistics/2010-statisticss/Charts/2010-top-5-cosmetic-surgery-procedures-graph.pdf]

[2] Lehnhardt M, Homann HH, Druecke D, Steinstraesser L, Steinau HU: [No problem with liposuction?]. Chirurg 2003, 74(9):808-814.
[3] Schrudde J: Suction curettage for body contouring. Plast Reconstr Surg 1982, 69(5):903-904.
[4] Rohrich RJ, Beran SJ, Fodor PB: The role of subcutaneous infiltration in suction-assisted lipoplasty: a review. Plast Reconstr Surg 1997, 99(2):514-519; discussion 520-516.
[5] Fodor PB, Watson JP: Wetting solutions in ultrasound-assisted lipoplasty. Clin Plast Surg 1999, 26(2):289-293; ix.
[6] Ahmad J, Eaves FF, 3rd, Rohrich RJ, Kenkel JM: The American Society for Aesthetic Plastic Surgery (ASAPS) survey: current trends in liposuction. Aesthet Surg J 2011, 31(2):214-224.
[7] Rohrich RJ, Muzaffar AR: Fatal outcomes from liposuction: census survey of cosmetic surgeons. Plast Reconstr Surg 2000, 105(1):436-446; discussion 447-438.
[8] (AACS) TAAOCS: 2006 Guidelines for Liposuction Surgery. In: 2006: A joint Ad Hoc Committee of the American Society of Lipo-Suction Surgery (ASLSS) and the American Academy of Cosmetic Surgery 2006.
[9] Haeck PC, Swanson JA, Gutowski KA, Basu CB, Wandel AG, Damitz LA, Reisman NR, Baker SB: Evidence-based patient safety advisory: liposuction. Plast Reconstr Surg 2009, 124(4 Suppl):28S-44S.
[10] de Jong RH: Mega-dose lidocaine dangers seen in "tumescent" liposuction. J Clin Monit Comput 2000, 16(1):77-79.
[11] Rubin JP, Bierman C, Rosow CE, Arthur GR, Chang Y, Courtiss EH, May JW, Jr.: The tumescent technique: the effect of high tissue pressure and dilute epinephrine on absorption of lidocaine. Plast Reconstr Surg 1999, 103(3):990-996; discussion 997-1002.
[12] Coleman WP, 3rd: The history of liposuction and fat transplantation in America. Dermatol Clin 1999, 17(4):723-727, v.
[13] Flynn TC, Coleman WP, 2nd, Field LM, Klein JA, Hanke CW: History of liposuction. Dermatol Surg 2000, 26(6):515-520.
[14] Illouz YG: History and current concepts of lipoplasty. Clin Plast Surg 1996, 23(4):721-730.
[15] Grazer FM, de Jong RH: Fatal outcomes from liposuction: census survey of cosmetic surgeons. Plast Reconstr Surg 2000, 105(1):436-446; discussion 447-438.
[16] Pitanguy I: Trochanteric Lipodystrophy. Plast Reconstr Surg 1964, 34:280-286.
[17] Iverson RE, Lynch DJ: Practice advisory on liposuction. Plast Reconstr Surg 2004, 113(5):1478-1490; discussion 1491-1475.
[18] Medical B: Byron Medical. In.; 2011.
[19] MicroAire: Online Product Catalog, Information on Cannulas. In.; 2011.
[20] Pitman GH: Liposuction and Aesthetic Surgery. In: St Louis, Mo: Quality Medical Publishing,. 1993: 87-93.
[21] Thornton LK, Nahai F: Equipment and instrumentation for ultrasound-assisted lipoplasty. Clin Plast Surg 1999, 26(2):299-304; x.
[22] Katz B, McBean J: Laser-assisted lipolysis: a report on complications. J Cosmet Laser Ther 2008, 10(4):231-233.

[23] Ribeiro Monteiro ML, Moura FC, Cunha LP: Bilateral visual loss complicating liposuction in a patient with idiopathic intracranial hypertension. J Neuroophthalmol 2006, 26(1):34-37.
[24] Gherardini G: An unusual complication after suction-assisted lipectomy and poor patient selection. Plast Reconstr Surg 2005, 115(2):664-665.